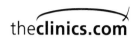

CLINICS IN
CHEST MEDICINE

Respiratory Disease in Older Patients

GUEST EDITOR
Margaret A. Pisani, MD

December 2007 • Volume 28 • Number 4

SAUNDERS

An Imprint of Elsevier, Inc.
PHILADELPHIA   LONDON   TORONTO   MONTREAL   SYDNEY   TOKYO

W.B. SAUNDERS COMPANY

A Division of Elsevier Inc.

Elsevier Inc. • 1600 John F. Kennedy Boulevard • Suite 1800 • Philadelphia, Pennsylvania 19103-2899

http://www.chestmed.theclinics.com

CLINICS IN CHEST MEDICINE
December 2007
Editor: Sarah E. Barth

Volume 28, Number 4
ISSN 0272-5231
ISBN-13: 978-1-4160-5047-6
ISBN-10: 1-4160-5047-7

Clinics in Chest Medicine (ISSN 0272-5231) is published quarterly by Elsevier Inc., 360 Park Avenue South, New York, NY 10010-1710. Months of issue are March, June, September, and December. Business and Editorial Offices: 1600 John F. Kennedy Blvd., Suite 1800, Philadelphia, PA 19103-2899. Customer Service Office: 6277 Sea Harbor Drive, Orlando, FL 32887-4800. Periodicals postage paid at New York, NY and additional mailing offices. Subscription prices are $232.00 per year (US individuals), $370.00 per year (US institutions), $113.00 per year (US students), $255.00 per year (Canadian individuals), $444.00 per year (Canadian institutions), $149.00 per year (Canadian students), $297.00 per year (international individuals) $444.00 per year (international institutions), and $149.00 per year (international students). International air speed delivery is included in all *Clinics* subscription prices. All prices are subject to change without notice. **POSTMASTER:** Send address changes to *Clinics in Chest Medicine,* Elsevier Periodicals Customer Service, 6277 Sea Harbor Drive, Orlando, FL 32887-4800. Customer Service: 1-800-654-2452 (US). From outside of the US, call 1-407-345-4000.

Clinics in Chest Medicine is covered in *Index Medicus, Current Contents/Clinical Medicine, EMBASE/Excerpta Medica, Science Citation Index,* and *ISI/BIOMED.*

Printed in the United States of America.

GUEST EDITOR

MARGARET A. PISANI, MD, MPH, Assistant Professor of Internal Medicine, Section of Pulmonary and Critical Care Medicine, Department of Internal Medicine, Yale University School of Medicine, New Haven, Connecticut

CONTRIBUTORS

MOHAMMAD M. AL-HAMED, MD, Division of Pulmonary and Critical Care Medicine, University of Arkansas for Medical Sciences, Little Rock, Arkansas

VERONICA BRITO, MD, Research Fellow, Pulmonary and Critical Care Medicine, Winthrop-University Hospital, Mineola, New York

SIDNEY S. BRAMAN, MD, Professor of Medicine; and Director, The Warren Alpert Medical School of Brown University, Division of Pulmonary and Critical Care Medicine, The Warren Alpert Medical School of Brown University and Rhode Island Hospital, Providence, Rhode Island

J. RANDALL CURTIS, MD, MPH, Professor, Division of Pulmonary and Critical Care Medicine, Department of Medicine, School of Medicine, University of Washington; Harborview Medical Center, Seattle, Washington

CAROLYN M. D'AMBROSIO, MD, MS, Assistant Professor of Medicine, Pulmonary, Critical Care and Sleep Medicine Division; and Center for Sleep Medicine, Tufts University School of Medicine, Tufts-New England Medical Center, Boston, Massachusetts

MARCIA L. ERBLAND, MD, Professor of Medicine, Division of Pulmonary and Critical Care Medicine, University of Arkansas for Medical Sciences; and Staff Physician, Central Arkansas Veterans Health Care System, Little Rock, Arkansas

SCOTT GETTINGER, MD, Assistant Professor of Medicine, Section of Medical Oncology, Yale School of Medicine, New Haven, Connecticut

NICOLA A. HANANIA, MD, MS, Associate Professor of Medicine, Section of Pulmonary and Critical Care Medicine; and Director, Asthma Clinical Research Center, Baylor College of Medicine, Houston, Texas

JOHN J. HARRINGTON, MD, MPH, Assistant Professor of Medicine, Division of Pulmonary Medicine, National Jewish Medical and Research Center; and Assistant Clinical Professor at Geriatric Medicine, University of Colorado Health Sciences, Denver, Colorado

ROHIT KATIAL, MD, Associate Professor of Medicine; and Program Director, Division of Adult Allergy and Immunology; and Director, Weinberg Clinical Research Unit, National Jewish Medical and Research Center, Denver, Colorado

TEOFILO LEE-CHIONG, Jr, MD, Associate Professor of Medicine, Division of Pulmonary Medicine, National Jewish Medical and Research Center; and Director, National Jewish Sleep Center; and Associate Professor of Medicine, Division of Pulmonary Medicine, University of Colorado Health Sciences, Denver, Colorado

KATHRYN LERZ, APRN, Division of Internal Medicine, Section of Pulmonary and Critical Care Medicine; and Clinical Coordinator, Pulmonary Hypertension Center, Yale University School of Medicine, New Haven, Connecticut

LAYOLA LUNGHAR, MD, Fellow, Pulmonary, Critical Care and Sleep Medicine Division, Tufts University School of Medicine, Boston, Massachusetts

JOHN R. McARDLE, MD, Assistant Professor of Medicine, Division of Internal Medicine, Section of Pulmonary and Critical Care Medicine, Yale University School of Medicine, New Haven, Connecticut

SHOAB A. NAZIR, MD, Assistant Professor of Medicine, Division of Pulmonary and Critical Care Medicine, University of Arkansas for Medical Sciences; and Staff Physician, Central Arkansas Veterans Health Care System, Little Rock, Arkansas

MICHAEL S. NIEDERMAN, MD, FACP, FCCP, Professor of Medicine; and Vice-Chairman, Department of Medicine, State University of New York at Stony Brook; Chairman, Department of Medicine, Winthrop-University Hospital, Mineola, New York

MARGARET A. PISANI, MD, MPH, Assistant Professor of Internal Medicine, Section of Pulmonary and Critical Care Medicine, Department of Internal Medicine, Yale University School of Medicine, New Haven, Connecticut

NEIL W. SCHLUGER, MD, Chief, Division of Pulmonary, Allergy, and Critical Care Medicine, Columbia University Medical Center; and Professor of Medicine, Epidemiology and Environmental Health Sciences, Columbia University, New York, New York

JONATHAN M. SINER, MD, Assistant Professor of Internal Medicine, Section of Pulmonary and Critical Care Medicine, Department of Internal Medicine, Yale University School of Medicine, New Haven, Connecticut

RENEE D. STAPLETON, MD, MSc, Assistant Professor of Medicine, Division of Pulmonary and Critical Care Medicine, Department of Medicine, School of Medicine, University of Washington; Harborview Medical Center, Seattle, Washington

LYNN T. TANOUE, MD, Professor of Medicine, Section of Pulmonary and Critical Care Medicine; and Medical Director, Yale Cancer Center Thoracic Oncology Program, Yale School of Medicine, New Haven, Connecticut

TERENCE K. TROW, MD, Assistant Professor of Medicine, Division of Internal Medicine, Section of Pulmonary and Critical Care Medicine; and Director, Pulmonary Hypertension Center, Yale University School of Medicine, New Haven, Connecticut

WEIHONG ZHENG, MD, Division of Adult Allergy and Immunology, National Jewish Medical and Research Center, Denver, Colorado

CONTENTS

Preface   ix

Margaret A. Pisani

Allergy and Immunology of the Aging Lung   663

Rohit Katial and Weihong Zheng

> The aging process is associated with progressively impaired immune surveillance and
> decreased ability to mount an appropriate immune response, which potentially leads to
> increased susceptibility to respiratory insults. In older patients, pneumonias rank high as
> a reason for hospitalization and cause significant morbidity and mortality. Currently,
> little is known about how the innate and adaptive immune responses change in the aged
> human lung or how the changes are linked to increasing susceptibility to respiratory
> disease. This article reviews the basics of pulmonary host defense and some recently
> published research on the immune response within the aging lung.

Sleep and Older Patients   673

John J. Harrington and Teofilo Lee-Chiong Jr

> Sleep disturbances are common among older adults. The elderly population reports
> more symptoms associated with poor sleep initiation and maintenance and increased
> daytime napping. Sleep problems may be caused by various factors, including
> medication use, medical and psychiatric illnesses, and primary sleep disorders. The
> consequences of poor sleep quality may include cognitive impairment, daytime
> sleepiness, and reduced quality of life. The evaluation and management of these
> disorders is discussed in this review.

Asthma in Older Adults   685

Sidney S. Braman and Nicola A. Hanania

> Asthma is underdiagnosed and undertreated in older adults. The classic symptoms,
> including episodic wheezing, shortness of breath, and chest tightness, are nonspecific in
> this age group. Older patients may underrate symptoms, and other diseases, such as
> chronic obstructive pulmonary disease, congestive heart failure, and angina, may have
> similar presentations. Objective measurements of lung function always should comple-
> ment the history taking and physical examination. Management of asthma in older
> adults should include careful monitoring, controlling triggers, optimizing and
> monitoring pharmacotherapy, and providing appropriate asthma education. Adverse
> effects to commonly used asthma medications are more common in older adults, and
> careful monitoring of their use and adverse effects is important.

Chronic Obstructive Pulmonary Disease in the Older Patient   703
Shoab A. Nazir, Mohammad M. Al-Hamed, and Marcia L. Erbland

Chronic obstructive pulmonary disease (COPD) is one of the most common chronic diseases in the world. It is a major cause of morbidity, mortality, and health care use, particularly in older adults. In the following sections, the authors review the diagnosis and management of COPD with a focus on special issues in older adults.

Pulmonary Hypertension in Older Adults   717
John R. McArdle, Terence K. Trow, and Kathryn Lerz

Pulmonary hypertension is a frequently encountered problem in older patients. True idiopathic pulmonary arterial hypertension can also be seen and requires careful exclusion in older patients. Institution of therapies must be tempered with an appreciation of individual comorbidities and functional limitations that may affect patients' ability to comply and benefit from the complex treatments available for pulmonary arterial hypertension. This article reviews the existing data on the various forms of pulmonary hypertension presenting in older patients and on appropriate therapy in this challenging population.

Treatment of Lung Cancer in Older Patients   735
Lynn T. Tanoue and Scott Gettinger

Lung cancer is a disease of older persons. It is the most common cause of cancer death in men and women in the United States. A comprehensive evaluation of medical comorbidities and functional status is important in all patients but perhaps more so in older adults, and it should be included in the assessment of older patients who have lung cancer. Age, per se, should not be a limiting factor to treatment, because a large body of evidence demonstrates that fit older patients who have lung cancer can safely undergo the same treatments as their younger counterparts with equally good results.

Pneumonia in the Older Patient   751
Michael S. Niederman and Veronica Brito

This article examines the bacteriology, clinical features, therapy for, and prevention of pneumonia in older patients. The discussion focuses on patients who develop pneumonia out of the hospital, including individuals with community-acquired pneumonia and health care–associated pneumonia. Health care–associated pneumonia incorporates patients who live in nursing homes when they develop pneumonia and in many instances requires management similar to nosocomial pneumonia. We have chosen not to discuss nosocomial pneumonia in older patients because it does not have distinctive features or a different management approach than when this illness arises in younger patients.

Tuberculosis and Nontuberculous Mycobacterial Infections in Older Adults   773
Neil W. Schluger

Tuberculosis is one of the world's great public health crises. It is estimated by the World Health Organization that roughly one third of the world's populations, or some 2 billion people, are infected with *Mycobacterium tuberculosis,* the causative agent. More than 8 million people every year develop active tuberculosis disease, and 2 million die as a result. This article reviews tuberculosis and nontuberculous mycobacterial infections in older adults.

Mechanical Ventilation and Acute Respiratory Distress Syndrome in Older Patients
Jonathan M. Siner and Margaret A. Pisani

783

As the population of the United States ages, an increasing number of elderly adults will be cared for in intensive care units. An understanding of how aging affects the respiratory system is important for patient care and ongoing research. The incidence rates of acute respiratory failure and of acute respiratory distress syndrome increase dramatically with age, and therefore understanding the relationship between age and ARDS is important. This article focuses on the age-specific changes in respiratory function. We present a discussion of the management of acute lung injury and acute respiratory distress syndrome with a focus on the role of mechanical ventilation. We conclude with what is known about age and its impact on mortality and functional outcomes after mechanical ventilation.

Non-Invasive Ventilation in the Older Patient Who Has Acute Respiratory Failure
Layola Lunghar and Carolyn M. D'Ambrosio

793

Older patients are at significantly increased risk of acute respiratory failure from multiple causes. Noninvasive positive pressure ventilation has been shown to dramatically improve care of patients with acute respiratory failure. Patient selection is important in all patients being treated with noninvasive positive pressure ventilation but is especially important in older patients. Delirium, confusion, and dementia can lead to difficulty for patients in tolerating this procedure and lead to a worsening respiratory status. The presence of a do-not-intubate order does not necessarily preclude the use of noninvasive positive pressure ventilation, and some patients may derive significant benefit from its use. Overall, noninvasive positive pressure ventilation is a reasonable and justifiable option in the treatment of acute respiratory failure in older patients.

End-of-Life Considerations in Older Patients Who Have Lung Disease
Renee D. Stapleton and J. Randall Curtis

801

The goal of palliative care is to prevent suffering and manage symptoms, maintain quality of life, and provide physical, emotional, and spiritual support for patients and their loved ones. Research suggests that patients with chronic lung disease receive suboptimal palliative care largely because of inadequate communication with their physicians. When patients have made decisions about life-sustaining therapies, physicians often either do not know patients' wishes or misunderstand them. Clinicians should realize that most patients want more information about end-of-life care and that efforts to initiate and improve communication with their patients are important. This article reviews the potential for enhanced palliative care for older patients with chronic lung disease.

Index

813

FORTHCOMING ISSUES

March 2008
Chest Imaging
David Lynch, MD, *Guest Editor*

June 2008
Controversies in Mechanical Ventilation
Neil MacIntyre, MD, *Guest Editor*

September 2008
Sarcoidosis
Robert Baughman, MD and
Marjolein Drent, MD, PhD, *Guest Editors*

RECENT ISSUES

September 2007
Chronic Obstructive Pulmonary Disease
Carolyn L. Rochester, MD, *Guest Editor*

June 2007
Cystic Fibrosis
Laurie A. Whittaker, MD, *Guest Editor*

March 2007
Pulmonary Arterial Hypertension
Harold I. Palevsky, MD, *Guest Editor*

ELSEVIER
SAUNDERS

Clin Chest Med 28 (2007) ix

CLINICS
IN CHEST
MEDICINE

Preface

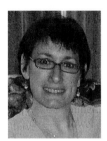

Margaret A. Pisani, MD, MPH
Guest Editor

People age 65 and older are the fastest growing segment of the United States' population. In the 2000 census, 12% of the population (35 million people) was age 65 and older. That number is projected to increase to 66 million, or 16% of the population, by the year 2050. Life expectancy also has increased; recent Centers for Disease Control and Prevention reports indicate life expectancy at 77.8 years. Age-adjusted death rates have decreased significantly with the largest changes occurring in older patients. Despite these trends, the 10 leading causes of death include several pulmonary etiologies including lung cancer, chronic respiratory diseases, influenza, and pneumonia.

This issue of *Clinics in Chest Medicine* is devoted to understanding the impact of respiratory diseases in older patients. It includes a review of allergy and immunology of the aging lung, sleep in older patients, and reviews on specific disease topics including asthma, chronic obstructive lung disease, pulmonary hypertension, lung cancer, pneumonia, tubuerculosis, and atypical mycobacteria. There are also reviews on the use of mechanical ventilation and noninvasive ventilation in older patients, and, importantly, end-of-life considerations.

Focusing on issues unique to older patients who have lung disease is important to improving their care, reducing morbidity, and improving their quality of life. This issue represents an excellent review of many lung diseases patients face as they age. I am grateful to the authors for their outstanding contributions to this issue. I owe a special thanks to Sarah Barth at Elsevier, who helped me at every step along the way. This issue is dedicated to my family, especially Alex and Sara, who kept me going on this and all of my projects.

Margaret A. Pisani, MD, MPH
*Section of Pulmonary
and Critical Care Medicine
Department of Internal Medicine
Yale University School of Medicine
300 Cedar Street
P.O. Box 208057
New Haven, CT 06520-8057, USA*

E-mail address: margaret.pisani@yale.edu

0272-5231/07/$ - see front matter © 2007 Elsevier Inc. All rights reserved.
doi:10.1016/j.ccm.2007.08.009

ELSEVIER
SAUNDERS

Clin Chest Med 28 (2007) 663–672

CLINICS
IN CHEST
MEDICINE

Allergy and Immunology of the Aging Lung

Rohit Katial, MD*, Weihong Zheng, MD

*Division of Adult Allergy and Immunology, National Jewish Medical and Research Center,
1400 Jackson Street, Denver, CO 80206, USA*

The alveolar membrane of the lung is one of the largest epithelial surface areas of the human body in contact with the external environment, and it is continuously exposed to various microorganisms and organic and inorganic particles. Like the skin or the gastrointestinal mucosa, the immune system of the lung is exposed to a host of foreign matters and differentiates potentially harmful agents from other innocuous materials.

The aging process is associated with progressively impaired immune surveillance and decreased ability to mount an appropriate immune response, which potentially leads to increased susceptibility to respiratory insults. Aged individuals are at increased risk for respiratory tract infections [1], interstitial lung disease [2], and pulmonary neoplasms [3]. Pneumonia ranks high as a cause for hospitalization and causes significant morbidity and mortality in older patients. The role of aged-based immune changes in increases in infection, interstitial lung disease, and neoplasms has not been linked clearly, but the increased incidence of infections in the older population does suggest a role for alterations in host immunity [4]. Although the senescence of the immune system in older adults is likely to play a contributing role in the pathogenesis of these disorders, little is known about how the innate and adaptive immune responses change in the aged human lung or how the changes are linked to increasing susceptibility to infections. Many previous assumptions about host defense of the aging human lung are based on either animal studies or ex vivo data from human peripheral blood. This article reviews the basics of pulmonary host defense and some recently published research on the immune response within the aging lung.

Overview of human immunity

The human immune system has cellular and soluble protein components that interact in a highly complex manner and lead to the basis for innate and adaptive responses. The innate immune system provides the first line of host defense, and its function does not depend on prior exposure to the microbe. The innate immune defense includes the epithelial barrier, leukocytes (neutrophils, macrophages, and natural killer cells), circulating effector proteins (complement, collectins, pentraxins), and numerous cytokines released from these cells (ie, interleukin [IL]-12, interferon-γ, tissue necrosis factor, chemokines).

Upon exposure to an antigen, the innate immune system responds by recruiting neutrophils, macrophages, and natural killer cells and activating the complement pathway. The products of complement activation can serve various roles in host defense, with the primary one being opsonization, a process whereby the complement components bind to the microbial cell surface and facilitate uptake by phagocytic cells. The complement system enhances the immune response by facilitating chemotaxis for other effector cells. For example, the complement-activated product C5a is a potent chemotactic factor for neutrophils and is involved in the activation of phagocytic cells [5] and release of oxidants and granule-based enzymes [6–8]. The collectins are another group of related proteins that serve as opsonins for bacterial products in plasma and tissues. The group includes mannose-binding lectin and the lung surfactant proteins SP-A and SP-D. The collectins have a common structure of a globular-like

* Corresponding author.
E-mail address: katialr@njc.org (R. Katial).

domain and a collagen-like tail, and the binding of the collectins to the bacterial surface promotes phagocytosis by macrophages and neutrophils. Mannose-binding lectin binds carbohydrates with terminal mannose and fucose, which are typically found on the microbial cell surface, which results in activation of the alternate complement pathway and leads to accumulation of C3b on the microbial surface.

Innate immunity depends highly on recognition of conserved pathogen-associated molecular patterns of micro-organisms (eg, lipopolysaccharide, lipoteichoic acids, mannans, peptidoglycans, glucans, or bacterial DNA), which are often essential for the survival of microbes but are not present on mammalian cells. The ability of the human immune system to detect pathogen-associated molecular patterns limits the capacity of microbes to evade immune surveillance and allows differentiation of self from non-self antigens.

The Toll-like receptors (TLRs) are a family of membrane proteins that binds pathogen-associated molecular patterns and are a subset of pattern recognition receptors. Ten mammalian TLRs have been identified [9]. They recognize an array of bacterial, fungal, and viral products, including gram-negative bacterial lipopolysaccharides, gram-positive bacterial peptidoglycans, bacterial lipoproteins, lipoteichoic acid, zymosan, flagellin, heat shock protein 60, unmethylated CpG motifs, and double-stranded viral RNA. Although a single TLR is responsible for stimulating inflammatory responses to a particular microbial ligand, the repertoire of specificities of the TLR system is apparently extended by the ability of TLRs to heterodimerize with one another, which minimizes the chance of immune evasion by microbial products.

After the initial identification and description of the mammalian TLR family, extensive studies have been performed to evaluate the susceptibility to infections by human microbial pathogens using mice with engineered deletions of each TLR molecule. In some bacterial infection models, mice with defective TLR signaling capacity succumb rapidly to *Staphylococcus aureus, Listeria monocytogenes, Mycobacterium tuberculosis,* and *Salmonella* infections [10–13]. Several human studies have confirmed the important role that TLRs play in a protective immune response by comparing the phenotypes of various polymorphisms of TLRs. Certain polymorphisms of TLRs render patients highly susceptible to pyogenic infections with *S aureus* [14], pneumonia caused by *Legionella*

pneumophila [15], or *M tuberculosis* [16]. Others have identified polymorphisms of TLR 4 to be associated with susceptibility to gram-negative infections [17] and gram-negative septic shock [18].

The innate immune system also plays a critical role in activating and coordinating the adaptive immune response by up-regulating costimulatory molecules and secreting cytokines, which influence lymphocytic function. Acquired immunity involves the activation and proliferation of antigen-specific B and T cells. Antigen-presenting cells (ie, macrophages and dendritic cells) from the innate arm of host defense process microbial antigens and present antigen proteins in association with major histocompatibility antigens class I and class II molecules to circulatory lymphocytes. Once an antigen-specific B cell recognizes the appropriate ligand, the cell transforms into a plasma cell and secretes antigen-specific antibodies, which serve numerous functions, including direct binding to antigen and opsonization. T cells augment B-cell development and can eradicate intracellular pathogens directly by cytotoxic activity against virally infected cells. The adaptive immune system has a memory component that is lacking in the innate immune system. Together, the innate and the adaptive immune systems enable the host to respond to various antigens encountered and preserve effector function for rechallenge against the same antigens at a future time.

Innate immunity in the lung

Nonspecific clearance mechanisms and components of innate immune surveillance are constantly active in the lung, eradicating pathogens and preventing infection. Innate immune defenses include epithelial cells, antimicrobial molecules generated in the airways, and the phagocytic defenses provided by the resident alveolar macrophages. Mechanical host defenses represent the first-line barrier to the invading substances. Particles larger than 5 μm are trapped in the upper airways and cleared by ciliary movement. Particles smaller than 5 μm potentially can be cleared by antibacterial molecules, including lysozymes, defensins, immunoglobulins, complement, and collectins. Lysozyme is lytic to many bacterial membranes, lactoferrin excludes iron from bacterial metabolism, and the defensins are antimicrobial peptides released from respiratory epithelial cells and leukocytes.

Recent studies have defined a critical role for airway epithelial cells in innate immune response in the lungs [19,20]. The epithelium lining the airway prevents the growth and colonization of inhaled microbes by several different mechanisms. A direct mechanical effect involves the ciliated cells moving trapped particulates upward and out of the lungs. The secretions produced in the airway contain lysozymes, lactoferrin, and antimicrobial defensins, which inhibit bacterial growth. Binding of pattern recognition receptors to pathogen-associated molecular patterns also stimulates epithelial cells to produce antimicrobial defensins and secrete chemokines, which serve to recruit neutrophils to the location of insult and provide further immune protection to the lung. Besides the mechanical factors and chemokines, epithelial-derived cytokines contribute to the host defense of the lung. Epithelial cells produce proinflammatory cytokines, including IL-1, -5, -6, and -8, RANTES, granulocyte-macrophage colony–stimulating factor, and transforming growth factor-β. One mechanism for production of epithelial cytokines is through lipopolysaccharide binding to TLR-9, which leads to nuclear factor (NF)-κB activation and a dose-dependent up-regulation of cytokines, specifically IL-6 and -8, and human β-defensin 2 in the airways [21,22].

Skerrett and coworkers [23] constructed a mouse model to express a dominant negative IκB construct in distal airway epithelial cells, preventing NF-κB activation, which led to impaired neutrophilic recruitment to the lung after lipopolysaccharide challenge and diminished levels of tissue necrosis factor-α, IL-1β, and macrophage inflammatory protein-2. This experiment confirmed the pathway of lipopolysaccharide recognition by distal airway epithelial cells and the importance of airway epithelial cells in the innate inflammatory response.

Alveolar macrophages are the first line of phagocytic defense against the infectious pathogens that escape mechanical and epithelial defenses [24]. These cells comprise up to 95% of the cellular constituents in bronchoalveolar fluid. Macrophages possess the ability to avidly phagocytose and are important for daily clearance of small microbial challenges and maintaining sterility of the lower airway. Some bacteria, such as *Mycobacterium* spp, *Nocardia* spp, *and Legionella* spp, can evade the standard microbicidal activity of the macrophagers and replicate intracellularly. In such a scenario or when pathogen load is too large, macrophages produce proinflammatory cytokines and initiate a localized inflammatory response by recruiting neutrophils from the lung capillary networks into the alveolar space. Neutrophils then eradicate the offending pathogens. In some instances, however, such as mycobacterial disease, the immune response may contain the infection but not lead to a sterilizing response. Alveolar macrophages in concert with other elements of innate defenses can clear foreign particles and bacterial pathogens from airspace surfaces; however, augmented innate and specific adaptive immune responses may come into play to clear virulent encapsulated bacteria, viruses, or intracellular pathogens that are capable of surviving within alveolar macrophages and ultimately lead to a pool of cells capable of memory function.

Adaptive immunity of the lung

The adaptive immune response is essential for pulmonary host defense and builds on the innate response. After exposure to a novel pathogen, the immune system within the lung generates humoral and cellular components. The primary cell for generating humoral immunity is the B cell; after antigen exposure, local antibody responses have been described. Using a mouse model with intratracheally administered sheep red blood cells, Kaltreider and Curtis' group demonstrated that particulate antigens are taken up in the alveolar space by macrophages or other antigen presenting cells. These cells then migrate via lymphatics to regional lymph nodes, where the primary immune response occurs. Once antigen-specific B cells are formed, they traffic back to the lung, where they terminally differentiate and expand into either antibody-secreting plasma cells or memory B cells [25–27]. If the pathogen is encountered again, the lung has the ability to respond quickly through recruitment of resident antigen-specific memory B cells, a process known as the amnestic response. The authors have shown that after oral mucosal and intranasal vaccine challenge, circulating antibody-secreting cells can be detected 1 week after vaccination. These cells transiently traffic between systemic and mucosal circulation. Adaptive responses seen systemically are linked to mucosal immunity but also differ in the manner in which antigen is handled [28]. In the upper respiratory tract, IgA predominates and IgG is present in lesser amounts. IgA serves as an immunologic barrier between organisms and mucosal surfaces and provides immune protection against mucosally presented antigens. Once pathogens are bound to IgA, they may be taken up by airway macrophages through the phagocytic process [29]. In the lower respiratory tract, immunoglobulins comprise the second largest class of proteins obtained from bronchoalveolar lavage (BAL) fluid after albumin [30], and IgG is of primary importance for its opsonizing and complement-activating properties [31]. Four IgG subclasses exist in BAL fluid in approximately the same proportions as found in serum. IgG1 represents approximately 60% to 70%, IgG2 represents 20% to 25%, and IgG3 and IgG4 represent less than 5% of the total IgG present in BAL fluid [31]. Protein antigens provoke IgG1 antibodies, whereas polysaccharide antigens predominantly give rise to the IgG2 subclass [32,33]. Smaller amounts of IgA and IgE are also found in the BAL fluid of normal persons [30].

Cell-mediated adaptive immunity in the lung is essential for clearing viruses, mycobacteria, and fungi. It is modulated by the humoral response and requires a coordinated action among T cells, natural killer cells, and dendritic cells [34]. Immature myeloid dendritic cells carry antigen from the pulmonary epithelial to regional lymph nodes and present them to naive T cells expressing the $\alpha\beta$ T-cell antigen receptor. Precursors of $\alpha\beta$ T cells are recruited from the bone marrow to the thymus, where they migrate from the cortex to the medulla and undergo positive and then negative selection, which ensures that their T-cell antigen receptor recognizes self peptide major histocompatibility complex but not with such strong affinity as to be autoreactive. During thymic maturation, T cells develop expression of CD8 or CD4, which is essential for antigen recognition in the context of class I or class II major histocompatibility. Most T cells in the lung are mature memory T cells [35] and mirror the predominance of memory B cells in the lung [25–27], which suggests that the lung is immediately available to respond to infections humorally and cellularly in an antigen-specific manner.

CD4 T cells can further be divided into T helper 1 (Th1) and T helper 2 (Th2) based on cytokine profiles involved. The differentiation of naïve CD4 T cells into Th1 and Th2 populations is controlled by cytokines produced by antigen presenting cells and by the T cells themselves. The differentiation of Th1 effectors is stimulated by virus, intracellular bacteria, such as *Listeria* and mycobacteria, and by some parasites, such as *Leishmania*. Th 1 responses are characterized by secretion of interferon-γ, IL-2, and tumor necrosis factor-α and they are especially crucial in the lungs because alveolar macrophages require exogenous interferons to activate STAT1-dependent killing of phagocytosed microbes [36]. Th2 differentiation occurs in response to helminthes and allergens. It is characterized by the production of IL-4, -5, -9, -10, and -13. These cytokines favor antibody production with class switching to IgE and IgG4. Exaggerated Th2 responses are thought to contribute to atopic diseases in the lung, such as asthma. IL-4 and -13 are thought to be IgE switch cytokines that may contribute to allergen-induced development of asthma. Data also have suggested that Th2 profile may favor fibrosis [37]. The protective role of T-cell immunity is essential in the lung regardless of the cytokine profile being exhibited, however. The tight regulation between Th1 and Th2 allows for a nonconflicting response. For example, if an intracellular pathogen such as *Myobacterium* induces secretion of IL-12 and interferon-γ for protective purposes, these same cytokines block Th2 induction, which ensures that a more appropriate antimicrobial response is generated to eradicate the offending microbe.

A third distinctive phenotype of T-cell response has been identified: regulatory T (T_{reg}) cells. They are a CD25+ CD4+ T-cell subset that expresses the Foxp3 transcription factor [38]. T_{reg} cells principally develop from thymocytes but also can be produced peripherally during chronic antigenic stimulation. T_{reg} cells can suppress CD4+ and CD8+ T-cell responses by an undefined contact-dependent mechanism [39]. T_{reg}-mediated suppression leads to immunologic self-tolerance and negative control of immune responses. Several explanations are possible for the mechanisms of T_{reg}-mediated suppression in vivo. First, expression of the high-affinity trimeric IL-2 receptor by T_{reg} cells might result in growth-factor competition and consumption of IL-2 [40,41]. Other than passive IL-2 deprivation, two major immunosuppressive cytokines (IL-10 and transforming growth factor-β) have been implicated as active effector mechanisms of T_{reg} cell-mediated suppression in vivo [42–44]. The primary purpose is to induce tolerance to an antigen and down-regulate an active response once a pathogen has been eradicated. This action ensures that no overactive immune response leads to increased cytokine activation beyond what is necessary, potentially preventing autoimmunity by controlling self-reacting T cells. One therapeutic approach using T_{reg} cells could include modulating the intensity of antimicrobial immune responses in acute and chronic infections to develop effective vaccines against microbes and prevent or treat allergic diseases. It is believed that one mechanism of down-regulating the allergic response with allergen immunotherapy involves invoking T_{reg} function.

Lung immunity and aging

Aging brings about changes in the structure and function of the lung, but immune responses also systemically wane and can impact lung host defense. Most data in this area center around adaptive responses because they have been studied more extensively than the innate response in the aged. TLR expression and cytokine secretion of macrophages from splenic and activated peritoneal cavities decline in aged mice [45]. It is also observed in mice that the phagocytic ability of macrophages from aged animals declines in parallel with decreased levels of macrophage-derived chemokines macrophage inmflammatory protein (MIP)-1α, MIP-1β, and MIP-2 and eotaxin [46]. In humans, the effect of aging on monocyte and macrophage function remains controversial and in many studies is unaffected. Monocyte/macrophage and lymphocyte recruitment to infected tissue was delayed in older individuals based on a study of cutaneous punch biopsies [47]. Monocytes from older patients are reported to display decreased cytotoxicity against tumor cells ex vivo after lipopolysaccharide activation, which is thought to be caused by decreased production of reactive oxygen intermediates [48]. Macrophage dysfunction with aging also may depress the feedback loop between macrophages and natural killer cells via factors such as IL-12. Superoxide production in neutrophils from aged individuals also decreases, which further compromises phagocytic function [49].

Recently, Van Duin and colleagues [50] demonstrated in humans that TLR1 surface expression in peripheral blood monocytes was reduced, whereas TLR2 was not affected. They also reported defective TLR-mediated tissue necrosis factor-α and IL-6 production in older subjects. Such observations could provide an explanation for increased infections in older patients and decreased vaccine response. A more detailed understanding of the impact of age on innate immunity is needed to overcome age-related defects and reduce disease morbidity in the aged population.

It is clear that the thymus involutes with age and is replaced by fatty tissue by 60 years of age, whereas the absolute numbers of CD3+, CD4+, and CD8+ cells decrease with age. The proportion of naïve T cells goes down and memory T cells increase. Although the number of memory cells increases, the cellular responses by these cells wane

[51]. Mouse data in aging animals have shown a diminished lymphocyte repertoire [52], reduced proliferative responses to mitogens and antigens [53,54], and a decline in Fas-mediated T-cell apoptosis [55]. In humans, increased CD45RO (memory marker) on T lymphocytes [56], shifting from a Th1 to Th2 cytokine profile [57], and declines in peripheral lymphocytes and soluble IL-2 receptors also have been reported [58]. These findings may explain why older adults often fail to elicit adequate immune responses to infection or immunization. In regard to B-cell function, antibody production is less efficient with advancing age and the antibodies produced tend to have reduced affinity for specific antigens as a result of age-related decline in somatic hypermutation because of defects in T and B cells [59].

The CD4/CD8 T-lymphocyte ratio in human peripheral blood tends to increase with advancing age [60,61], and similar changes have been reported in the lung. Myer and colleagues [62] investigated the BAL and peripheral blood subsets in clinically normal nonsmoking volunteers of two different age groups (19–36 and 64–83 years). The total cells per milliliter in BAL fluid were significantly increased in the older age group. The mean percentage of lymphocytes in BAL fluid was also increased in this group compared with the younger cohort. The ratio of CD4+ to CD8+ T lymphocytes in BAL fluid was significantly increased (with an absolute increase in CD4+ cells) in the older group and it was considerably higher than the peripheral blood CD4/CD8 ratio. Activated CD4+/human leukocyte antigen-DR+ lymphocytes were also increased. The authors speculated that the relative increase in CD4+ lymphocytes for older healthy subjects probably represented an accumulation of memory cells and primed T cells caused by cumulative antigenic stimulation at mucosal surfaces. As a result, activated lymphocyte subsets may play a role in age-related low-grade inflammation in the aging lung and contribute to alterations in lung matrix and function that are associated with the aging process. Although lymphocytes and lymphocyte subsets retrieved from the lung by BAL have been studied in disease and, to some degree, in normal individuals, little information exists as it relates to aging [63–65].

The model of low-grade chronic inflammation in the lung correlating with the immunologic changes seen in the aged individuals was furthered when Myer and colleagues [66] studied the BAL profile of normal individuals in discordant age groups (20–36, 45–55, and 65–78 years). The authors measured the level of immunoglobulin (IgG, IgA, IgM), albumin, IL-6 and -10, cell surface antigen expression, and superoxide anion production in BAL fluid. A significant increase in total cell concentration, neutrophils, and BAL immunoglobulin content was observed in the oldest age group. They also demonstrated that mean lymphocyte subset (CD4+/CD8+) ratios were significantly increased in blood and, to a greater degree, in BAL for the oldest versus youngest age groups. Similarly, BAL-derived cells displayed increased phorbol myristate acetate-stimulated release of superoxide anion for the oldest versus youngest subject group, and mean BAL IL-6 concentrations were significantly elevated in aged individuals compared with younger individuals. These observations suggested that even in asymptomatic and clinically normal aged volunteers, altered inflammatory cell profiles reflect the presence of low-grade inflammation in the lower respiratory tracts based on significantly increased numbers of phagocytic cells, immunoglobulins, IL-6 concentration, and superoxide anion release.

Franceschi and coworkers [67,68] put forward a similar hypothesis. They studied centenarians as a model to address the immunologic and genetic basis of aging and suggested that immunosenescence was a remodeling of the immune system in which sustained, lifelong exposure to antigenic stresses leads to a gradual decline of naive T cells, an accumulation of memory T cells and effector CD8+/CD28− T cells, and decline in T-cell repertoire. In contrast, many aspects of innate immunity, such as phagocytosis, natural killer cell cytotoxicity, chemotaxis, and complement activities, showed less decline. Innate immunity was believed to become progressively more important to aged individuals as a means to fill the "immunologic gap" that appears as a result of declining adaptive immunity. The consequence of these changes was interpreted as a state of chronic low-grade inflammation driven by IL-6 production from the overrepresented effector cells. Such a state was termed "inflammaging." Similar processes may be the common and most important driving forces of age-related pathologies, such as neurodegeneration, atherosclerosis, and diabetes [68].

Longevity correlates with fairly well-preserved immune responses in older patients [69]. Conversely, immune parameters were measured in a longitudinal study of a very old population of Swedish people, and decreased survival was associated with low numbers of CD4+ T cells and CD19+ B cells, impaired T-cell proliferative response to mitogenic stimulation, and increased numbers of CD8+ cytotoxic-suppressor cells [70].

Likely there is no simple explanation for the increased susceptibility of older individuals to lung infection, but age-associated changes are thought to increase the risk to older patients for pulmonary infections. Other factors that place older adults at higher risk for respiratory infections include systemic diseases, impaired oral [71] and mucociliary clearance [72], predisposition to aspiration [73], malnutrition [74], and residence in long-term care facilities [75]. The pathogens that are frequently involved include atypical pathogens, such as *Legionella* spp, *Chlamydiae pneumoniae*, and influenza A and B, parainfluenza virus, respiratory syncytial virus, *Bordetella pertussis*, *Haemophilus influenzae*, and *M tuberculosis*.

Allergy of the aging lung

The incidence of asthma—primarily allergic asthma—is highest among young children: approximately 3000 in 100,000 individuals in the first year of life and 900 in 100,000 in years 1 to 4. The incidence rate remains at approximately 100 in 100,000 after the age of 20 years [76,77]. Epidemiologic studies have focused largely on children and young adults. Much less information has been available about the epidemiology of allergic asthma in older individuals. Studies have shown that asthma is common in older adults and may be associated with severe symptoms that require unscheduled physician visits and hospitalizations. Chronic airway obstruction seen in this population rarely goes into complete remission [76,78].

Factors responsible for development of asthma in older patients have not been defined fully. Usually there is no familial correlation for these groups of patients. Occupational exposures are important during the working years. Otherwise, common environmental allergens are thought to be less important with increasing age, because individuals at risk of becoming sensitized probably will have done so by the time they reach the later years. Asthma is associated with elevated serum IgE levels from childhood into old age, but skin test or specific IgE antibody test responses are often negative in adult-onset asthma [79–84]. In a large number of patients, their first asthmatic symptoms are frequently described as having been preceded by a concomitant upper respiratory viral infection. This factor suggests that an infectious trigger may play a role in the onset of asthma in older patients

[76]. The role of air pollution in the incidence of adult asthma is still controversial [85,86].

Lung function depends on precision and accuracy of the equipment, and longitudinal data may have some inherent measurement bias. Lung volumes being influenced by body size have shown some consistent patterns in normal cohorts. All lung volumes increase to a point of maximal development in childhood [87]. The total lung capacity after adjusting for height does not seem to change beyond this point [88]. Interestingly, functional residual capacity and residual volume seem to increase in cross-sectional studies [89–91], and FEV_1 begins to decline in adulthood. The age at which FEV_1 declines has changed as successive birth cohorts are being studied. Estimates of age of decline in cross-sectional studies suggest the early 20s [92,93], but longitudinal data report that the decline does not begin until age 36 [94,95]. Gottlieb and colleagues [96] conducted a longitudinal study in approximately 1000 middle-aged and older men with no history of asthma participating in the Normative Aging Study to investigate the relationship between allergy and decline in lung function. They examined the immediate cutaneous hypersensitivity to common aeroallergens, chronic respiratory symptoms, peripheral eosinophil counts, methacholine responsiveness, and subsequent rate of decline of lung function. The results suggested that cutaneous hypersensitivity to common aeroallergens is a significant independent predictor of lung function decline in this population. The rate of decline of FEV_1 in the nonallergic nonsmoking group was 30.4 mL/year, whereas in the allergic nonsmoking group it was 38.9 mL/year [96]. O'Connor and colleagues [97] did not find a relationship between atopy and level of FEV_1 in a similar Normative Aging Study cohort, however. The latter group defined atopy as skin test reactivity more than 5 mm, whereas the former study used the parameter of more than 2 mm. Other data have examined the relationship between atopy and lung function and shown mixed results. The discordance in the literature may be explained by methodologic differences to include the number of allergens used for testing, the type of allergens, and the scale on which atopy is measured.

Summary

Recent research on bronchoalveolar fluid has shed some light on the immune cell profile and acellular components of the aging lung, but the exact impact of these changes on host defense against respiratory infections is largely unknown. A better understanding of the age-associated changes in pulmonary host defense mechanisms is imperative before we can focus on manipulating age-related immune defects to reduce the susceptibility of older patients to respiratory tract disease. Only then can we possibly reduce morbidity and mortality and the considerable health care burden posed by the increased incidence of pneumonia and other inflammatory diseases of the lung in this at-risk population.

References

[1] Marston BJ, Plouffe JF, File TM Jr, et al. Incidence of community-acquired pneumonia requiring hospitalization: results of a population-based active surveillance study in Ohio. The community-based pneumonia incidence study group. Arch Intern Med 1997;157:1709–18.

[2] Coultas DB, Zumwalt RE, Black WC, et al. The epidemiology of interstitial lung diseases. Am J Respir Crit Care Med 1994;150:967–72.

[3] Hendrick AM, Hendrick DJ. Thoracic tumors in the elderly patient. In: Connolly MJ, editor. Respiratory disease in the elderly patient. London: Chapman and Hall; 1996. p. 141–69.

[4] National Center for Health Statistics. Health, United States, 2006 with chartbook on trends in the health of Americans. Available at: http://www.cdc.gov/nchs/hus.htm.

[5] Marder SR, Chenoweth DE, Goldstein IM, et al. Chemotactic responses of human peripheral blood monocytes to the complement-derived peptides C5a and C5a des Arg. J Immunol 1985;134:3325–31.

[6] Goldstein IM, Weissmann G. Generation of C5-derived lysosomal enzyme-releasing activity (C5a) by lysates of leukocyte lysosomes. J Immunol 1974; 113:1583–8.

[7] Sacks T, Moldow CF, Craddock PR, et al. Oxygen radicals mediate endothelial cell damage by complement-stimulated granulocytes: an in vitro model of immune vascular damage. J Clin Invest 1978;61: 1161–7.

[8] Mollnes TE, Brekke OL, Fung M, et al. Essential role of the C5a receptor in *E. coli*-induced oxidative burst and phagocytosis revealed by a novel lepirudin-based human whole blood model of inflammation. Blood 2002;100:1869–77.

[9] Schnare M, Rollinghoff M, Qureshi S. Toll-like receptors: sentinels of host defence against bacterial infection. Int Arch Allergy Immunol 2006;139(1): 75–85 [e-pub 2005 Nov 25].

[10] Takeuchi O, Hoshino K, Akira S. Cutting edge: TLR2-deficient and MyD88-deficient mice are highly susceptible to *Staphylococcus aureus* infection. J Immunol 2000;165:5392–6.

[11] Torres D, Barrier M, Bihl F, et al. Toll-like receptor 2 is required for optimal control of *Listeria monocytogenes* infection. Infect Immun 2004;72:2131–9.

[12] Drennan M-B, Nicolle D, Quesniaux VJ, et al. Toll-like receptor 2-deficient mice succumb to *Mycobacterium tuberculosis* infection. Am J Pathol 2004; 164:49–57.

[13] Vazquez-Torres A, Vallance BA, Bergman MA, et al. Toll-like receptor 4 dependence of innate and adaptive immunity to *Salmonella*: importance of the Kupffer cell network. J Immunol 2004;172:6202–8.

[14] Lorenz E, Mira JP, Cornish KL, et al. A novel polymorphism in the Toll-like receptor 2 gene and its potential association with staphylococcal infection. Infect Immun 2000;68:6398–401.

[15] Hawn TR, Verbon A, Lettinga KD, et al. A common dominant TLR5 stop codon polymorphism abolishes flagellin signaling and is associated with susceptibility to Legionnaires' disease. J Exp Med 2003; 198:1563–72.

[16] Ogus A-C, Yoldas B, Ozdemir T, et al. The Arg753GLn polymorphism of the human toll-like receptor 2 gene in tuberculosis disease. Eur Respir J 2004;23:219–23.

[17] Agnese D-M, Calvano E, Hahm SJ, et al. Human Toll-like receptor 4 mutations but not CD14 polymorphisms are associated with an increased risk of gram-negative infections. J Infect Dis 2002;186: 1522–5.

[18] Lorenz E, Mira JP, Frees KL, et al. Relevance of mutations in the TLR4 receptor in patients with gram-negative septic shock. Arch Intern Med 2002; 162:1028–32.

[19] Diamond G, Legarda D, Ryan LK. The innate immune response of the respiratory epithelium. Immunol Rev 2000;173:27–38.

[20] Martin TR, Frevert CW. Innate immunity in the lungs. Proc Am Thorac Soc 2005;2:403–11.

[21] Beutler B. Innate immunity: an overview. Mol Immunol 2004;40(12):845–59.

[22] Platz J, Beisswenger C, Dalpke A, et al. Microbial DNA induces a host defense reaction of human respiratory epithelial cells. J Immunol 2004;173: 1219–23.

[23] Skerrett SJ, Liggitt HD, Hajjar AM, et al. Respiratory epithelial cells regulate lung inflammation in response to inhaled endotoxin. Am J Physiol Lung Cell Mol Physiol 2004;287:L143–52.

[24] Zhang P, Summer WR, Bagby GJ, et al. Innate immunity and pulmonary host defense. Immunol Rev 2000;173:39–51.

[25] Curtis JL, Kaltreider HB. Characterization of bronchoalveolar lymphocytes during a specific antibody-forming cell response in the lungs of mice. Am Rev Respir Dis 1989;139:393–400.

[26] Kaltreider HB, Caldwell JL, Byrd PK. The capacity of normal murine alveolar macrophages to function as antigen-presenting cells for the initiation of primary antibody-forming cell responses to sheep erythrocytes in vitro. Am Rev Respir Dis 1986;133: 1097–104.

[27] Kaltreider HB, Curtis JL, Arraj SM. The mechanism of appearance of specific antibody-forming cells in lungs of inbred mice after immunization with sheep erythrocytes intratracheally. II. Dose-dependence and kinetics of appearance of antibody-forming cells in hilar lymph nodes and lungs of unprimed and primed mice. Am Rev Respir Dis 1987;135:87–92.

[28] Katial RK, Brandt BL, Moran EE, et al. Immunogenicity and safety testing of a group B meningococcal native outer membrane vesicle vaccine. Infect Immun 2002;70:702–7.

[29] Twigg HL. Humoral immune defense (antibodies): recent advances. Proc Am Thorac Soc 2005;2: 417–21.

[30] Group TBC. Proteins in bronchoalveolar lavage fluid. Am Rev Respir Dis 1990;141:S183–8.

[31] Merrill WW, Naegel GP, Olchowski JJ, et al. Immunoglobulin G subclass proteins in serum and lavage fluid of normal subjects: quantitation and comparison with immunoglobulins A and E. Am Rev Respir Dis 1985;131:584–7.

[32] Siber GR, Schur PH, Aisenberg AC, et al. Correlation between serum IgG-2 concentrations and the antibody response to bacterial polysaccharide antigens. N Engl J Med 1980;303:178–82.

[33] Stevens R, Dichek D, Keld B, et al. IgG1 is the predominant subclass of in vivo- and in vitro-produced anti-tetanus toxoid antibodies and also serves as the membrane IgG molecule for delivering inhibitory signals to anti-tetanus toxoid antibody-producing B cells. J Clin Immunol 1983;3:65–9.

[34] Curtis JL. Cell-mediated adaptive immune defense of the lungs. Proc Am Thorac Soc 2005;2:412–6.

[35] Saltini C, Kirby M, Trapnell BC, et al. Biased accumulation of T lymphocytes with "memory"-type CD45 leukocyte common antigen gene expression on the epithelial surface of the human lung. J Exp Med 1990;171:1123–40.

[36] Punturieri A, Alviani RS, Polak T, et al. Specific engagement of TLR4 or TLR3 does not lead to IFN-ß– mediated innate signal amplification and STAT1 phosphorylation in resident murine alveolar macrophages. J Immunol 2004;173:1033–42.

[37] Jakubzick C, Kunkel SL, Puri RK, et al. Therapeutic targeting of IL-4- and IL-13-responsive cells in pulmonary fibrosis. Immunol Res 2004;30(3):339–49.

[38] Kronenberg M, Rudensky A. Regulation of immunity by self-reactive T cells. Nature 2005;435: 598–604.

[39] Shevach EM. CD4$^+$ CD25$^+$ suppressor T cells: more questions than answers. Nat Immun 2002;2: 389–400.

[40] Barthlott T, Kassiotis G, Stockinger B. T cell regulation as a side effect of homeostasis and competition. J Exp Med 2003;197:451–60.

[41] Barthlott T, Moncrieff H, Veldhoen M, et al. CD25$^+$CD4$^+$ T cells compete with naive CD4$^+$ T

cells for IL-2 and exploit it for the induction of IL-10 production. Int Immunol 2005;17:279–88.

[42] Sakaguchi S. Naturally arising CD4$^+$ regulatory T cells for immunologic self-tolerance and negative control of immune responses. Annu Rev Immunol 2004;22:531–62.

[43] Asseman C, Mauze S, Leach MW, et al. An essential role for interleukin 10 in the function of regulatory T cells that inhibit intestinal inflammation. J Exp Med 1999;190:995–1004.

[44] Powrie F, Carlino J, Leach MW, et al. A critical role for transforming growth factor but not interleukin 4 in the suppression of T helper type 1-mediated colitis by CD45RB(low) CD4+ T cells. J Exp Med 1996; 183:2669–74.

[45] Renshaw M, Rockwell J, Engleman C, et al. Cutting edge: impaired toll-like receptor expression and function in aging. J Immunol 2002;169: 4697–701.

[46] Swift ME, Burns AL, Gray KL, et al. Age-related alterations in the inflammatory response to dermal injury. J Invest Dermatol 2001;117:1027–35.

[47] Ashcroft GS, Horan MA, Ferguson MW. Aging alters the inflammatory and endothelial cell adhesion molecule profiles during human cutaneous wound healing. Lab Invest 1998;78:47–58.

[48] McLachlan J. Antitumor properties of aged human monocytes. J Immunol 1995;154:832–43.

[49] Polingnano A. Age-associated changes of neutrophils: responsiveness in a human healthy elderly population. Cytobios 1994;80:145–53.

[50] van Duin D, Mohanty S, Thomas V, et al. Age-associated defect in human TLR-1/2 function. J Immunol 2007;178:970–5.

[51] Flurkey K, Stadecker M, Miller RA. Memory T lymphocyte hyporesponsiveness to non-cognate stimuli: a key factor in age-related immunodeficiency. Eur J Immunol 1992;22:931–5.

[52] Nicoletti C, Borghesi-Nicoletti C, Yang X, et al. Repertoire diversity of antibody response to bacterial antigens in aged mice. II. Phosphorylcholine-antibody in young and aged mice differs in both V_H/V_L gene repertoire and in specificity. J Immunol 1991;147:2750–5.

[53] Linton PJ, Haynes L, Tsui L, et al. From naive to effector: alterations with aging. Immunol Rev 1997;160:9–18.

[54] Miller RA, Garcia G, Kirk CJ, et al. Early activation defects in T lymphocytes from aged mice. Immunol Rev 1997;160:79–90.

[55] Zhou T, Edwards CK, Mountz JK. Prevention of age-related T cell apoptosis defect in CD2-*fas* transgenic mice. J Exp Med 1995;182:129–37.

[56] Jackola DR, Ruger JK, Miller RA. Age-associated changes in human T cell phenotype and function. Aging (Milano) 1994;6:25–34.

[57] Cakman I, Rohr J, Schutz RM, et al. Dysregulation between TH$_1$ and TH$_2$ T cell subpopulations in the elderly. Mech Ageing Dev 1996;87:197–209.

[58] Liu J, Wang S, Liu H, et al. The monitoring biomarker for immune function of lymphocytes in the elderly. Mech Ageing Dev 1997;94:177–82.

[59] Song H, Price PW, Cerny J. Age-related changes in antibody repertoire: contribution from T-cells. Immunol Rev 1997;160:55–62.

[60] Masanori U, Hirokawa K, Kurashima C, et al. Differential age-change in the numbers of CD4+CD45RA+ and CD4+CD29+ T cell subsets in human peripheral blood. Mech Ageing Dev 1992;63:57–68.

[61] Amadori A, Zamarchi R, de Silvestro G, et al. Genetic control of the CD4/CD8 T-cell ratio in humans. Nat Med 1995;1:1279–83.

[62] Meyer KC, Ershler W, Rosenthal N, et al. Immune dysregulation in the aging human lung. Am J Respir Crit Care Med 1996;153:1072–9.

[63] Agostini C, Chilosi M, Zambello R, et al. Pulmonary immune cells in health and disease: lymphocytes. Eur Respir J 1993;6:1378–401.

[64] Berman JS, Beer DJ, Theodore AC, et al. Lymphocyte recruitment to the lung. Am Rev Respir Dis 1990;142:238–57.

[65] The BAL Cooperative Group Steering Committee. Bronchoalveolar lavage constituents in healthy individuals, idiopathic pulmonary fibrosis, and selected comparison groups. Am Rev Respir Dis 1990; 141(Suppl):S169–202.

[66] Meyer KC, Soergel P. Bronchoalveolar lymphocyte phenotypes change in the normal aging human lung. Thorax 1999;54:697–700.

[67] Franceschi C, Bonafe M, Valensin S. Human immunosenescence: the prevailing of innate immunity, the failing of clonotypic immunity, and the filling of immunological space. Vaccine 2000;18:1717–20.

[68] Franceschi C, Bonafe M. Centenarians as a model for healthy aging. Biochem Soc Trans 2003;31: 457–61.

[69] Francheschi C, Monti D, Samsoni P, et al. The immunology of exceptional individuals: the lesson of centenarians. Immunol Today 1995;16:12–6.

[70] Ferguson FG, Wikby A, Maxon P, et al. Immune parameters in a longitudinal study of a very old population of Swedish people: a comparison between survivors and nonsurvivors. J Gerontol 1995;50:B378–82.

[71] Smaldone GC. Deposition and clearance: unique problems in the proximal airways and oral cavity in the young and elderly. Respir Physiol 2001;128:33–8.

[72] Ho JC, Chan KN, Hu WH, et al. The effect of aging on nasal mucociliary clearance, beat frequency, and ultrastructure of respiratory cilia. Am J Respir Crit Care Med 2001;163:983–8.

[73] Kikuchi R, Watabe N, Konno T, et al. High incidence of silent aspiration in elderly patients with community-acquired pneumonia. Am J Respir Crit Care Med 1994;150:251–3.

[74] Riquelme R, Torres A, El-Ebiary M, et al. Community-acquired pneumonia in the elderly: a multivariate

analysis of risk and prognostic factors. Am J Respir Crit Care Med 1996;154:1450–5.

[75] Strausbaugh LJ, Sukumar SR, Joseph CL. Infectious disease outbreaks in nursing homes: an unappreciated hazard for frail elderly persons. Clin Infect Dis 2003;36:870–6.

[76] Bauer BA, Reed CE, Yunginger JW. Incidence and outcomes of asthma in the elderly: a population-based study in Rochester, Minnesota. Chest 1997; 111:303–10.

[77] Yunginger JW, Reed CE, O'Connell EJ, et al. A community-based study of the epidemiology of asthma: incidence rates, 1964. Am Rev Respir Dis 1992;146:888–94.

[78] Burrows B, Barbee RA, Cline MG, et al. Characteristics of asthma among elderly adults in a sample of the general population. Chest 1991;100:935–42.

[79] Dodge RR, Burrows B. The prevalence and incidence of asthma and asthma-like symptoms in a general population sample. Am Rev Respir Dis 1980; 122:567–75.

[80] Burrows B, Lebowitz MD, Barbee RA, et al. Findings before diagnoses of asthma among the elderly in a longitudinal study of a general population sample. J Allergy Clin Immunol 1991;88:870–7.

[81] Sunyer J, Anto JM, Castellsagué J, et al. Total serum IgE is associated with asthma independently of specific IgE levels: the Spanish Group of the European Study of Asthma. Eur Respir J 1996;9:1880–4.

[82] Tollerud DJ, O'Connor GT, Sparrow D, et al. Asthma, hay fever, and phlegm production associated with distinct patterns of allergy skin test reactivity, eosinophilia, and serum IgE levels: the Normative Aging Study. Am Rev Respir Dis 1991;144:776–81.

[83] Almind M, Viskum K, Evald T, et al. A seven-year follow-up study of 343 adults with bronchial asthma. Dan Med Bull 1992;39:561–5.

[84] Sunyer J, Anto JM, Sabria J, et al. Relationship between serum IgE and airway responsiveness in adults with asthma. J Allergy Clin Immunol 1995; 95:699–706.

[85] Eschenbacher WL, Holian A, Campion RJ. Air toxics and asthma: impacts and end points. Environ Health 1995;103(Suppl 6):209–11.

[86] Castellsague J, Sunyer J, Saez M, et al. Short-term association between air pollution and emergency room visits for asthma in Barcelona. Thorax 1995; 50:1051–6.

[87] Zeleznik J. Normative aging of the respiratory system. Clin Geriatr Med 2003;19(1):1–18.

[88] McClaran SR, Babcock MA, Pegelow DF, et al. Longitudinal effects of aging on lung function at rest and exercise in healthy active fit elderly adults. J Appl Physiol 1995;78:1957–68.

[89] Mittman C, Edelman NH, Norris AH, et al. Relationship between chest wall and pulmonary compliance with age. J Appl Physiol 1965;20:1211–6.

[90] Knudson RJ, Clark DF, Kennedy TC, et al. Effect of aging alone on mechanical properties of the normal adult human lung. J Appl Physiol 1977;43: 1054–62.

[91] Gibson GJ, Pride NB, O'Cain C, et al. Sex and age differences in pulmonary mechanics in normal nonsmoking subjects. J Appl Physiol 1976;41:20–5.

[92] Crapo RO, Morris AH, Gardner RM. Reference spirometric values using techniques and equipment that meet ATS recommendations. Am Rev Respir Dis 1981;123:659–64.

[93] Knudson RJ, Lebowitz MD, Holberg CJ, et al. Changes in the normal maximal expiratory flow volume curve with growth and aging. Am Rev Respir Dis 1983;127:725–34.

[94] Burrows B, Lebowitz MD, Camilli AE, et al. Longitudinal changes in forced expiratory volume in one second in adults. Am Rev Respir Dis 1986;133: 974–80.

[95] Tager IB, Segal MR, Speizer FE, et al. The natural history of forced expiratory volumes: effect of cigarette smoking and respiratory symptoms. Am Rev Respir Dis 1988;138:837–49.

[96] Gottlieb DJ, Sparrow D, O'Connor GT, et al. Skin test reactivity to common aeroallergens and decline of lung function: the Normative Aging Study. Am J Respir Crit Care Med 1996;153(2):561–6.

[97] O'Connor GT, Sparrow D, Segal M, et al. Risk factors for ventilatory impairment among middle-aged and elderly men: the Normative Aging Study. Chest 1993;103:376–82.

ELSEVIER
SAUNDERS

Clin Chest Med 28 (2007) 673–684

CLINICS
IN CHEST
MEDICINE

Sleep and Older Patients

John J. Harrington, MD, MPH[a,b,*], Teofilo Lee-Chiong Jr, MD[a,b]

[a]Division of Pulmonary Medicine, National Jewish Medical and Research Center,
1400 Jackson Street, Denver, CO 80206, USA
[b]University of Colorado Health Sciences, 4200 East 9th Avenue and Colorado Boulevard,
Denver, CO 80262, USA

Sleep complaints are common among the elderly. Older adults often take longer to fall asleep and have more frequent nighttime awakenings. In a study of more than 9000 participants aged 65 years or older, more than 50% of respondents reported at least one chronic sleep complaint. The most commonly reported problem was the inability to stay asleep [1]. Elderly people also tend to be sleepier during the day compared with younger adults. Complaints of sleep problems in the geriatric population are often secondary to other medical comorbidities and not simply related to aging [2].

Sleep architecture

The progression of sleep stages throughout the night is predictable and is commonly represented in the form of hypnograms (Fig. 1). Based on poly-somnographic (PSG) data (ie, electro-encephalography [EEG], eye movement, and muscle tone), sleep can be divided into two distinct states, namely, non-rapid eye movement (non-REM) and rapid eye movement (REM) sleep. Non-REM sleep is further subdivided into light sleep, stages 1 and 2, and deep sleep, stage 3 (formerly stages 3 and 4), also known as slow wave sleep (SWS) or delta sleep. Normal sleep cycles transition through stages 1 to 3 and REM approximately every 90 to 120 minutes. In general, SWS is more abundant during the early portion of

the night, whereas REM stage sleep tends to increase during the latter half of nocturnal sleep.

Age-related sleep changes

Aging is associated with changes in sleep architecture. Older persons typically have more frequent nighttime arousals, awakenings, and sleep stage shifts [3]. The duration of nighttime awakenings also is increased. Age-related changes include reductions in total sleep time, sleep efficiency (ie, time asleep/time spent in bed), and SWS [4]. There is often a reduction in percentage of REM sleep along with a shortened REM sleep latency and an increase in the duration of the first REM sleep episode. In a recent study by van Cauter and colleagues [5], stage REM sleep was reduced by as much as 50% in late life subjects compared with younger adults. Intra-night distribution of REM sleep seems to be more uniform among the elderly compared with younger persons, who tend to have a greater proportion of REM sleep in the latter half of the night [6]. Some evidence also suggests that the density of rapid eye movements during REM sleep is reduced in older subjects [7]. Other changes during sleep among elderly people include increased time spent awake at night [5,8] and longer latencies to sleep [8].

Aging and circadian rhythms

Aging is associated with dampening of the circadian sleep–wake rhythms [9]. This in turn may result in greater sleepiness during the daytime and reduced nocturnal sleep efficiency. There are concurrent reductions in the amplitude of

* Corresponding author. National Jewish Medical and Research Center, 1400 Jackson Street, Denver, CO 80206.
E-mail address: harringtonj@njc.org (J.J. Harrington).

0272-5231/07/$ - see front matter © 2007 Elsevier Inc. All rights reserved.
doi:10.1016/j.ccm.2007.07.002

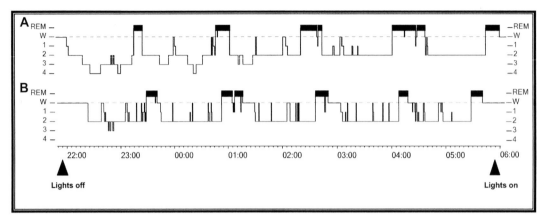

Fig. 1. Two sample hypnograms from overnight polysomnograms comparing representative sleep architecture of (*A*) a young adult and (*B*) an older adult. REM, rapid eye movement; W, awake; 1–4, sleep stages 1, 2, 3, and 4.

melatonin secretion and core body temperature. Phase advancement of circadian rhythms is common, leading to greater likelihood of early morning awakenings and excessive sleepiness earlier in the evening [3]. Recent research indicates that reductions in circadian rhythm amplitude [9,10], increased susceptibility to arousing circadian signals, and reduced homeostatic pressure for sleep [11] may all play a role in this age-related phenomenon.

Causes of sleep disturbance with aging

Several factors could contribute to the greater sleep fragmentation seen with aging. In addition to the dampening of circadian sleep–wake rhythms and decreased homeostatic sleep drive described previously, other factors such as a greater sensitivity to adverse environmental factors (eg, noise) may be important. Sleep problems among older adults are often caused by other primary sleep disorders (such as obstructive sleep apnea, periodic limb movements in sleep, restless legs syndrome [RLS], and REM sleep behavior disorder), medical, neurologic, and psychiatric illnesses, or the adverse effects on sleep of medications used to treat them. Important factors associated with sleep disturbance in this population group include nocturia, chronic pain syndromes, menopause in women, and stress (eg, bereavement).

Insomnia

Insomnia is a disorder marked by one or more of the following complaints: difficulty initiating or maintaining sleep, waking too early in the morning, or sleep that is chronically nonrestorative or poor in quality. In addition, these complaints are present despite adequate circumstances and opportunities for sleep, and they result in impairment of daytime function (eg, mood disturbances, attention and memory impairments, or fatigue) [12]. Older adults who have insomnia more often describe symptoms of poor sleep maintenance rather than problems with sleep initiation [8].

Insomnia is the most common sleep complaint among older adults, and its prevalence in this age group has been estimated to be between 20% and 40% [1,13] with an annual incidence of approximately 5% [14]. Nearly 50% of elderly subjects reported symptoms of insomnia at least a few nights per week in a large sample of community-dwelling elders, but few reported receiving treatment for these complaints [2]. Furthermore, not only is increasing age associated with a higher risk for developing insomnia, but there is also a greater likelihood that these symptoms will become chronic.

There are multiple potential consequences of chronic insomnia among older adults. Sleep complaints may be associated with excessive daytime sleepiness, fatigue, cognitive dysfunction [15], falls [16], depression [2], increased mortality [17], decreased quality of life [2], economic burden [18], and possibly early institutionalization. Potential adverse effects of sedative-hypnotics, such as amnesia, increased risk for accidents and falls, and residual daytime somnolence, are also important considerations [19], especially because of a disproportionate use of these medications in this population [20].

Although primary insomnia occurs, secondary forms are common and are caused by various medical and psychiatric comorbidities [21]. Insomnia may be related to pain syndromes, neurologic disorders (eg, dementia and Parkinson disease), and pulmonary and cardiac disorders [22]. Also, other primary sleep disorders, such as sleep-disordered breathing and RLS, should be considered as potential etiologies [13]. Finally, medication use, abuse, or withdrawal can cause sleep disruption, as can psychologic stressors such as retirement and bereavement.

Initial treatment strategies for insomnia complaints in this population should include lifestyle modifications, such as practicing good sleep hygiene, limiting alcohol [23] and caffeine intake [24], increasing daytime light exposure [25], and encouraging physical activity [26]. Although there is recent evidence to support exercise as an intervention for late-life insomnia [27], further research is needed to clarify its role in insomnia treatment [26], especially when considering physical frailties of this population. Studies evaluating the possible benefits of timed bright light exposure for sleep maintenance insomnia have demonstrated differing results [25,28,29]. Because of a lack of standards regarding timing and duration of light exposure, further research is needed to better evaluate this therapy in older persons [30,31].

Cognitive-behavioral therapy (CBT) should be offered to those patients who fail to respond to these lifestyle modifications. The fundamental components of CBT include sleep hygiene [32], sleep restriction [33], stimulus control [34], cognitive restructuring [35], and muscle relaxation [36,37]. Recent studies evaluating these techniques in older persons suffering from insomnia have demonstrated effectiveness [38] comparable to that for younger subjects [39] and that they may be at least as or more effective than pharmacologic therapy in this age group [40,41]. Because several weekly sessions of CBT may be inaccessible or impractical for some patients, studies evaluating modified regimens of this treatment have been performed and have shown good results [42,43]. CBT can also be used to assist in medication withdrawal or tapering among long-term hypnotic users [44,45].

Pharmacotherapy for insomnia could be considered in certain patients with the following caveats. Pharmacodynamics and pharmacokinetics are different in older patients [46] and should be considered when prescribing medications in this population. The effect a medication may have

on other disease states or even primary sleep disorders should be considered [47]. For instance, benzodiazepines can potentially worsen hypoxemia related to sleep-disordered breathing. Development of tolerance, risk for dependency and abuse, memory impairment, and possible rebound insomnia after medication withdrawal also may be problematic [48]. Patients who develop tolerance may self-escalate their dose of benzodiazepines to attain comparable therapeutic benefit. In addition to rebound insomnia, discontinuation after chronic use can result in various withdrawal symptoms, such as anxiety, irritability, and restlessness. The use of hypnotics is generally considered in appropriate cases of acute insomnia, but may also be of benefit for chronic insomnia that has not responded adequately to CBT [49].

Non-benzodiazepine benzodiazepine receptor agonist (NBBRA) sedative-hypnotics may be safer alternatives to benzodiazepines because of their more selective binding, shortened half-lives, and fewer drug interactions [50–52]. The hypnosedative action of NBBRAs is comparable with that of benzodiazepines. Unlike conventional benzodiazepines, they possess no significant anxiolytic, myorelaxant, or anticonvulsant activity. Medications in this class include zaleplon, zolpidem, and eszopiclone. There are studies supporting their safety and efficacy in this population [52–54], but few have been long-term in design [54]. The risks for tolerance and dependency with chronic use seem low, and abuse potential is generally minimal. They are less likely to impair daytime performance and memory than are longer-acting benzodiazepines.

Ramelteon, a selective melatonin (MT1/MT2) receptor agonist, with its greater receptor affinity compared to melatonin, improved subjective latency as documented by sleep diaries. In a study of 829 insomnia patients aged 65 years or older, use was not associated with rebound insomnia on withdrawal [55]. Ramelteon has also been shown to improve sleep efficiency and increase total sleep time. In addition, in subjects who had mild to moderate obstructive sleep apnea (OSA), there seemed to be minimal adverse respiratory effects, such as number of respiratory events or oxygen desaturations with ramelteon compared with placebo [56].

Despite their common use for patients who have sleep disturbance, there are limited data on the efficacy and safety of off-label prescription of sedating antidepressants, such as trazodone, for primary insomnia among patients without comorbid mood disorders. Trazodone can give rise to arrhythmias, blurring of vision, delirium, dizziness, hypotension, and priapism, and is not recommended for use in patients who have significant cardiac disease or arrhythmias. Cardiac arrhythmias and orthostatic hypotension also can be seen with the older tricyclic antidepressants, such as amitriptyline and nortriptyline.

Self-administration of nonprescription hypnotic agents is common. Many such agents contain first generation histamine H-1 antagonists (eg, diphenhydramine and chlorpheniramine), melatonin or botanical compounds, or combinations thereof. As a class, however, these nonprescription agents possess weak hypnotic properties and are generally effective only for mild sleep disturbance.

Diphenhydramine is associated with rapid development of tolerance to its soporific effects, adverse anticholinergic effects (blurring of vision, dry mouth, urinary retention, and constipation), and detrimental effect on daytime alertness, cognition, and psychomotor performance. The use of melatonin for insomnia complaints is based on findings of decreased pineal melatonin secretion in older persons [57,58] and is supported by sleep improvements noted with replacement therapy in elderly melatonin-deficient subjects [59]. Melatonin supplementation in this population, however, is not Federal Drug Administration (FDA)-approved. Few of the herbal preparations that have been described for treating sleep disturbance have been studied in older adults who have chronic insomnia. Significant adverse effects have occurred with their use. Valerian, especially in cases of overdose, can cause abdominal pain, chest tightness, tremor, lightheadedness, mydriasis, and fine hand tremors. Kava has been removed from the market in several countries because of concerns about hepatotoxicity.

Selection among the numerous available hypnotic agents should take into account the nature and chronicity of the sleep disturbance, characteristics of the patient, and specific drug profile (absorption and elimination kinetics, abuse potential, and possible drug interactions). Changes in drug dosing are often required for older adults because of the presence of comorbid neurocognitive impairment and altered hepatic and renal clearance mechanisms, both of which might enhance the sensitivity of elderly patients to the hypnotic effects of medications. Patients should be advised against operating motor vehicles when using these medications.

The combined use of CBT and pharmacologic therapy for chronic insomnia may be considered in appropriate older patients. In one study evaluating the effectiveness of behavioral, pharmacologic, or a combination intervention, short-term sleep quality improvements were demonstrated with combined therapy [60]. During a 24-month follow-up period, however, behavioral therapy alone, in contrast to pharmacologic therapy, resulted in more sustained sleep improvements and was perceived as more satisfying to the participating subjects.

Sleep-disordered breathing

Sleep apnea is characterized by recurrent 10-second airway flow restriction (hypopneas) or obstruction (apneas). These partial or complete upper airway occlusions may cause sleep disruption, frequent arousals from sleep, and oxygen desaturation (Fig. 2). Obstructive sleep apnea is a disorder marked by upper airway obstruction, often at the level of the tongue base or retropalatal space, despite continued respiratory effort. In contrast, central sleep apnea (CSA) is associated with diminished or absent airflow but without a compensatory respiratory effort.

As in younger individuals, male predominance of sleep apnea persists in older patients. The estimated prevalence of OSA among older adults may range from 13% to 28% in men and from 4% to 20% in women [61,62]. The reason for prevalence discrepancies among these and other studies [63–68] may be related to differences in study methodologies (eg, subjective versus objective data) and diagnostic criteria used [69]. The increased prevalence of OSA in older women may be related to postmenopausal status [70,71]. In the Wisconsin Sleep Cohort Study, a population-based sample of 589 women, after adjusting for known confounders, the likelihood of sleep-disordered breathing was significantly increased in postmenopausal women compared with those who were premenopausal [72].

Age-related alterations of respiratory anatomy and physiology may contribute to sleep apnea in the elderly population. Increased upper airway adipose deposition, pharyngeal bony changes possibly related to remodeling, and a longer pharyngeal airway (noted in women) [73] may predispose to upper airway collapse. Protective dilator reflexes against airway collapse [74] are diminished with age [73]. In addition, reduced

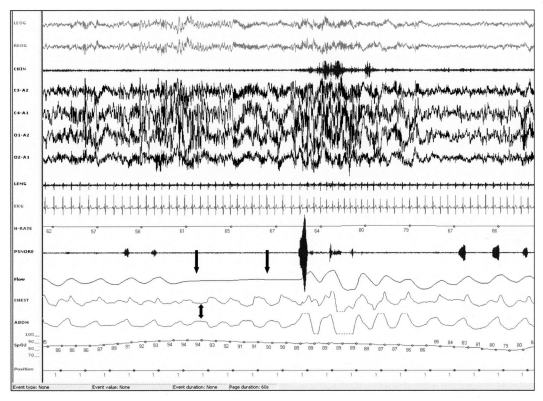

Fig. 2. This 60-second sleep epoch illustrates an example of an obstructive apnea. Note the absence of nasal airflow (*arrows*) with evidence of continued respiratory effort and paradoxic motion of the chest and abdominal tracings (*double arrow*). Channels are as follows: electro-oculogram (left: LEOG; right: REOG), chin EMG (CHIN), EEG (left central [C3–A2], right central [C4–A1], left occipital [O1–A2], right occipital [O2–A1]), electrocardiogram (EKG), limb EMG (left leg [LEMG]), snoring (PSNORE), nasal–oral airflow (Flow), respiratory effort (thoracic [CHEST]), abdominal (ABDM), and oxygen saturation (SpO2).

respiratory responsiveness to upper airway occlusion during obstructive apneas [75] may further contribute to the occurrence of sleep apnea in the elderly population. Unlike in younger individuals, body habitus as a risk factor for apnea is less important with advancing age.

Obstructive sleep apnea in older adults may result in complaints of daytime sleepiness [76]. Long-term consequences of sleep-disordered breathing, specifically cognitive deficiencies, were noted in some [69,77] but not all studies [78]. Other trials have demonstrated outcomes of ischemic strokes [79] and mood disorders [62,80,81]. The association of OSA and nocturia may also be clinically important in this population [82–84]. Although there are cardiovascular effects, such as systemic hypertension, associated with OSA, the severity may differ from younger persons. In the Sleep Heart Health Study, subjects younger than 65 years of age who had OSA

were more likely to have hypertension than were older participants [85]. In a recent study of 353 older veterans, neither OSA nor CSA shortened survival; however, those subjects who had congestive heart failure and CSA did have reduced life spans [86].

Older patients complaining of symptoms suggestive of OSA, such as excessive daytime sleepiness, should warrant further evaluation. Other commonly reported symptoms, including witnessed apneas and snoring, may be less often reported in this population, especially if there is no bed partner. The presence of clinical symptoms, such as excessive daytime sleepiness, seems to be less common, and if present, seems less severe compared with younger patients who have OSA.

The diagnosis of sleep apnea requires an overnight polysomnogram to determine the presence and severity of sleep apnea and is based on a resultant apnea–hypopnea index (AHI), which represents the frequency of respiratory events per hour of sleep. Respiratory events are scored as either obstructive or central, depending on whether respiratory effort is noted.

The decision whether or not to treat sleep apnea in older adults is typically based on various factors, but should include disease severity, associated symptoms, and other illnesses. As in younger patients, older patients who have OSA should be encouraged to maintain optimal weight and to avoid alcohol and sedative medications close to bedtime. Persons who have sleep apnea that is more prominent in the supine position should be educated about techniques to avoid this sleeping position.

The primary treatment for OSA in elderly persons is continuous positive airway pressure (CPAP). This therapy, which is applied by way of either a nasal or a full-face mask, generates positive airway pressure that acts as a pneumatic splint to reduce airway collapsibility. Although CPAP compliance is less than optimal in the general population, its acceptability in older persons is not significantly different than in younger patients [87,88], and simple interventions may improve compliance in this population [89,90]. Because of potential benefits related to CPAP therapy in regard to cognition [91] and subjective daytime sleepiness [92], this therapy should be considered in those patients who have neurocognitive disorders. In a recent study by Ayalon and colleagues [93], subjects who had Alzheimer-type dementia were noted to have adherence comparable to other patients who had OSA.

Oral appliances that enlarge the oropharyngeal airway by advancing the mandible are another treatment option for patients who refuse or cannot tolerate CPAP therapy. Options for dental devices may be severely limited, however, in patients who are edentulous. In addition, OSA severity may be significantly worse in edentulous patients who do not wear their dentures while sleeping [94]. This association with tooth loss and sleep-disordered breathing may be related to tongue and jaw repositioning [95] and to decrements in retropharyngeal airspace and vertical occlusal dimensions [96].

Surgical procedures, such as a uvulopalatopharyngoplasty (UPPP) [97], are designed to lessen or eliminate sleep-disordered breathing by increasing the oropharyngeal dimensions by excising excessive soft palatal and tonsillar tissue. Other procedures, such as radiofrequency tongue base ablation, used alone or in conjunction with UPPP [98], may be safe and effective in selected older patients intolerant to CPAP therapy [99,100]. More complex procedures, such as maxillomandibular reconstruction, are not recommended in this population because of their associated complications. Although bariatric surgery improved OSA in a small sample of morbidly obese patients aged 65 years or older [101], its role in the management of sleep-disordered breathing needs further study.

Restless legs syndrome and periodic limb movements in sleep

RLS is a diagnosis based on symptoms of unpleasant or uncomfortable leg sensations that are accompanied by an intense urge to move the legs. These symptoms, which are often described as "creepy-crawly sensations," occur during periods of rest or inactivity, are worse at night, and are either completely relieved or lessened with movement [102]. The underlying mechanisms of RLS are not entirely clear, but iron metabolism and dopaminergic neural functioning seem to be involved [103,104]. The prevalence of RLS in the geriatric population ranges from 8.3% to 19% [105,106] and is twice as common among older women [107]. In contrast to early-onset RLS, which is often familial and less associated with serum iron status, late-onset RLS is more rapidly progressive and is often related to iron deficiency [108,109]. Other conditions commonly associated with RLS include uremia, peripheral neuropathies, diabetes mellitus, and Parkinson disease [110].

Periodic limb movements in sleep (PLMS) is a common condition among older adults. These periodic episodes of repetitive rhythmic limb contractions are characterized by big toe extension and ankle, knee, and occasionally hip flexion [111]. These movements may be associated with arousals from sleep and may result in complaints of daytime sleepiness or insomnia [112]. The prevalence of PLMS in community-dwelling elderly subjects may be as high as 45% [113]. The diagnosis of PLMS is based on PSG findings of recurrent limb movements (Fig. 3). The occurrence of these movements may be unknown to the elderly patient, especially if they lack a bed partner. PLMS are often associated with sleep apnea [67] and are frequently noted in patients who have RLS [105].

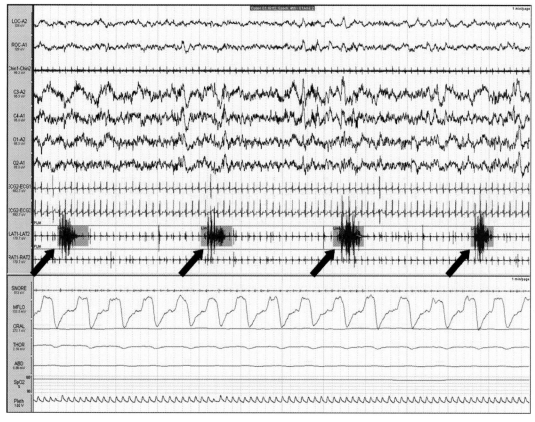

Fig. 3. A 60-second sleep epoch demonstrating a succession of four periodic limb movements (*arrows*) occurring in the left anterior tibialis muscle.

Treatment for RLS and PLMS may require nonpharmacologic and pharmacologic strategies. Iron supplementation is recommended if serum iron studies indicate low iron stores. A trial of abstinence from alcohol, caffeine, and nicotine intake also could be considered. A thorough assessment of prescribed and over-the-counter medication should be performed, because antidepressants, neuroleptic agents, and dopamine antagonists may contribute to RLS symptoms [114]. Medical therapy with levodopa-carbidopa and newer dopaminergic agonists, including pramipexole and ropinirole, are frequently used in the treatment of PLMS and RLS. Benzodiazepines, typically low-dose clonazepam, and low-potency opiates have been used, but side effects (eg, excess sedation, constipation, and nausea) may limit their efficacy in this population. Gabapentin may be an option for elderly patients who have more painful RLS or those who have concomitant peripheral neuropathy. Because of concerns regarding falls and increased somnolence associated with this medication, starting doses of 100 to 300 mg may be appropriate [114].

Rapid eye movement sleep behavior disorder

REM sleep behavior disorder (RBD) is a parasomnia that is characterized by dream-enacting behaviors during REM sleep resulting from a loss of usual skeletal muscle atonia during this sleep stage [115]. Nocturnal behaviors reported can be violent or aggressive in nature and may include yelling, grabbing, punching, kicking, and running [116]. Sleep-related injury, such as ecchymoses, lacerations, and fractures, to the patient or their bed partner were the presenting complaint in nearly 80% of cases in one series [116]. RBD prevalence increases with age and is much more common in men, with nearly 90% of patients being men older than age 50 years [116,117]. The exact prevalence of this disorder in the geriatric population remains unknown, but may approach 0.4% [118].

RBD is frequently associated with neurodegenerative diseases, such as Parkinson disease, multiple system atrophy, and dementia, and its presence often predates these diagnoses [117,119]. An acute form of RBD may be precipitated by alcohol or barbiturate withdrawal, caffeine intake, or the use of some antidepressant medications [21,116]. Multiple disorders may mimic RBD, including delirium, nocturnal seizures, and confusional arousals associated with respiratory events in OSA [120].

Diagnostic evaluation should include a detailed history from the patient and bed partner. PSG features of RBD consist of an attenuation of normal REM sleep atonia represented by excessive phasic electromyographic (EMG) activity during REM sleep (Fig. 4) [120]. PSG recordings should also include time-synchronized video monitoring, which may document abnormal behaviors.

RBD treatment should include environmental recommendations to increase safety while in the bedroom. Discontinuation of medications that may precipitate or aggravate RBD should be considered [121]. Low-dose clonazepam (0.5 to 2.0 mg) is most often prescribed for this disorder and is effective in most patients [116]. Abrupt discontinuation of clonazepam should be avoided because of potential rebound. If there are contraindications, such as cognitive impairment or OSA, or if tolerance develops to this medication, a trial of melatonin may be considered [122–124]. The use of alternative medications, including pramipexole [125] and donepezil [126], has also been studied, but their role is as yet less well established.

Summary

Older patients experience changes in their sleep architecture with aging, with more frequent arousals and a reduction in total sleep time and sleep efficiency. Multiple factors contribute to sleep disturbance with aging, including underlying medical and psychiatric disorders, which should

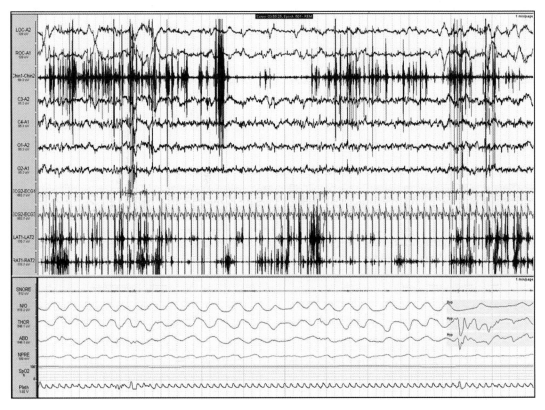

Fig. 4. This 60-second sleep epoch demonstrates evidence of excessive chin and limb EMG tone during REM sleep.

be evaluated for in older patients who have sleep complaints. Sleep-disordered breathing is also common among older patients and may be related to physiologic changes, such as age-related alterations in respiratory anatomy and postmenopausal state in women. Physicians caring for older patients need to take a careful sleep history to discern etiologies of sleep disturbances and provide appropriate evaluation and treatment.

References

[1] Foley DJ, Monjan AA, Brown SL, et al. Sleep complaints among elderly persons: an epidemiologic study of three communities. Sleep 1995;18(6): 425–32.

[2] Foley D, Ancoli-Israel S, Britz P, et al. Sleep disturbances and chronic disease in older adults: results of the 2003 National Sleep Foundation Sleep in America Survey. J Psychosom Res 2004;56(5): 497–502.

[3] Phillips B, Ancoli-Israel S. Sleep disorders in the elderly. Sleep Med 2001;2:99–114.

[4] Ohayon MM, Carskadon MA, Guilleminault C, et al. Meta-analysis of quantitative sleep parameters from childhood to old age in healthy individuals: developing normative sleep values across the human lifespan. Sleep 2004;27(7):1255–73.

[5] Van Cauter E, Leproult R, Plat L. Age-related changes in slow wave sleep and REM sleep and relationship with growth hormone and cortisol levels in healthy men. JAMA 2000;284(7):861–8.

[6] Reynolds CF 3rd, Kupfer DJ, Taska LS, et al. Sleep of healthy seniors: a revisit. Sleep 1985;8(1):20–9.

[7] Darchia N, Campbell IG, Feinberg I. Rapid eye movement density is reduced in the normal elderly. Sleep 2003;26(8):973–7.

[8] Floyd JA, Medler SM, Ager JW, et al. Age-related changes in initiation and maintenance of sleep: a meta-analysis. Res Nurs Health 2000;23(2): 106–17.

[9] Haung YL, Liu RY, Wang QS, et al. Age-associated difference in circadian sleep-wake and rest-activity rhythms. Physiol Behav 2002;76:597–603.

[10] Buysse DJ, Browman KE, Monk TH, et al. Napping and 24-hour sleep/wake patterns in healthy elderly and young adults. J Am Geriatr Soc 1992; 40(8):779–86.

[11] Dijk DJ, Duffy JF, Czeisler CA. Contribution of circadian physiology and sleep homeostasis to age-related changes in human sleep. Chronobiol Int 2000;17(3):285–311.

[12] Edinger JD, Bonnet MH, Bootzin RR, et al. Derivation of research diagnostic criteria for insomnia: report of an American Academy of Sleep Medicine Work Group. Sleep 2004;27(8):1567–96.

[13] Sateia MJ, Doghramji K, Hauri PJ, et al. Evaluation of chronic insomnia. An American Academy of Sleep Medicine review. Sleep 2000;23(2): 243–308.

[14] Foley DJ, Monjan A, Simonsick EM, et al. Incidence and remission of insomnia among elderly adults: an epidemiologic study of 6,800 persons over three years. Sleep 1999;22(Suppl 2): S366–72.

[15] Cricco M, Simonsick EM, Foley DJ. The impact of insomnia on cognitive functioning in older adults. J Am Geriatr Soc 2001;49(9):1185–9.

[16] Brassington GS, King AC, Bliwise DL. Sleep problems as a risk factor for falls in a sample of community-dwelling adults aged 64–99 years. J Am Geriatr Soc 2000;48(10):1234–40.

[17] Manabe K, Matsui T, Yamaya M, et al. Sleep patterns and mortality among elderly patients in a geriatric hospital. Gerontology 2000;46(6): 318–22.

[18] Ozminkowski RJ, Wang S, Walsh JK. The direct and indirect costs of untreated insomnia in adults in the United States. Sleep 2007;30(3):263–73.

[19] Conn DK, Madan R. Use of sleep-promoting medications in nursing home residents: risks versus benefits. Drugs Aging 2006;23(4):271–87.

[20] Wysowski DK, Baum C. Outpatient use of prescription sedative-hypnotic drugs in the United States, 1970 through 1989. Arch Intern Med 1991; 151(9):1779–83.

[21] Ayalon L, Liu L, Ancoli-Israel S. Diagnosing and treating sleep disorders in the older adult. Med Clin North Am 2004;88(3):737–50, ix–x.

[22] Ancoli-Israel S. Insomnia in the elderly: a review for the primary care practitioner. Sleep 2000; 23(Suppl 1):S23–30 [discussion: S36–8].

[23] Ancoli-Israel S, Roth T. Characteristics of insomnia in the United States: results of the 1991 National Sleep Foundation Survey. I. Sleep 1999; 22(Suppl 2):S347–53.

[24] Curatolo PW, Robertson D. The health consequences of caffeine. Ann Intern Med 1983;98(5 Pt 1): 641–53.

[25] Campbell SS, Dawson D, Anderson MW. Alleviation of sleep maintenance insomnia with timed exposure to bright light. J Am Geriatr Soc 1993; 41(8):829–36.

[26] Morgan K. Daytime activity and risk factors for late-life insomnia. J Sleep Res 2003;12(3): 231–8.

[27] Li F, Fisher KJ, Harmer P, et al. Tai chi and self-rated quality of sleep and daytime sleepiness in older adults: a randomized controlled trial. J Am Geriatr Soc 2004;52(6):892–900.

[28] Campbell SS, Dawson D. Bright light treatment of sleep disturbance in older subjects. Sleep Res 1991; 20:448.

[29] Suhner AG, Murphy PJ, Campbell SS. Failure of timed bright light exposure to alleviate age-related sleep maintenance insomnia. J Am Geriatr Soc 2002;50(4):617–23.

[30] Montgomery P, Dennis J. Cognitive behavioural interventions for sleep problems in adults aged 60+. Cochrane Database Syst Rev 2003;1:CD003161.

[31] McCurry SM, Logsdon RG, Teri L, et al. Evidence-based psychological treatments for insomnia in older adults. Psychol Aging 2007;22(1):18–27.

[32] Hauri P, editor. Case studies in insomnia. New York: Plenum Medical Book Company; 1991.

[33] Spielman AJ, Saskin P, Thorpy MJ. Treatment of chronic insomnia by restriction of time in bed. Sleep 1987;10:45–56.

[34] Bootzin R, Nicassio P. Behavioral treatments for insomnia. New York: Academic Press, Inc.,; 1978.

[35] Morin CM, Kowatch RA, Barry T, et al. Cognitive-behavior therapy for late-life insomnia. J Consult Clin Psychol 1993;61(1):137–46.

[36] Woolfolk R, McNulty T. Relaxation Treatment for insomnia: a component analysis. J Consult Clin Psychol 1983;51(4):495–503.

[37] Jacobson E, editor. Progressive relaxation. Chicago: University of Chicago Press; 1974.

[38] Morin CM, Bootzin RR, Buysse DJ, et al. Psychological and behavioral treatment of insomnia: update of the recent evidence (1998–2004). Sleep 2006;29(11):1398–414.

[39] Irwin MR, Cole JC, Nicassio PM. Comparative meta-analysis of behavioral interventions for insomnia and their efficacy in middle-aged adults and in older adults 55+ years of age. Health Psychol 2006;25(1):3–14.

[40] Perlis ML, Smith MT, Cacialli DO, et al. On the comparability of pharmacotherapy and behavior therapy for chronic insomnia. Commentary and implications. J Psychosom Res 2003;54(1):51–9.

[41] Sivertsen B, Omvik S, Pallesen S, et al. Cognitive behavioral therapy vs zopiclone for treatment of chronic primary insomnia in older adults: a randomized controlled trial. JAMA 2006;295(24):2851–8.

[42] Germain A, Moul D, Franzen P, et al. Effects of a brief behavioral treatment for late-life insomnia: preliminary findings. J Clin Sleep Med 2006;2(4):407–8.

[43] Rybarczyk B, Lopez M, Schelble K, et al. Home-based video CBT for comorbid geriatric insomnia: a pilot study using secondary data analyses. Behav Sleep Med 2005;3(3):158–75.

[44] Morin CM, Bastien C, Guay B, et al. Randomized clinical trial of supervised tapering and cognitive behavior therapy to facilitate benzodiazepine discontinuation in older adults with chronic insomnia. Am J Psychiatry 2004;161(2):332–42.

[45] Morgan K, Dixon S, Mathers N, et al. Psychological treatment for insomnia in the regulation of long-term hypnotic drug use. Health Technol Assess 2004;8(8):iii–v, 1–68.

[46] Hicks R, Dysken M, Davis J, et al. The pharmacokinetics of psychotropic medication in the elderly: a review. J Clin Psychiatry 1981;42:374–85.

[47] Gillin J, Ancoli-Israel S. The impact of age on sleep and sleep disorders. Baltimore (MD): Williams & Wilkins; 1992.

[48] Gillin JC, Spinweber CL, Johnson LC. Rebound insomnia: a critical review. J Clin Psychopharmacol 1989;9(3):161–72.

[49] McCall WV. Diagnosis and management of insomnia in older people. J Am Geriatr Soc 2005; 53(Suppl 7):S272–7.

[50] Salva P, Costa J. Clinical pharmacokinetics and pharmacodynamics of zolpidem. Therapeutic implications. Clin Pharmacokinet 1995;29(3):142–53.

[51] Melton ST, Wood JM, Kirkwood CK. Eszopiclone for insomnia. Ann Pharmacother 2005;39(10):1659–66.

[52] Ancoli-Israel S, Walsh JK, Mangano RM, et al. Zaleplon, a novel nonbenzodiazepine hypnotic, effectively treats insomnia in elderly patients without causing rebound effects. Prim Care Companion J Clin Psychiatry 1999;1(4):114–20.

[53] Krystal AD, Walsh JK, Laska E, et al. Sustained efficacy of eszopiclone over 6 months of nightly treatment: results of a randomized, double-blind, placebo-controlled study in adults with chronic insomnia. Sleep 2003;26(7):793–9.

[54] Ancoli-Israel S, Richardson GS, Mangano RM, et al. Long-term use of sedative hypnotics in older patients with insomnia. Sleep Med 2005;6(2):107–13.

[55] Roth T, Seiden D, Sainati S, et al. Effects of ramelteon on patient-reported sleep latency in older adults with chronic insomnia. Sleep Med 2006; 7(4):312–8.

[56] Kryger M, Wang-Weigand S, Roth T. Safety of ramelteon in individuals with mild to moderate obstructive sleep apnea. Sleep Breath 2007;11(3):159–64.

[57] Magri F, Sarra S, Cinchetti W, et al. Qualitative and quantitative changes of melatonin levels in physiological and pathological aging and in centenarians. J Pineal Res 2004;36(4):256–61.

[58] Haimov I, Laudon M, Zisapel N, et al. Sleep disorders and melatonin rhythms in elderly people. BMJ 1994;309(6948):167.

[59] Haimov I, Lavie P, Laudon M, et al. Melatonin replacement therapy of elderly insomniacs. Sleep 1995;18(7):598–603.

[60] Morin CM, Colecchi C, Stone J, et al. Behavioral and pharmacological therapies for late-life insomnia: a randomized controlled trial. JAMA 1999; 281(11):991–9.

[61] Enright PL, Newman AB, Wahl PW, et al. Prevalence and correlates of snoring and observed apneas in 5201 older adults. Sleep 1996;19(7):531–8.

[62] Ancoli-Israel S, Kripke DF, Klauber MR, et al. Sleep-disordered breathing in community-dwelling elderly. Sleep 1991;14(6):486–95.

[63] Carskadon MA, Dement WC. Respiration during sleep in the aged human. J Gerontol 1981;36(4):420–3.

[64] Coleman RM, Miles LE, Guilleminault CC, et al. Sleep-wake disorders in the elderly: polysomnographic analysis. J Am Geriatr Soc 1981;29(7): 289–96.

[65] Roehrs T, Zorick F, Sicklesteel J, et al. Age-related sleep-wake disorders at a sleep disorder center. J Am Geriatr Soc 1983;31(6):364–70.

[66] Yesavage J, Bliwise D, Guilleminault C, et al. Preliminary communication: intellectual deficit and sleep-related respiratory disturbance in the elderly. Sleep 1985;8:30–3.

[67] Ancoli-Israel S, Kripke DF, Mason W, et al. Sleep apnea and periodic movements in an aging sample. J Gerontol 1985;40(4):419–25.

[68] Mosko SS, Dickel MJ, Paul T, et al. Sleep apnea and sleep-related periodic leg movements in community resident seniors. J Am Geriatr Soc 1988; 36(6):502–8.

[69] Janssens JP, Pautex S, Hilleret H, et al. Sleep disordered breathing in the elderly. Aging (Milano) 2000;12(6):417–29.

[70] Resta O, Caratozzolo G, Pannacciulli N, et al. Gender, age and menopause effects on the prevalence and the characteristics of obstructive sleep apnea in obesity. Eur J Clin Invest 2003;33(12):1084–9.

[71] Resta O, Bonfitto P, Sabato R, et al. Prevalence of obstructive sleep apnoea in a sample of obese women: effect of menopause. Diabetes Nutr Metab 2004;17(5):296–303.

[72] Young T, Finn L, Austin D, et al. Menopausal status and sleep-disordered breathing in the Wisconsin Sleep Cohort Study. Am J Respir Crit Care Med 2003;167(9):1181–5.

[73] Malhotra A, Huang Y, Fogel R, et al. Aging influences on pharyngeal anatomy and physiology: the predisposition to pharyngeal collapse. Am J Med 2006;119(1):72 e9–14.

[74] Mezzanotte WS, Tangel DJ, White DP. Waking genioglossal electromyogram in sleep apnea patients versus normal controls (a neuromuscular compensatory mechanism). J Clin Invest 1992;89(5):1571–9.

[75] Krieger J, Sforza E, Boudewijns A, et al. Respiratory effort during obstructive sleep apnea: role of age and sleep state. Chest 1997;112(4):875–84.

[76] Cohen-Zion M, Stepnowsky C, Marler, et al. Changes in cognitive function associated with sleep disordered breathing in older people. J Am Geriatr Soc 2001;49(12):1622–7.

[77] Dealberto M, Pajot N, Courbon D, et al. Breathing disorders during sleep and cognitive performance in an older community sample: the EVA study. J Am Geriatr Soc 1996;44:1287–94.

[78] Foley DJ, Masaki K, White L, et al. Sleep-disordered breathing and cognitive impairment in elderly Japanese–American men. Sleep 2003;26(5): 596–9.

[79] Munoz R, Duran-Cantolla J, Martinez-Vila E, et al. Severe sleep apnea and risk of ischemic stroke in the elderly. Stroke 2006;37(9):2317–21.

[80] Peppard PE, Szklo-Coxe M, Hla KM, et al. Longitudinal association of sleep-related breathing disorder and depression. Arch Intern Med 2006;166(16): 1709–15.

[81] Sharafkhaneh A, Giray N, Richardson P, et al. Association of psychiatric disorders and sleep apnea in a large cohort. Sleep 2005;28(11):1405–11.

[82] Endeshaw YW, Johnson TM, Kutner MH, et al. Sleep-disordered breathing and nocturia in older adults. J Am Geriatr Soc 2004;52(6):957–60.

[83] Oztura I, Kaynak D, Kaynak HC. Nocturia in sleep-disordered breathing. Sleep Med 2006;7:362–7.

[84] Bliwise DL, Adelman CL, Ouslander JG. Polysomnographic correlates of spontaneous nocturnal wetness episodes in incontinent geriatric patients. Sleep 2004;27(1):153–7.

[85] Nieto FJ, Young TB, Lind BK, et al. Association of sleep-disordered breathing, sleep apnea, and hypertension in a large community-based study. Sleep heart health study. JAMA 2000;283(14):1829–36.

[86] Ancoli-Israel S, DuHamel ER, Stepnowsky C, et al. The relationship between congestive heart failure, sleep apnea, and mortality in older men. Chest 2003;124(4):1400–5.

[87] Parish JM, Lyng PJ, Wisbey J. Compliance with CPAP in elderly patients with OSA. Sleep Med 2000;1(3):209–14.

[88] Pelletier-Fleury N, Rakotonanahary D, Fleury B. The age and other factors in the evaluation of compliance with nasal continuous positive airway pressure for obstructive sleep apnea syndrome. A Cox's proportional hazard analysis. Sleep Med 2001;2(3): 225–32.

[89] Aloia MS, Di Dio L, Ilniczky N, et al. Improving compliance with nasal CPAP and vigilance in older adults with OAHS. Sleep Breath 2001;5(1): 13–21.

[90] Russo-Magno P, O'Brien A, Panciera T, et al. Compliance with CPAP therapy in older men with obstructive sleep apnea. J Am Geriatr Soc 2001;49(9):1205–11.

[91] Aloia MS, Ilniczky N, Di Dio P, et al. Neuropsychological changes and treatment compliance in older adults with sleep apnea. J Psychosom Res 2003;54(1):71–6.

[92] Chong MS, Ayalon L, Marler M, et al. Continuous positive airway pressure reduces subjective daytime sleepiness in patients with mild to moderate Alzheimer's disease with sleep disordered breathing. J Am Geriatr Soc 2006;54(5):777–81.

[93] Ayalon L, Ancoli-Israel S, Stepnowsky C, et al. Adherence to continuous positive airway pressure treatment in patients with Alzheimer's disease and obstructive sleep apnea. Am J Geriatr Psychiatry 2006;14(2):176–80.

[94] Bucca C, Cicolin A, Brussino L, et al. Tooth loss and obstructive sleep apnoea. Respir Res 2006;7:8.

[95] Erovigni F, Graziano A, Ceruti P, et al. Cephalometric evaluation of the upper airway in patients

with complete dentures. Minerva Stomatol 2005;
54(5):293–301.

[96] Gassino G, Cicolin A, Erovigni F, et al. Obstructive sleep apnea, depression, and oral status in elderly occupants of residential homes. Int J Prosthodont 2005;18(4):316–22.

[97] Fujita S, Conway W, Zorick F, et al. Surgical correction of anatomic abnormalities in obstructive sleep apnea syndrome: uvulopalatopharyngoplasty. Otolaryngol Head Neck Surg 1981;89(6): 923–34.

[98] Friedman M, Ibrahim H, Lee G, et al. Combined uvulopalatopharyngoplasty and radiofrequency tongue base reduction for treatment of obstructive sleep apnea/hypopnea syndrome. Otolaryngol Head Neck Surg 2003;129(6):611–21.

[99] Kezirian EJ, Powell NB, Riley RW, et al. Incidence of complications in radiofrequency treatment of the upper airway. Laryngoscope 2005;115(7):1298–304.

[100] Steward DL, Weaver EM, Woodson BT. Multilevel temperature-controlled radiofrequency for obstructive sleep apnea: extended follow-up. Otolaryngol Head Neck Surg 2005;132(4):630–5.

[101] Nelson LG, Lopez PP, Haines K, et al. Outcomes of bariatric surgery in patients > or = 65 years. Surg Obes Relat Dis 2006;2(3):384–8.

[102] Allen RP, Picchietti D, Hening WA, et al. Restless legs syndrome: diagnostic criteria, special considerations, and epidemiology. A report from the restless legs syndrome diagnosis and epidemiology workshop at the National Institutes of Health. Sleep Med 2003;4(2):101–19.

[103] O'Keeffe ST, Gavin K, Lavan JN. Iron status and restless legs syndrome in the elderly. Age Ageing 1994;23(3):200–3.

[104] Milligan SA, Chesson AL. Restless legs syndrome in the older adult: diagnosis and management. Drugs Aging 2002;19(10):741–51.

[105] Ohayon MM, Roth T. Prevalence of restless legs syndrome and periodic limb movement disorder in the general population. J Psychosom Res 2002; 53(1):547–54.

[106] Phillips B, Young T, Finn L, et al. Epidemiology of restless legs symptoms in adults. Arch Intern Med 2000;160(14):2137–41.

[107] Rothdach AJ, Trenkwalder C, Haberstock J, et al. Prevalence and risk factors of RLS in an elderly population: the MEMO study. Memory and Morbidity in Augsburg Elderly. Neurology 2000;54(5): 1064–8.

[108] Allen RP, Earley CJ. Defining the phenotype of the restless legs syndrome (RLS) using age-of-symptom-onset. Sleep Med 2000;1:11–9.

[109] O'Keeffe ST. Secondary causes of restless legs syndrome in older people. Age Ageing 2005;34(4): 349–52.

[110] Zucconi M, Ferini-Strambi L. Epidemiology and clinical findings of restless legs syndrome. Sleep Med 2004;5(3):293–9.

[111] Hornyak M, Trenkwalder C. Restless legs syndrome and periodic limb movement disorder in the elderly. J Psychosom Res 2004;56(5):543–8.

[112] Ancoli-Israel S, Poceta JS, Stepnowsky C, et al. Identification and treatment of sleep problems in the elderly. Sleep Med Rev 1997;1(1):3–17.

[113] Ancoli-Israel S, Kripke DF, Klauber MR, et al. Periodic limb movements in sleep in community-dwelling elderly. Sleep 1991;14(6):496–500.

[114] Silber MH, Ehrenberg BL, Allen RP, et al. An algorithm for the management of restless legs syndrome. Mayo Clin Proc 2004;79(7):916–22.

[115] Mahowald MW, Schenck CH. REM sleep behavior disorder. In: Kryger MH, Dement W, Roth T, editors. Principles and practice of sleep medicine. 2nd edition. Philadelphia: Saunders; 1994. p. 574–88.

[116] Schenck CH, Mahowald MW. REM sleep behavior disorder: clinical, developmental, and neuroscience perspectives 16 years after its formal identification in SLEEP. Sleep 2002;25(2):120–38.

[117] Olson EJ, Boeve BF, Silber MH. Rapid eye movement sleep behaviour disorder: demographic, clinical and laboratory findings in 93 cases. Brain 2000; 123(Pt 2):331–9.

[118] Chiu HF, Wing YK, Lam LC, et al. Sleep-related injury in the elderly—an epidemiological study in Hong Kong. Sleep 2000;23(4):513–7.

[119] Schenck CH, Bundlie SR, Mahowald MW. Delayed emergence of a parkinsonian disorder in 38% of 29 older men initially diagnosed with idiopathic rapid eye movement sleep behaviour disorder. Neurology 1996;46(2):388–93.

[120] Mahowald M, Schenck C. REM sleep parasomnias. In: Kryger MH, Dement W, editors. Principles and practice of sleep medicine. 3rd edition. Philadelphia: W.B. Saunders; 2000. p. 724–37.

[121] Wolkove N, Elkholy O, Baltzan M, et al. Sleep and aging: 2. Management of sleep disorders in older people. CMAJ 2007;176(10):1449–54.

[122] Kunz D, Bes F. Melatonin as a therapy in REM sleep behavior disorder patients: an open-labeled pilot study on the possible influence of melatonin on REM-sleep regulation. Mov Disord 1999; 14(3):507–11.

[123] Takeuchi N, Uchimura N, Hashizume Y, et al. Melatonin therapy for REM sleep behavior disorder. Psychiatry Clin Neurosci 2001;55(3): 267–9.

[124] Boeve BF, Silber MH, Ferman TJ. Melatonin for treatment of REM sleep behavior disorder in neurologic disorders: results in 14 patients. Sleep Med 2003;4(4):281–4.

[125] Gagnon JF, Postuma RB, Montplaisir J. Update on the pharmacology of REM sleep behavior disorder. Neurology 2006;67(5):742–7.

[126] Ringman JM, Simmons JH. Treatment of REM sleep behavior disorder with donepezil: a report of three cases. Neurology 2000;55(6):870–1.

ELSEVIER
SAUNDERS

Clin Chest Med 28 (2007) 685–702

CLINICS
IN CHEST
MEDICINE

Asthma in Older Adults

Sidney S. Braman, MD[a],*, Nicola A. Hanania, MD, MS[b]

[a]The Warren Alpert Medical School of Brown University, Division of Pulmonary and Critical Care Medicine,
The Warren Alpert Medical School of Brown University and Rhode Island Hospital, 593 Eddy Street,
Providence, RI 02903, USA
[b]Section of Pulmonary and Critical Care Medicine, Asthma Clinical Research Center, Baylor College of Medicine,
1504 Taub Loop, Houston, Texas 77030, USA

Asthma is characterized by chronic airway inflammation that is driven by a complex interaction of inflammatory cells, mediators, and cytokines that leads to airway hyperresponsiveness and airflow obstruction [1]. According to the National Center for Health Statistics, the overall prevalence of asthma in the US population is approximately 6% to 7% [2]. Although the diagnosis and treatment of asthma often focuses on a younger population, it is estimated that more than 1 million adults older than age 65 in the United States carry a diagnosis of asthma. In a survey of older persons from four communities in the United States, the prevalence of physician-diagnosed asthma was 4%, with another 4% having probable asthma (symptoms of asthma without a diagnosis) [3]. Other estimates of prevalence have shown a broad range from 4% to 9% [3–5].

Asthma in older adults is associated with a significant number of hospitalizations and emergency department visits, which lead to substantial amounts of health care costs. In 1999, the United States rate for asthma hospitalization for patients older than 65 years of age was 21.1 per 10,000 [2]. Older patients with asthma are more likely to die from their disease than younger individuals, and although mortality rates in some age groups have decreased, this is not true of older adults [6]. According to the US Centers for Disease Control and Prevention(CDC), asthma deaths in older adults account for more than 50%

of asthma fatalities annually, with approximately 5.8 asthma deaths per 100,000 in this group reported in the years 2001 to 2003 [2,7]. The National Health Interview survey reported that current asthma prevalence in older adults is highest among Puerto Rican Americans. Like other chronic diseases in this age group, asthma in older adults population has a major impact on patient well-being and causes significant impairment in health status, symptoms of depression, and significant limitation of daily activity [3,8–10].

Although most older patients with asthma have long-standing asthma that may have developed early in life, some develop asthma late in life (late-onset disease). Late-onset asthma may occur at any age, even in the eighth and ninth decades of life. When it does occur, moderate to severe symptoms are more likely [11]. Despite the frequent occurrence of asthma in older adults, it is a diagnosis that has been overlooked frequently. Even when discovered, it is often undertreated [3,12–16]. Several important reasons that may explain the underdiagnosis and undertreatment of asthma in older adults are discussed in this article. This article also focuses on the epidemiologic, clinical, and pharmacologic aspects of asthma in the geriatric population.

The definition of asthma

An expert panel of the National Institutes of Health has provided us with the most widely accepted current definition of asthma for any age [17]. Asthma is a chronic inflammatory disease of the airways in which many cells play a role, in particular, mast cells, eosinophils, and T lymphocytes.

* Corresponding author.
  E-mail address: sidney_braman@brown.edu
(S.S. Braman).

In susceptible individuals, this inflammation causes recurrent episodes of wheezing, breathlessness, chest tightness, and cough, particularly at night or in the early morning or both. These symptoms are usually associated with widespread but variable airflow limitation that is at least partially reversible either spontaneously or with treatment. This inflammation also causes an associated increase in airway hyperresponsiveness to various stimuli. This definition highlights the three cardinal features of asthma: airflow obstruction, reversibility of obstruction, and bronchial hyperresponsiveness.

Epidemiology of asthma in older adults

It has been difficult to assign precise figures to the prevalence and incidence of asthma in the general population because often studies do not clearly distinguish asthma from other obstructive lung diseases in this population. Men and women who develop typical asthma after age 40 usually have prior symptoms of cough and sputum production and often have pulmonary function abnormalities before the diagnosis of asthma [7,18]. In many older patients it is not possible to distinguish asthma from chronic bronchitis, especially in current or former cigarette smokers. A label of "asthmatic bronchitis" may be more appropriate for such patients, but this term has not gained widespread use. In population surveys that inquire about asthma and chronic obstructive pulmonary disease (COPD), subjects frequently reported more than one disease. For example, in the NHANES III survey, 25% of subjects with current bronchitis reported that they also had current asthma and 34.3% subjects with current asthma reported that they had current chronic bronchitis. Similarly, 19.4% of the subjects with emphysema reported that they had current asthma [7].

Community surveys, in which a physician diagnosis of asthma was required, have provided data on asthma in older adults. The prevalence of active asthma in these studies, which represented new cases excluding those in remission, peaked in early childhood at approximately 8% to 10% of the population, declined to approximately 5.5% during late adolescence, and rose again to approximately 7% to 9% during late adulthood (older than age 70). In 1987, data from the National Center for Health Statistics showed that in the 65- to 74-year-old age group, the rate for active asthma or wheeze was 10.4% compared with 5.7% in younger teenagers, 6.9% in the 18- to 44-year-old age group, and 9.6% in the 45- to 64-year-old age group [19]. In another report from a population-based cohort of older individuals living in Rochester, Minnesota, a group of patients who had asthma were identified with the onset of asthma after age 65 [13]. The age-specific incidence of asthma in individuals aged 65 to 74 years was 103 per 100,000; it was 81 per 100,000 in persons aged 75 to 84 and 58 per 100,000 in persons older than 85 years.

Current statistics regarding morbidity and mortality in older patients are concerning. In 1985, 58% of the men and 71% of the women whose deaths were attributed to asthma in England and Wales were older than 70 years. In a US study of asthma deaths that occurred in hospitals or nursing homes, 80% of the deaths occurred in patients aged 55 years and older [20]. Seventy-five percent of these patients were known to be smokers or ex-smokers. A careful analysis of these cases revealed that many younger patients who had asthma did clearly have asthma and died of a severe sudden attack. In persons over age 55, confounding factors were much more prevalent. These patients frequently had underlying chronic bronchitis or COPD, were admitted to the hospital for nonrespiratory problems, and died of chronic respiratory failure. Less aggressive therapy was given to these older patients, both in the outpatient setting and during hospitalization. There was often a delay in seeking medical care, which was thought to be a major factor in their deaths. This study also suggested that many older patients with asthma-like symptoms and a history of previous smoking have COPD as an underlying or even dominant feature of their disease. This factor undoubtedly overestimated the true mortality from asthma in this age group. More recent data from an analysis of US death certificates have shown that unlike younger age groups, mortality rates for older patients who have asthma continue to rise, especially in women [6]. There is likely to be a serious death certificate misclassification of cause of death in older people with asthma, however, often as result of confounding medical conditions. Factors that may increase risk of death in this population include delay in seeking diagnosis and treatment, poor cardiopulmonary reserve, impaired perception of increasing airway obstruction, blunted hypoxic ventilator drive, and psychosocial and cognitive problems, which are common in this age group.

Pathophysiology of asthma in older adults

Asthma is caused by a complex interaction of cells, mediators, and cytokines that results in airway inflammation [1,21]. The characteristic cellular changes involve (1) constitutive cells, such as epithelial cells, mucous glands, endothelial cells, and myofibroblasts, (2) resident cells, such as bone marrow–derived mast cells and macrophages, and (3) infiltrating cells, such as eosinophils, CD4 (helper cell) T lymphocytes, neutrophils, basophils, and platelets. These inflammatory cells are capable of generating a wide variety of mediators that can induce bronchoconstriction. Several typical histopathologic findings can be found in the airways of patients who have asthma.

Histopathologic findings in asthma

Infiltration of the airways by inflammatory cells, such as mast cells, eosinophils, activated T lymphocytes, and neutrophils, can be demonstrated by bronchial biopsies and inferred by demonstrating increased numbers of these cells on bronchoalveolar lavage. The number of activated lymphocytes found in bronchial biopsies has been correlated with the number of local activated eosinophils and the severity of asthma. Specific cytokines, most of which are products of lymphocytes and macrophages, seem to direct the movement of cells to the site of airway inflammation. They also activate the cells and cause them to release their mediators. Mast cells, usually as a result of IgE-mediated stimulation, also release preformed mediators, such as histamine and proteases, and further act as regulators of inflammation by producing cytokines that promote eosinophil infiltration and activation. Several mast cell products induce bronchoconstriction and cause increased mucus secretion.

Edema of the airway mucosa occurs secondary to increased capillary permeability with leakage of serum proteins into the interstitium. Several cell-derived mediators are capable of inducing edema formation, including histamine, prostaglandin E, leukotriene-C4 (LTC4), LTD4, LTE4, platelet-activating factor, and bradykinin. Denudation of the airway epithelium can lead to airway edema and loss of substances in the mucosa that protect the airway. Epithelial damage promotes bronchial hyperresponsiveness because access by irritating substances to sensory nerve endings is increased. Another characteristic finding in severe asthma is the presence of tenacious mucus plugs in the airways. Death from asthma usually occurs from blockage of the airways by diffuse mucus plugging.

Thickening of the reticular basement membrane, the laminar reticularis, is observed with light microscopy and is a constant feature of asthma. There is also evidence of increased bronchial smooth muscle mass, which contributes considerably to the thickness of the airway wall. The airway architecture is also changed by the deposition of types III and V collagen and fibronectin beneath the basement membrane, which has been referred to as "subepithelial fibrosis." The architectural changes seen in and beneath the basement membrane and in the bronchial smooth muscle are referred to as airway remodeling and are thought to cause permanent changes that result in fixed airflow obstruction.

Histopathologic findings in asthma in older adults

Sputum, bronchoalveolar lavage, and bronchial mucosal biopsy specimens from older patients who have stable asthma have confirmed the presence of prominent eosinophilia and CD4+ T lymphocytes, as seen with younger patients who have asthma [22]. Thickening of the reticular basement membrane and disruption of the epithelial lining also have been described. Pathologic findings have been compared in young and older subjects who have died of fatal attacks of asthma [23]. Old and young patients who have asthma have thickened airway smooth muscle compared with normal subjects. Older patients who have asthma with a longer duration of disease demonstrate increase in airway wall thickness, however, predominantly because of an increase in the adventitial area. Greater postmortem reduction in airway lumen is also found in older patients who have asthma. The luminal content and subepithelial collagen deposition are similar in both asthma groups. The presence of greater wall thickness in older patients who have asthma supports the concept that aging and asthma duration result in airway remodeling, which causes "fixed" or irreversible airflow obstruction in this population.

Neurogenic influences

In addition to the structural changes that occur in the airway lining and wall in patients who have asthma, there is evidence that the neural control of the airways is abnormal. Neurogenic mechanisms may augment or modulate the inflammatory response seen in these patients [1]. The autonomic nervous system regulates many aspects of airway function, such as airway tone, airway secretions, blood flow, microvascular permeability, and the release of inflammatory cells. It is likely that autonomic dysfunction is caused by inflammation because inflammatory mediators can modulate the release of neurotransmitters from airway nerves.

Bronchial hyperresponsiveness

Airway inflammation is thought to be a key factor in producing a cardinal feature of asthma-bronchial hyperresponsiveness [1], which can be described as an exaggerated bronchoconstrictive response by the airways to various stimuli, such as aeroallergens, histamine, methacholine, cold air, and environmental irritants. It is not clear whether bronchial hyperresponsiveness is acquired or is genetically determined to appear with the appropriate stimulus. In general, it is thought that airway inflammation is the stimulus for bronchial hyperresponsiveness because it may be induced by several inciting events, including viral respiratory infections, allergic reactions, and exposure to noxious agents, such as ozone and sulfur dioxide. The degree of bronchial hyperresponsiveness can be determined in the pulmonary function laboratory by standard inhalation bronchoprovocation challenge testing. The methacholine inhalation challenge is the most frequently used clinical tool to determine the presence and degree of bronchial hyperresponsiveness.

Bronchoprovocation testing is a safe, effective method to uncover asthma in older adults [24,25]. Evidence exists, however, that some sympathetic and parasympathetic nervous system functions are diminished with age [26,27]. This decline in autonomic nervous system function is consistent with a generalized diminution of peripheral somatic nerve function with aging. Although the protective laryngeal gag reflex seems to be diminished in normal older subjects, however [28], there is evidence that the cholinergically mediated cough reflex may not be similarly affected [29]. Measurements of cholinergic bronchoconstrictive reflexes have shown mixed results, although most studies have shown a positive correlation between aging and airway hyperresponsiveness [30]. There is a relationship between the degree of bronchial hyperresponsiveness and prechallenge pulmonary function; a low FEV_1 (forced expiratory volume in one second) predicts heightened responsiveness [31]. Although this relationship may explain why some studies have shown that bronchial responsiveness is heightened in older adults, aging may be an independent factor that influences airway responsiveness [32]. Other factors that may contribute to heightened airway responsiveness in the older population are atopy and current or previous smoking history.

Airway obstruction

Airway obstruction is another cardinal feature of asthma. The causes of airflow limitation in asthma are listed in Box 1. Inflammation of the bronchial wall may uncouple the mechanical linkage between the parenchyma and the airway, which may contribute to airway narrowing and bronchial hyperresponsiveness. During an acute attack of asthma, airway resistance increases and measures of airflow are abnormal.

There is growing evidence that the airway function of young and middle-age persons who have asthma declines at a greater rate than normal subjects [33–35]. The rate of decline increases with increasing age and in individuals who smoke cigarettes [34,36]. In late-onset asthma, there is evidence that lung function is reduced even before a diagnosis is made and declines rapidly shortly after diagnosis [37,38]. Thereafter, it remains fairly stable. These effects on patients who have asthma are variable because not all individuals show a steep rate of decline. The precise reasons for this individual variability have not been defined, although there is evidence that atopy and marked bronchial hyperresponsiveness are two important risk factors for airflow obstruction [39]. The long duration and severity of previous disease are also important factors [40,41], although many older patients who have asthma with severe airflow obstruction report having had a relatively short duration of symptoms of months to a few years. In one random survey from the Mayo Clinic of 1200 patients over age

---

Box 1. Causes of airflow limitation in asthma

Acute bronchoconstriction
Mucus plugging of airways
Bronchial wall edema
Inflammatory cell infiltration
Airway wall remodeling (fibrosis)
Smooth muscle hypertrophy
Uncoupling of elastic recoil forces

65 who have asthma, only 1 in 5 patients had normal pulmonary function ($FEV_1 > 80\%$ predicted), whereas a similar number showed moderate to severe airflow obstruction ($FEV_1 < 50\%$ predicted) even after administration of an inhaled short-acting bronchodilator [42]. The cause of chronic persistent airflow obstruction in asthma has not been explained. Structural changes of emphysema are minimal, and airway remodeling is thought to be the main cause.

The presence of airflow obstruction is usually confirmed by documenting a reduced FEV_1 and ratio of FEV_1/FVC (forced vital capacity) on spirometry. Traditionally, a ratio of less than 70% increases the probability of asthma in older patients with asthma symptoms, although the use of the statistically derived lower limit of normal values may be more accurate for defining obstruction in older adults [43]. A brisk response to a short-acting bronchodilator may demonstrate the second cardinal feature of asthma: reversible airflow obstruction ("a responder"). When airflow obstruction is found in older patients, attempts should be made to demonstrate reversibility after the inhalation of a short-acting β-adrenergic agent such as albuterol. Age is not a significant predictor of the acute bronchodilator response in asthma. Using American Thoracic Society criteria, demonstration of significant reversibility (postbronchodilator FEV_1 or FVC increases more than 12% and 200 mL) increases the probability of the diagnosis. Although the response to an inhaled bronchodilator is generally greater with asthma, many patients who have COPD also meet the American Thoracic Society reversibility criteria on any given testing day. The response to bronchodilator in these patients may not persist, however. More than 50% of patients change "responder" status between visits, which makes the test less than reliable for confirming the diagnosis of asthma, especially in older adults.

In general, when complete reversibility of airflow obstruction is documented, COPD, a disease of fixed airway obstruction, is excluded. A negative bronchodilator response to a short-acting β-agonist, on the other hand, does not rule out a diagnosis of asthma, and as many as 30% of patients with fixed airflow obstruction have a past history of asthma. Reduced beta2-adrenoreceptor responsiveness has been demonstrated in normal older men and women. When compared with young and normal older subjects, older patients who have late-onset asthma have been shown to have reductions in β-adrenergic receptor affinity

while maintaining normal receptor density. There is also evidence that postreceptor events are impaired in the aged because cyclic AMP production by pathways that are independent of adrenergic receptor stimulation is depressed [44–46]. As one would predict, the bronchodilator response to inhaled β-agonists declines with age [47–49], although this is not the case with anticholinergic agents.

Atopy and asthma in older adults

Atopic asthma

Allergic and atopic reactions in the upper and lower airways are important in the pathogenesis of asthma in childhood and young adulthood. Their role in older adults is less clear. The term "extrinsic asthma" has been used to describe patients whose asthma is triggered by exposure to inhaled aeroallergens. Atopy is defined by the presence of abnormal amounts of IgE antibodies in response to contact with environmental antigens and can be manifested as asthma, eczema, or seasonal and perennial allergic rhinitis. This can be demonstrated clinically by the presence of elevated total or specific serum IgE levels in the blood or by demonstrating positive skin prick tests to various standardized aeroallergens. In older patients with or without asthma, an elevated level of IgE may be an important risk factor for the development of chronic airflow obstruction [50]. This finding is especially true in current smokers but also is seen in former smokers. Although the cause of elevated IgE in smokers is not known, research has shown that these antibodies are not directed against common aeroallergens [51]. The association of IgE and airflow obstruction also has been shown to be independent of smoking; the two are thought to act synergistically.

Atopy is an age-related phenomenon; in community surveys, the peak prevalence of immediate skin test reactivity occurs during the third decade and falls rapidly after age 50 [52]. The proportion of persons who have asthma who have atopy varies with age. I childhood the rate is approximately 80%; between ages 20 and 40 it is 50%, and after age 50, the rate is less than 20%. Elevated serum IgE levels are closely related to the likelihood of a subsequent asthma diagnosis in younger patients who have asthma, which is also true for older patients who have asthma [37]. The reported prevalence of allergic asthma after age 65 has varied considerably. In one study of older persons who have asthma who were followed in a pulmonary clinic, patients who had acquired their asthma at an early age had a greater likelihood of previous allergic disease, such as eczema or seasonal allergic rhinitis [53]. None of the patients who had acquired asthma after age 60 had a previous atopic history. Immediate hypersensitivity skin tests to 43 aeroallergens in this group were uniformly negative, and IgE levels were elevated in approximately 20% of patients. This rate compares with a 36% positive skin test rate in a community-based survey [38].

Other studies have explored the relationship between allergy and asthma in older adults [3,54–56]. One study was conducted on patients over age 65 years with moderate and severe persistent asthma who were recruited from the medical, geriatric, and allergy clinics of a tertiary health care center [54]. Allergy skin test results were positive to at least one allergen in 75% of patients. The most prevalent reactions were to indoor allergens, such as cat and dog dander and cockroach dust mite. Bermuda grass produced the second most prevalent positive skin test result. Home visits were done to sample for indoor allergens. Although most homes had high levels of indoor allergens, there was no correlation between home allergens above significant levels and severity of asthma measured by lung function testing. No evidence was presented that exposure to these aeroallergens caused worsening of asthma symptoms. Another study was reported with data collected from the Cardiovascular Health Study, a clinical study conducted by randomly sampling older individuals from four US communities [3]. This study showed that many older patients who had asthma reported that their respiratory problems started in childhood. Although skin testing and IgE levels were not available in the study patients, approximately half reported that wheezing was triggered by contact with plants, animals, or pollens and was seasonal. In a study of older urban patients who have asthma, the presence of cockroach-specific IgE antibody has been shown to be associated with more severe asthma and an increase in airflow obstruction [56].

A history of atopy is the strongest predictor of asthma in older adults [57]. Individuals who are capable of becoming sensitized will have done so by the time they are older. There is a complex interplay between allergens and asthma; some allergens cause sensitization, some enhance the allergic response, and some actually induce asthma attacks. Although atopy may be important in the pathogenesis of asthma of some older patients who have asthma, in general it is rare to find clinical provocation of asthma by common aeroallergens—a dominant feature in this age group. Avoidance of potential allergens in the environment of older adult patients who have asthma should be advised.

Nonatopic asthma

The term "intrinsic asthma" is used to describe patients who have none of the typical features of atopy, including a positive family history of allergy and asthma, positive immediate hypersensitivity reactions to skin prick-tests, and an elevated serum IgE level. As noted, such patients are generally older than persons who have atopic asthma and have a later onset of their asthma. Bronchial biopsy studies on patients who have intrinsic asthma have been compared with a group of patients who have extrinsic asthma with a comparable severity of symptoms [21]. There is a more intense inflammatory cell infiltrate in the bronchial mucosa of the patients who have intrinsic asthma with leukocytes, macrophages, and CD3 and CD4 cells. Patients who have intrinsic asthma have an exaggerated T-cell response to maintain the same degree of symptoms and bronchial hyperresponsiveness. This finding may mean that intrinsic asthma may involve activation by an as-yet unidentified antigen. Putative nonallergic antigens that may cause such reactions include viral antigens or inappropriately recognized "self-antigens." In support of the former causative agent, it is noteworthy that most older patients who develop asthma after age 65 years have their first asthmatic symptom preceded immediately by or concomitant with an upper respiratory tract infection [13].

Clinical characteristics of asthma in older adults

Data on the clinical features of asthma in older adults have been derived from longitudinal community surveys and case studies [3,13,38,53,58,59]. Two distinct presentations, which are based on the onset and duration of the disease state, have been described for asthma in older adults [41,53,58]. Patients who have late-onset asthma start having asthma symptoms for the first time when they are aged 65 or older. Some studies of older persons who have asthma have shown that as a group, as many as 40% have their first attack after the age of 40 years. [38,53,60]. Patients who belong to this group tend to have fewer atopic manifestations, higher baseline FEV_1, and a more pronounced bronchodilator response than patients who have long-standing asthma, who start having asthma symptoms early in life. Patients who belong to this group tend to have higher incidence of atopic diseases, more severe and irreversible or partially reversible airway obstruction, and more hyperinflation. The duration of the disease in this group is an important determinant of severity and development of irreversible airflow obstruction [61].

Classic symptoms of asthma, including episodic wheezing, shortness of breath, and chest tightness, are not uncommon in older adults. These symptoms are generally worse at night and with exertion and are often precipitated by an upper respiratory tract infection. Symptoms of asthma in older adults are nonspecific, however, and may be caused by various other conditions.

Dyspnea is a common symptom and may be attributed to different underlying pathologic abnormalities, including heart or lung diseases. Exertional dyspnea and paroxysmal nocturnal dyspnea are present in a smaller number of older patients who have asthma. Many older patients limit their activity to avoid getting dyspneic; others assume that their dyspnea is a result of aging and avoid seeking medical attention early in their disease process. Aging, per se, does not cause dyspnea, however, and a cause must be pursued in assessing an older patient who complains of breathlessness. Cough is a prominent symptom and occasionally may be the only presenting symptom [62]. Wheezing, on the other hand, may not be as prominent, and its presence is not specific and does not correlate with severity of obstruction. Asthma is often triggered by environmental exposures but may be related to other concomitant disorders or therapies (Table 1). History of atopy is a strong predictor of asthma in this age group, and allergic rhinitis, sinusitis, and nasal polyps are not uncommon. Respiratory symptoms are often triggered by medications, such as aspirin, nonsteroidal anti-inflammatory agents, or β-blockers, commonly used by older patients. This possibility mandates that physicians perform a comprehensive review of medications taken by patients upon presentation. Physical examination in older patients who have asthma is usually nonspecific and may misguide the diagnosis.

Table 1
Triggers of asthma in older adults

Environmental exposures	Aeroallergens
	Irritants (Cigarette Smoke, household aerosols, paints)
	Strong Odors (Perfumes)
Comorbid conditions	Viral upper respiratory infections
	Gastroesophageal reflux
	Allergic rhinitis/sinusitis
Food/drinks	Metabisulfite ingestion (wine, beer, food preservatives)
Medications	Aspirin
	Nonsteroidal anti-inflammatory drugs (eg, ibuprofen, indomethacin, naproxen)
	Beta-blockers

Studies have shown consistently that symptoms caused by asthma are frequently overlooked by older patients and their physicians. Several factors contribute to the underdiagnosis and misdiagnosis of asthma in this age group (Box 2). One reason why asthma has been an overlooked diagnosis in older adults is that the symptoms are common to other comorbidities present in older patients. The hallmark symptoms of asthma, including shortness of breath, wheeze, and cough, are nonspecific in older adults and are mimicked by other diseases, such as congestive heart failure, emphysema and chronic bronchitis (COPD), chronic aspiration, gastroesophageal reflux disease, and tracheobronchial tumors. Distinguishing asthma from COPD may be challenging; in some patients asthma cannot be distinguished from COPD with current diagnostic tests. The management of these patients should be similar to that of patients who have asthma. It has been known for more than a century that early morning wheezing is a prominent symptom of congestive heart failure; it has been called cardiac asthma because it can mimic the clinical picture of asthma. Typical symptoms of gastroesophageal reflux in older adults, such as vomiting and heartburn, may be absent. In a study of older patients with esophageal reflux proven by intraesophageal pH monitoring, chronic cough, hoarseness, and wheezing were present in 57% of patients [63,64]. In addition to causing asthma-like symptoms, evidence also indicates that gastroesophageal reflux disease

Box 2. Factors that contribute to the underdiagnosis of asthma in older patients

Patient factors (poor recognition by patient)
- Do not present early for diagnosis
- Underrate symptoms
- Poor access to care

Physician factors (difficulty in diagnosis)
- Diagnosis of exclusion
- Diagnosis is complicated by discrepancy between symptoms and the degree of airway obstruction
- Inadequate use of lung function tests

may be a cause of worsening asthma. Unlike younger adults who have asthma, a family or personal history of atopy is usually absent. Blood and sputum eosinophilia are common but not universal.

Older patients also have been shown to have a reduced perception of bronchoconstriction, which further delays medical intervention. Many older patients are fearful of having an illness and dying and are reluctant to admit that they have symptoms. Even when they do so, they may underestimate the symptoms or consider them a result of normal aging. Underreporting of symptoms in older adults may have many causes, including depression, cognitive impairment, social isolation, denial, and confusing symptoms with those of other comorbid illnesses.

Objective measures of lung function, such as spirometry and peak flow measurements, are generally underused in older patients, which also contributes to the delay or absence of diagnosis [13,65]. Lung function testing is especially important in this age group because there is an age-related reduction in the perception of dyspnea seen in older adults [66]. Spirometry may be difficult to perform in some situations, however, because of physical and cognitive impairment. It is hard to define the lower limits of predicted normal values in this age group, however, which may vary in different patients. Older patients who have asthma also may demonstrate an impaired acute bronchodilator response, which can lead to a misdiagnosis of COPD. This poor response may result from the decreased number of β-adrenergic receptors on smooth airway muscles that has

been described with the aging process. Airway obstruction may be absent at the time of testing in approximately 8% of older patients, and further testing, which may include methacholine challenge testing or even cardiopulmonary exercise stress testing, may be needed to confirm the diagnosis.

Measurement of airway hyperresponsiveness to methacholine may not be an accurate test in older adults [67]. Peak expiratory flow variability may be helpful in the diagnosis and follow-up of patients with obstructive airway diseases, but poor coordination and muscle weakness in some patients may lead to an inaccurate reading [68,69]. A recent prospective study failed to demonstrate any advantage of peak flow monitoring over symptom monitoring as an asthma management strategy for older adults who have moderate-severe asthma when used in a comprehensive asthma management program [70]. Other tests, such as measuring the carbon monoxide diffusing capacity of the lung, may help distinguish between asthma and COPD.

The rate of smoking among older patients who have asthma is 10% to 13% and is approximately half that of the general adult population. Lung function is generally lower in individuals who smoke compared with those who do not smoke because of concomitant COPD [38]. Even in individuals who do not smoke, most older patients who have asthma have moderate or severe persistent asthma. For instance, the Tucson Epidemiological Study of Obstructive Lung Disease identified 46 patients who had asthma who were 65 years or older at the time of enrollment [38]. Many of these older patients had severe disease with marked ventilatory impairment. Almost one half admitted to frequent wheezing attacks or wheezing on most days, whereas only 30% of the group had rare episodes of shortness of breath with wheezing.

Management of asthma in older adults

The goals of asthma therapy in older patients are to treat the acute symptoms, prevent chronic symptoms, decrease emergency department visits and hospitalizations, preserve normal activity level, and optimize pulmonary function with minimal adverse effects from medications [62,71]. Optimal management also should focus on improving health status and quality of life in these patients, which is greatly impaired by respiratory symptoms and depressive symptoms [3]. A proper evaluation of asthma symptoms can lead to early diagnosis, effective treatment, and avoidance of unnecessary emergency department visits and hospitalizations.

General considerations

Population studies of asthma in older adults have shown that unlike many younger adults, who often require no medications or only need β-agonist therapy for occasional symptoms, most older patients need continuous treatment programs to control their disease. Undertreatment is common, however, and several factors contribute to this undertreatment of older patients who have asthma (Box 3) [3,16,72–74].

At a time when memory loss is common and financial resources are often limited, many older patients require complicated and frequent dosing with multiple expensive drugs. Unfortunately, this has led to a significant rate of noncompliance among older patients. Aging has been shown to be a significant predictor for poor adherence to medication therapy [75]. Attempts to identify patients at high risk for noncompliance have failed. Gender, socioeconomic factors, educational level, marital status, and severity of disease do not seem to be good predictors of compliance [62]. It is common for older patients to live alone, which creates additional barriers to appropriate care. Such patients often lack adequate nutrition and immediate physical and emotional comfort.

Box 3. Factors that contribute to the undertreatment of asthma in older adults

Poor knowledge of the disease
- Poor understanding of pathophysiology and asthma self-management
- Belief in the myth that the condition is caused by aging and is untreatable
- Misdiagnosis

Obstacles to asthma therapy
- Poor access to health care
- Medication cost
- Fear of corticosteroids
- Poor medication delivery device technique

Compassionate and sympathetic support from the physician and office staff often can be as beneficial as pharmacologic intervention. Sensitivity to economic issues can lead to less costly prescriptions. Written lists of medications and dosing schedules are especially helpful, and frank, open discussions about such issues as loneliness, finance, and loss of autonomy from chronic illness are appreciated. Because of a patient's advanced age, the illness may prove an exaggerated threat of dying, which may lead to denial and undermedication or high anxiety and overreliance on medication, physician visits, and office phone calls.

There are short- and long-term therapeutic objectives for every patient who has asthma [62]. Short-term objectives involve control of immediate symptoms. Long-term objectives are directed at disease prevention because there are well-proven strategies for avoiding serious exacerbations of acute bronchospasm, which often lead to emergency room visits or hospitalization. To meet these therapeutic objectives, four components of asthma care should be considered, as discussed in the following sections.

Assessment and monitoring

Optimal treatment of asthma depends on a careful assessment of a patient's symptoms and objective monitoring by office spirometry and home peak expiratory flow rate measurements. Older patients who have asthma have been shown to deteriorate for longer periods before hospital admission for severe acute asthma than younger patients. In a study of hospital admissions for asthma that compared patients over age 65 to patients younger than age 40, 65% of older patients had worsening symptoms for more than 14 days before admission compared with 29% for the younger group [76]. One reason for this delay may be the blunted perception of breathlessness that has been found in older patients compared with younger patients [66]. Monitoring of lung function with peak flow meters or office spirometry is essential in caring for many older patients who have asthma.

Controlling triggers

Measures should be taken to avoid triggers that can cause worsening of symptoms. As with asthma at any age, education concerning avoidance of aggravating factors that can lead to severe bronchospasm is useful. Although aeroallergens are less important in provoking symptoms in older adults than young subjects, a program that implements environmental control measures, such as avoiding or minimizing aeroallergen exposure, should be instituted in patients with documented sensitivity to specific allergens. Such programs may not always be successful, however, especially because lifestyle changes in older adults may be difficult. All patients should receive annual influenza vaccine prophylaxis. Pneumococcal vaccine administration is also recommended. The most important provocative factors include viral respiratory infections, irritants (eg, cigarette smoke, paints, varnish, household aerosols), and pharmacologic agents that are often prescribed for concomitant illnesses. β-Adrenoreceptor antagonists (β-blockers) commonly used for ischemic heart disease, arrhythmias, and hypertension may precipitate bronchoconstriction in any patient who has asthma [77]. This list includes noncardioselective agents (eg, propranolol, pindolol, and timolol) and to a lesser extent cardioselective agents (eg, metoprolol and acebutolol). Topical β-blockers are also widely used in older patients to reduce intraocular pressure in wide-angle glaucoma. With such treatment, sufficient systemic absorption may occur to cause fatal status asthmaticus [78]. The severity of β-blocker–induced bronchoconstriction correlates with the severity of underlying airflow obstruction and the degree of bronchial reactivity and may be reduced by the use of a cardioselective topical β-blocking agent, such as betaxolol [79]. Aspirin and nonsteroidal anti-inflammatory agents may precipitate acute asthma and should be avoided when possible. Angiotensin-converting enzyme inhibitors may cause dry cough and worsening of symptoms of asthma and should be avoided. Gastroesophageal reflux disease is one of the most common triggers of asthma and is often silent. If gastroesophageal reflux disease is suspected, patients should be given proper instructions to elevate the head of their bed, avoid certain food items that may exacerbate the reflux, and avoid eating 2 hours before retiring to bed. Most of these patients also benefit from empirical treatment with standard therapies.

Pharmacologic therapy

Therapeutic approach to asthma in older patients does not differ from what is recommended for young patients. Statements on standard of care for treating asthma have been published by the National Institutes of Heath in the United States and others around the world [17,62]. Treatment protocols use step-care pharmacologic therapy based on the intensity of asthma symptoms and the clinical response to these interventions. As symptoms and lung function worsen, step-up or add-on therapy is given. As symptoms improve, therapy can be "stepped down." Several considerations must be taken into consideration when considering appropriate pharmacologic therapy in older patients who have asthma (Table 2). Special attention also should be given to the potential adverse effects of commonly used medications (Table 3) [80].

Anti-inflammatory agents

Anti-inflammatory agents are capable of reducing airway inflammation, thereby improving lung function, decreasing bronchial hyperreactivity, reducing symptoms, and improving the overall quality of life. Corticosteroids are the most useful anti-inflammatory agents. They act by preventing migration and activation of inflammatory cells, interfering with the production of prostaglandins and leukotrienes, reducing microvascular leakage, and enhancing the action of β-adrenergic receptors on airway smooth muscle. They are available for oral, parenteral, and inhaled use.

Inhaled corticosteroids are a safe and effective treatment for persistent asthma whether it is mild, moderate, or severe. Metered dose inhalers (MDIs) or dry powder formulations are available

Table 2
Special considerations for pharmacologic therapy for asthma in older adults

Consideration	Contributing factor(s)
Delivery of medication	Poor inhaler technique
Effectiveness of medication	Difference in pharmacodynamics and pharmacokinetics than in the younger population, diminished response to β2-agonists, comorbidities
Compliance with medication	Complex regimen, prohibitive cost, poor memory, and delivery technique
Safety of medication	Increased risk from comorbid conditions (eg, cardiac, osteoporosis), interaction with other medications

Table 3
Adverse effects of asthma medications in older patients

Medications	Adverse reactions
β2-agonists	Tremors, palpitations, arrhythmias, hypokalemia
Ipratropium bromide	Urinary retention, mucosal dryness
Corticosteroids	
Inhaled	Thrush, dysphonia, potential for systemic effects if used in high dose
Systemic	Osteoporosis, adrenal suppression, skin thinning, diabetes mellitus, myopathy, increased blood pressure, glaucoma
Theophylline	Tachyarrhythmias, nausea, vomiting insomnia, seizures, interaction with other medications

as beclomethasone, triamcinolone, flunisolide, fluticasone, budesonide, and mometasone. They can reduce airway inflammation after several months of treatment, but long-term treatment is usually necessary. Long-term use of inhaled corticosteroids has been associated with a good safety profile. Higher doses of inhaled steroids (eg, >1000 μg/d) are capable of causing hypophyseal-pituitary-adrenal axis suppression. Local adverse effects, such as hoarseness, dysphonia, cough, and oral candidiasis, do occur but usually can be avoided by the use of a spacer or holding chamber and rinsing the mouth after each use.

Despite the pivotal role of inhaled corticosteroids in asthma [81], many older patients are undertreated with this group of medications [72]. In the Cardiovascular Health Study, 39% of older patients who had asthma were not taking any medications, and less than one third used inhaled corticosteroids, although most of them had moderate-to-severe asthma [3]. On the other hand, 19% of patients were taking oral corticosteroids, despite the fact that these medications can profoundly raise the risk of bone fracture and increase likelihood of cataracts, muscle weakness, back pain, bruising, and oral candidiasis in this age group [82].

Oral preparations, such as prednisone, are useful for acute exacerbations of asthma that is unresponsive to bronchodilator therapy. Doses of 40 to 60 mg/d are given until the patient responds

and then the dosage can be tapered. Poorly controlled asthma often requires daily or alternate-day maintenance with prednisone in dosages of 10 to 15 mg. Intravenous corticosteroids, usually given as methylprednisolone, 60 to 80 mg, every 6 to 8 hours for 1 or 2 days, are effective within 4 to 6 hours of administration in preventing further progression of the severe asthma exacerbation that requires hospitalization. Attempts to reduce dependence on oral corticosteroids should be made, especially by the use of inhaled agents. Asthma in older patients is often a severe unrelenting disease, however. Although the goal of asthma therapy is always to control the disease without systemic steroids, this is often not possible in older patients. The side effects of corticosteroid therapy may be severe. Attempts should be made to (1) maximize therapy with inhaled steroids, (2) keep oral steroids to the minimum dose possible, (3) use relatively short-acting oral preparations such as prednisone and methylprednisolone, and (4) attempt to control symptoms with alternate-day dosing.

Leukotriene-modifying agents are also asthma controllers. There are two subclasses: the 5-lipoxygenase inhibitors, which inhibit the cysteinyl leukotrienes and leukotriene B4, and the leukotriene D4 receptor antagonists of the cysteinyl leukotrienes C4, D4, and E4. These agents have been shown to be effective in preventing allergen-induced asthma, exercise-induced asthma, and aspirin-induced bronchospasm. Studies on their use in older patients are limited. The leukotriene-modifying agents also may reduce asthma exacerbation rates and the need for steroid bursts. These agents are generally safe. Rare cases of Churg-Strauss vasculitis have occurred in patients with severe steroid-dependent asthma who have had a recent steroid taper.

Bronchodilators

Bronchodilators are important medications in the acute and chronic management of asthma. Older patients who have asthma may be less responsive to certain bronchodilators compared with younger patients [44,45,83]. Aging-related modifications might be responsible for the different effectiveness of bronchodilators in older patients as compared with younger individuals [84]. These differences must be explored further in future clinical trials.

Inhaled short-acting β2-adrenergic agonists are the treatment of choice for the acute exacerbation of asthma symptoms. Inhaled agents can be delivered by MDI, dry-powder capsules, and compressor-driven nebulizers. Despite the minimal systemic absorption seen with these agents, slight tachycardia may be observed, which is presumably caused by vasodilatation that results from the stimulation of β2 receptors in vascular smooth muscle. Tremor also may occur and is especially troublesome in geriatric patients. It is thought to be caused by stimulation of β2 receptors in skeletal muscle. In general, short-acting β-agonists have been proven to be safe and effective in all age groups [85]. The use of regularly scheduled as opposed to as-needed dosing of short-acting β2-agonists has been associated with diminished control of asthma and heightened bronchial reactivity, however, and there have been reports that asthma medications—particularly β-agonist therapy—are contributing to increased morbidity and mortality around the world. This is especially seen in persons who use more than two MDIs per month [86]. If the observed increase in mortality is caused by the drug, it would have special relevance to older patients because it has been postulated that at least some excessive deaths are primarily cardiac and many older individuals have coronary disease. Several mechanisms for cardiac toxicity have been outlined [87]. β-Agonists can cause a dose-dependent drop in serum potassium and a dose-dependent increase in the QT interval on the electrocardiogram. Because sudden death from ventricular arrhythmia can be caused by both of these mechanisms and be a complication of ischemic heart disease, use in older patients should be monitored closely. Ideally short-acting β2-adrenergic agonists should be prescribed for acute symptom relief on an as-needed basis. The need for regularly scheduled doses should alert the physician to the need for more intense anti-inflammatory medication.

Long-acting β2-agonists are helpful for long-term maintenance therapy and are used to control nocturnal symptoms. Recent studies on inadequately controlled asthma have shown superior benefit to adding a long-acting β-agonist to a moderate-dose inhaled corticosteroid regimen rather than doubling the dose of the inhaled corticosteroid, adding theophylline, or adding a leukotriene pathway modifier. Two agents are available: salmeterol and formoterol, both of which have a duration of action of 12 hours. Formoterol has the advantage of a more rapid onset of action, similar to the short-acting agents. Salmeterol is available in a dry powder formulation in combination with fluticasone, which gives the advantage of providing bronchodilation with anti-inflammatory benefits. It improves compliance because of prompt relief of symptoms and enables lower dosing of the inhaled steroid because of the complementary action of the two agents.

Although there is evidence that β-receptor function diminishes with age [44,45,48,49], these agents should be used because of their proven track record. The use of other agents, such as inhaled ipratropium, which has an excellent safety profile in older patients, should be considered when additional bronchodilator therapy is necessary. It must be remembered that ipratropium has a slower onset of action and requires 30 to 60 minutes until maximal effect. Inhaled anticholinergic agents produce bronchodilation by reducing vagal tone. They are widely used in patients who have COPD; however, their role in long-term maintenance of asthma in older patients has not been established.

Theophylline is an effective bronchodilator and has some anti-inflammatory properties. Its use has diminished over the past decade, however, because of safety concerns, especially in older patients. Sustained-released formulations of theophylline may be useful as maintenance therapy in moderate and severe persistent asthma for persons who are on inhaled steroid and long-acting β-agonist therapy and are still symptomatic. The narrow therapeutic range of theophylline, frequency of concomitant illnesses that alter theophylline kinetics, and many drug interactions that affect the clearance of theophylline make it important to monitor closely the blood theophylline level in older patients who have asthma. The clinical manifestations of theophylline toxicity have been correlated with blood levels of the drug. With high serum concentrations (>30 µg/mL), life-threatening events may occur, including seizures and cardiac arrhythmias, such as atrial fibrillation, supraventricular tachycardia, ventricular ectopy, and ventricular tachycardia. The most common cause for theophylline toxicity is a self-administered increase in medication. There is a step-wise increase in the frequency of life-threatening events caused by theophylline toxicity with advancing age. At comparable theophylline blood levels, patients older than 75 years have a 16-fold greater risk of life-threatening events or death compared to patients younger than 25 years [88]. The risk of theophylline toxicity can be minimized with careful patient monitoring and education. When using theophylline in older patients, monitoring blood levels is important to avoid toxicity, and a range of 8 to 15 μg/mL is generally considered therapeutic.

Asthma education

The complexity of prescription regimen, coupled with the memory loss and cognitive dysfunction that may be present in older patients, partially contributes to poor compliance with therapy. Health care workers always should consider implementing different strategies to overcome some of these barriers in the hopes of achieving better compliance (Table 4).

Patient education is an effective tool and should be an integral part in the management of asthma [89]. It improves patients' skills and motivates them to gain better control of the disease. Physicians should encourage open communications with their patients and should define realistic goals of therapy to avoid noncompliance. Active participation by patients and family members in monitoring lung function, avoiding provocative agents, and making decisions regarding

medications gives patients the confidence to control their own disease. It is important to assist patients in developing a reasonable medication schedule, because they may have relatively unusual wake/sleep patterns. All patients should recognize the rationale behind using the different medications, the correct way to use them, and their side effects [62,71]. Polypharmacy also should be avoided.

Mastering the technique of inhaled medication delivery device is a challenging problem in older patients, and most older patients are unable to properly use the MDI, even after proper instruction [90–96]. Inadequate timing of actuation and inhalation is the most frequent error made. Impaired mental function, weakened or deformed hands, and motor or musculoskeletal diseases are other reasons for inadequate MDI use. To minimize this problem, MDI technique should be observed at every visit, and patients should be reinstructed as needed. There are several solutions to this problem. One may deliver short-acting β-agonists, ipratropium, and the inhaled corticosteroid budesonide as aerosolized solutions by pressurized hand-held nebulizers [97]. Alternatively, there is a breath-actuated pressurized MDI, which obviates the need to synchronize actuation with inhalation [98]. The use of spacer devices fitted to the mouthpiece of the MDI has been shown to overcome most of the drawbacks of MDI therapy [99]. Spacers have been shown to decrease oropharyngeal deposition, increase intrapulmonary deposition, reduce the incidence of oropharyngeal candidiasis, and improve the pulmonary function of patients who have asthma who use the conventional MDI inappropriately. Because drug deposition into the lungs with spacers is greater, the spacers also have the advantage of reducing the number of inhalations of drug needed and, therefore, the cost of drug therapy. Their use in older patients is highly desirable. Finally, newer dry powder delivery devices, such as the turbohaler, diskus, twisthaler, and aerolizer, which deliver inhaled corticosteroids or long-acting β-agonists, have provided simple, easy-to-use preparations that do not require coordination or muscle strength [100].

Table 4
Strategies for overcoming barriers to compliance in older patients

Barriers to compliance	Therapeutic strategies
Arthritis of hands and fingers	Avoid MDIs
	Use breath-actuated inhalers, DPIs, or nebulizers
Poor medication delivery device technique	Use spacer devices
	Use breath-actuated inhalers, DPIs, or nebulizers
Depression	Identify and treat affective disorders
Poor memory	Simplify medication regimen
	Limit dosing frequency, if possible
	Use written action plans in large-type fonts
Limited or fixed income	Bear drug cost in mind when prescribing
Poor perception of bronchospasm	Use objective measures of pulmonary function to monitor therapy
Visual impairment	Use color-coding
	Use enlarged type fonts on medications

Abbreviation: DPI, dry powder device.

Clinical outcome and prognosis

In adulthood, there is a steady incidence of new-onset asthma through all ages, even in older adults. Many patients begin with recurrent wheezing after respiratory viral infections. This pattern may gradually or abruptly develop into persistent wheezing and often severe, poorly responsive disease. At other times, asthma develops explosively, with no previous respiratory symptoms, immediately after the onset of a typical viral respiratory infection. Longitudinal studies of patients who have asthma have shown that remission from asthma is common in the second decade of life and may be as high as 60% to 70% but is much less common in older age groups, occurring in approximately 20%. Older patients who have asthma with severe symptoms, long-standing disease, reduced pulmonary function, or a concomitant diagnosis of COPD are much less likely to have a remission. In one study of non-smoking older patients who had asthma over a 7-year period, not a single patient went into complete remission [101]. Two patients (8%) died from progressive chronic respiratory insufficiency, as if they had cigarette-induced COPD; both had extremely low baseline FEV_1 at entry into this study. Nearly all the patients remained dependent on steroids, with persistent symptoms during the study period. These findings were similar to those described in a community-based survey [38].

The number of unscheduled ambulatory visits, emergency visits, and hospitalizations are high in older patients who have asthma, which confirms the high degree of morbidity in this age group [102,103]. When an assessment is done by community-based sampling, quality-of-life scores have been reported to be low in patients who have persistent asthma when compared with older patients who have mild asthma or no asthma at all [3]. Patients frequently report poor health, depression, and a significant limitation of activities of daily living [10]. In a study of adult patients who had asthma in 15 managed care organizations, patients over the age of 65 were twice as likely to be hospitalized than younger patients. The prevalence of comorbidities was also higher: sinusitis (50% versus 38%), heartburn (35% versus 23%), chronic bronchitis (43% versus 16%), emphysema (19% versus 1%), and congestive heart failure (8% versus 1%). Because care seemed to be better for older patients, it is likely that these comorbidities and age itself were the causes of increased hospital use. In fact, if older patients who have severe or difficult-to-treat asthma have been identified by physician assessment, they seem to do better than younger patients. In the

Epidemiology and Natural History of Asthma: Outcomes and Treatment Regimens (TENOR) study, despite lower lung function, older patients who had asthma (mean age, 72 years) had lower rates of unscheduled office visits, emergency department visits, and corticosteroid bursts [104]. Patients reported in this TENOR study received more aggressive care than younger adults, including higher use of inhaled and oral corticosteroids, which undoubtedly had an impact on outcomes.

Summary

Asthma is frequently overlooked in the geriatric population. Objective measures of pulmonary function can aid in a prompt diagnosis and lead to effective treatment and improved quality of life. Because smoking is an important risk factor for asthma-like symptoms of wheeze, cough, and sputum production, asthma is frequently confused with COPD. The onset of wheezing, shortness of breath, and cough in an older patient is likely to cause concern. Although the adage "all that wheezes is not asthma" is true at any age, it is especially true in older adults. Diagnosis based on objective measures is essential. Objective measures of lung function are usually helpful in confirming the diagnosis and staging the severity of the disease. In patients with asthma symptoms and no airflow obstruction, methacholine testing is helpful. When a normal methacholine challenge is present, a diagnosis of asthma can be excluded and the physician can pursue other diagnostic considerations, such as heart failure, chronic aspiration syndrome, pulmonary embolic disease, and carcinoma of the lung. Management of asthma in older adults does not differ from that of younger patients, although careful monitoring of compliance with therapy and adverse events to medication is essential in this population. Despite severe symptoms and physiologic impairment, most older patients who have asthma improve with therapy and can lead active, productive lives.

References

[1] Bousquet J, Jeffery PK, Busse WW, et al. Asthma: from bronchoconstriction to airways inflammation and remodeling. Am J Respir Crit Care Med 2000; 161:1720–45.

[2] Mannino DM, Homa DM, Akinbami LJ, et al. Surveillance for asthma: United States, 1980–1999. MMWR Surveill Summ 2002;51:1–13.

[3] Enright PL, McClelland RL, Newman AB, et al. Underdiagnosis and undertreatment of asthma in the elderly: Cardiovascular Health Study Research Group. Chest 1999;116:603–13.

[4] Enright PL, Kronmal RA, Higgins MW, et al. Prevalence and correlates of respiratory symptoms and disease in the elderly: Cardiovascular Health Study. Chest 1994;106:827–34.

[5] Burr ML, Charles TJ, Roy K, et al. Asthma in the elderly: an epidemiological survey. Br Med J 1979; 1:1041–4.

[6] Moorman JE, Mannino DM. Increasing U.S. asthma mortality rates: who is really dying? J Asthma 2001;38:65–71.

[7] Mannino DM, Gagnon RC, Petty TL, et al. Obstructive lung disease and low lung function in adults in the United States: data from the National Health and Nutrition Examination Survey, 1988–1994. Arch Intern Med 2000;160:1683–9.

[8] Slavin RG. The elderly asthmatic patient. Allergy Asthma Proc 2004;25:371–3.

[9] Dyer CA, Hill SL, Stockley RA, et al. Quality of life in elderly subjects with a diagnostic label of asthma from general practice registers. Eur Respir J 1999; 14:39–45.

[10] Nejjari C, Tessier JF, Barberger-Gateau P, et al. Functional status of elderly people treated for asthma-related symptoms: a population based case-control study. Eur Respir J 1994;7:1077–83.

[11] Savage-Brown A, Mannino DM, Redd SC. Lung disease and asthma severity in adults with asthma: data from the Third National Health and Nutrition Examination. J Asthma 2005;42:519–23.

[12] Banerjee DK, Lee GS, Malik SK, et al. Underdiagnosis of asthma in the elderly. Br J Dis Chest 1987; 81:23–9.

[13] Bauer BA, Reed CE, Yunginger JW, et al. Incidence and outcomes of asthma in the elderly: a population-based study in Rochester, Minnesota. Chest 1997;111:303–10.

[14] Boezen HM, Rijcken B, Schouten JP, et al. Breathlessness in elderly individuals is related to low lung function and reversibility of airway obstruction. Eur Respir J 1998;12:805–10.

[15] Dow L, Fowler L, Phelps L, et al. Prevalence of untreated asthma in a population sample of 6000 older adults in Bristol, UK. Thorax 2001;56: 472–6.

[16] Parameswaran K, Hildreth AJ, Chadha D, et al. Asthma in the elderly: underperceived, underdiagnosed and undertreated. A community survey. Respir Med 1998;92:573–7.

[17] National Heart, Lung and Blood Institute, National Institute of Health. National Asthma Education and Prevention Program: expert panel report 2. Guidelines for the diagnosis and management of asthma. Bethesda (MD): NIH Publication; 2001. 97–4051.

[18] Dodge RR, Burrows B. The prevalence and incidence of asthma and asthma-like symptoms in a general population sample. Am Rev Respir Dis 1980;122:567–75.

[19] Evans R III, Mullally DI, Wilson RW, et al. National trends in the morbidity and mortality of asthma in the US. Prevalence, hospitalization and death from asthma over two decades: 1965–1984. Chest 1987;91:65S–74S.

[20] Barger LW, Vollmer WM, Felt RW, et al. Further investigation into the recent increase in asthma death rates: a review of 41 asthma deaths in Oregon in 1982. Ann Allergy 1988;60:31–9.

[21] Kay AB. Pathology of mild, severe, and fatal asthma. Am J Respir Crit Care Med 1996;154: S66–9.

[22] Fabbri LM, Romagnoli M, Corbetta L, et al. Differences in airway inflammation in patients with fixed airflow obstruction due to asthma or chronic obstructive pulmonary disease. Am J Respir Crit Care Med 2003;167:418–24.

[23] Bai TR, Cooper J, Koelmeyer T, et al. The effect of age and duration of disease on airway structure in fatal asthma. Am J Respir Crit Care Med 2000; 162:663–9.

[24] Braman SS, Corrao WM. Bronchoprovocation testing. Clin Chest Med 1989;10:165–76.

[25] Connolly MJ, Kelly C, Walters EH, et al. An assessment of methacholine inhalation tests in elderly asthmatics. Age Ageing 1988;17:123–8.

[26] Davis PB, Byard PJ. Relationships among airway reactivity, pupillary alpha-adrenergic and cholinergic responsiveness, and age. J Appl Physiol 1988; 65:200–4.

[27] Pfeifer MA, Weinberg CR, Cook D, et al. Differential changes of autonomic nervous system function with age in man. Am J Med 1983;75:249–58.

[28] Pontoppidan H, Beecher HK. Progressive loss of protective reflexes in the airway with the advance of age. JAMA 1960;174:2209–13.

[29] Braman SS, Amico CA, Steigman D, et al. Cough and bronchoconstrictive reflexes in normal elderly subjects. Am.Rev.Respir.Dis 1987;135(4):A476.

[30] Scichilone N, Messina M, Battaglia S, et al. Airway hyperresponsiveness in the elderly: prevalence and clinical implications. Eur Respir J 2005;25:364–75.

[31] O'Connor GT, Sparrow D, Weiss ST. Normal range of methacholine responsiveness in relation to prechallenge pulmonary function: the Normative Aging Study. Chest 1994;105:661–6.

[32] Rijcken B, Schouten JP, Weiss ST, et al. The relationship of nonspecific bronchial responsiveness to respiratory symptoms in a random population sample. Am Rev Respir Dis 1987;136:62–8.

[33] Jedrychowski W, Krzyzanowski M, Wysocki M. Are chronic wheezing and asthma-like attacks related to FEV1 decline? The Cracow Study. Eur J Epidemiol 1988;4:335–42.

[34] Peat JK, Woolcock AJ, Cullen K. Rate of decline of lung function in subjects with asthma. Eur J Respir Dis 1987;70:171–9.

[35] Ulrik CS, Lange P. Decline of lung function in adults with bronchial asthma. Am J Respir Crit Care Med 1994;150:629–34.

[36] Jedrychowski W, Maugeri U, Gomola K, et al. Effects of domestic gas cooking and passive smoking on chronic respiratory symptoms and asthma in elderly women. Int J Occup Environ Health 1995;1: 16–20.

[37] Burrows B, Lebowitz MD, Barbee RA, et al. Findings before diagnoses of asthma among the elderly in a longitudinal study of a general population sample. J Allergy Clin Immunol 1991;88:870–7.

[38] Burrows B, Barbee RA, Cline MG, et al. Characteristics of asthma among elderly adults in a sample of the general population. Chest 1991;100:935–42.

[39] van Schayck CP, Dompeling E, van Herwaarden CL, et al. Interacting effects of atopy and bronchial hyperresponsiveness on the annual decline in lung function and the exacerbation rate in asthma. Am Rev Respir Dis 1991;144:1297–301.

[40] Brown PJ, Greville HW, Finucane KE. Asthma and irreversible airflow obstruction. Thorax 1984; 39:131–6.

[41] Cassino C, Berger KI, Goldring RM, et al. Duration of asthma and physiologic outcomes in elderly nonsmokers. Am J Respir Crit Care Med 2000;162: 1423–8.

[42] Reed CE. The natural history of asthma in adults: the problem of irreversibility. J Allergy Clin Immunol 1999;103:539–47.

[43] Roberts SD, Farber MO, Knox KS, et al. FEV1/FVC ratio of 70% misclassifies patients with obstruction at the extremes of age. Chest 2006;130: 200–6.

[44] Connolly MJ. Ageing, late-onset asthma and the beta-adrenoceptor. Pharmacol Ther 1993;60: 389–404.

[45] Connolly MJ, Crowley JJ, Charan NB, et al. Impaired bronchodilator response to albuterol in healthy elderly men and women. Chest 1995;108: 401–6.

[46] Connolly MJ, Crowley JJ, Nielson CP, et al. Peripheral mononuclear leukocyte beta adrenoceptors and non-specific bronchial responsiveness to methacholine in young and elderly normal subjects and asthmatic patients. Thorax 1994; 49:26–32.

[47] Kendall MJ, Woods KL, Wilkins MR, et al. Responsiveness to beta-adrenergic receptor stimulation: the effects of age are cardioselective. Br J Clin Pharmacol 1982;14:821–6.

[48] Ullah MI, Newman GB, Saunders KB. Influence of age on response to ipratropium and salbutamol in asthma. Thorax 1981;36:523–9.

[49] van Schayck CP, Folgering H, Harbers H, et al. Effects of allergy and age on responses to salbutamol and ipratropium bromide in moderate asthma and chronic bronchitis. Thorax 1991;46:355–9.

[50] Dow L, Coggon D, Campbell MJ, et al. The interaction between immunoglobulin E and smoking in airflow obstruction in the elderly. Am Rev Respir Dis 1992;146:402–7.

[51] Burrows B, Halonen M, Barbee RA, et al. The relationship of serum immunoglobulin E to cigarette smoking. Am Rev Respir Dis 1981;124:523–5.

[52] Barbee RA, Lebowitz MD, Thompson HC, et al. Immediate skin-test reactivity in a general population sample. Ann Intern Med 1976;84:129–33.

[53] Braman SS, Kaemmerlen JT, Davis SM. Asthma in the elderly: a comparison between patients with recently acquired and long-standing disease. Am Rev Respir Dis 1991;143:336–40.

[54] Huss K, Naumann PL, Mason PJ, et al. Asthma severity, atopic status, allergen exposure and quality of life in elderly persons. Ann Allergy Asthma Immunol 2001;86:524–30.

[55] Renwick DS, Connolly MJ. Persistence of atopic effects on airway calibre and bronchial responsiveness in older adults. Age Ageing 1997;26:435–40.

[56] Rogers L, Cassino C, Berger KI, et al. Asthma in the elderly: cockroach sensitization and severity of airway obstruction in elderly nonsmokers. Chest 2002;122:1580–6.

[57] Parameswaran K, Hildreth AJ, Taylor IK, et al. Predictors of asthma severity in the elderly: results of a community survey in Northeast England. J Asthma 1999;36:613–8.

[58] Weiner P, Magadle R, Waizman J, et al. Characteristics of asthma in the elderly. Eur Respir J 1998;12: 564–8.

[59] Busse PJ. Allergic respiratory disease in the elderly. Am J Med 2007;120:498–502.

[60] Braman SS. Asthma in the elderly. Exp Lung Res 2005;(31 Suppl 1):6–7.

[61] Quadrelli SA, Roncoroni A. Features of asthma in the elderly. J Asthma 2001;38:377–89.

[62] National Institutes of Health. NAEPP working group: consideration for diagnosing and managing asthma in the elderly. Bethesda (MD): NIH; 1996. Publication # 96–3662.

[63] Raiha I, Impivaara O, Seppala M, et al. Determinants of symptoms suggestive of gastroesophageal reflux disease in the elderly. Scand J Gastroenterol 1993;28:1011–4.

[64] Raiha I, Hietanen E, Sourander L. Symptoms of gastro-oesophageal reflux disease in elderly people. Age Ageing 1991;20:365–70.

[65] Bellia V, Pistelli R, Catalano F, et al. Quality control of spirometry in the elderly: the SA.R.A. study. SAlute respiration nell'Anziano = Respiratory Health in the Elderly. Am J Respir Crit Care Med 2000;161:1094–100.

[66] Connolly MJ, Crowley JJ, Charan NB, et al. Reduced subjective awareness of bronchoconstriction provoked by methacholine in elderly asthmatic and

normal subjects as measured on a simple awareness scale. Thorax 1992;47:410–3.

[67] Cuttitta G, Cibella F, Bellia V, et al. Changes in FVC during methacholine-induced bronchoconstriction in elderly patients with asthma: bronchial hyperresponsiveness and aging. Chest 2001;119:1685–90.

[68] Enright PL, Burchette RJ, Peters JA, et al. Peak flow lability: association with asthma and spirometry in an older cohort. Chest 1997;112:895–901.

[69] Enright PL, McClelland RL, Buist AS, et al. Correlates of peak expiratory flow lability in elderly persons. Chest 2001;120:1861–8.

[70] Buist AS, Vollmer WM, Wilson SR, et al. A randomized clinical trial of peak flow versus symptom monitoring in older adults with asthma. Am J Respir Crit Care Med 2006;174:1077–87.

[71] Smyrnios NA. Asthma: a six-part strategy for managing older patients. Geriatrics 1997;52:36–4.

[72] Sin DD, Tu JV. Underuse of inhaled steroid therapy in elderly patients with asthma. Chest 2001; 119:720–5.

[73] Sin DD, Tu JV. Are elderly patients with obstructive airway disease being prematurely discharged? Am J Respir Crit Care Med 2000;161:1513–7.

[74] Hartert TV, Togias A, Mellen BG, et al. Underutilization of controller and rescue medications among older adults with asthma requiring hospital care. J Am Geriatr Soc 2000;48:651–7.

[75] Barr RG, Somers SC, Speizer FE, et al. Patient factors and medication guideline adherence among older women with asthma. Arch Intern Med 2002;162:1761–8.

[76] Petheram IS, Jones DA, Collins JV. Assessment and management of acute asthma in the elderly: a comparison with younger asthmatics. Postgrad Med J 1982;58:149–51.

[77] Tafreshi MJ, Weinacker AB. Beta-adrenergic-blocking agents in bronchospastic diseases: a therapeutic dilemma. Pharmacotherapy 1999;19: 974–8.

[78] Prince DS, Carliner NH. Respiratory arrest following first dose of timolol ophthalmic solution. Chest 1983;84:640–1.

[79] Dunn TL, Gerber MJ, Shen AS, et al. The effect of topical ophthalmic instillation of timolol and betaxolol on lung function in asthmatic subjects. Am Rev Respir Dis 1986;133:264–8.

[80] Braman SS. Drug treatment of asthma in the elderly. Drugs 1996;51:415–23.

[81] Sin DD, Tu JV. Inhaled corticosteroid therapy reduces the risk of rehospitalization and all-cause mortality in elderly asthmatics. Eur Respir J 2001; 17:380–5.

[82] Walsh LJ, Wong CA, Oborne J, et al. Adverse effects of oral corticosteroids in relation to dose in patients with lung disease. Thorax 2001;56: 279–84.

[83] Banerji A, Clark S, Afilalo M, et al. Prospective multicenter study of acute asthma in younger versus older adults presenting to the emergency department. J Am Geriatr Soc 2006;54:48–55.

[84] Bellia V, Battaglia S, Matera MG, et al. The use of bronchodilators in the treatment of airway obstruction in elderly patients. Pulm Pharmacol Ther 2006; 19:311–9.

[85] Devoy MA, Fuller RW, Palmer JB. Are there any detrimental effects of the use of inhaled long-acting beta 2-agonists in the treatment of asthma? Chest 1995;107:1116–24.

[86] Spitzer WO, Suissa S, Ernst P, et al. The use of beta-agonists and the risk of death and near death from asthma. N Engl J Med 1992;326:501–6.

[87] Robin ED, McCauley R. Sudden cardiac death in bronchial asthma, and inhaled beta-adrenergic agonists. Chest 1992;101:1699–702.

[88] Shannon M, Lovejoy FH Jr. The influence of age vs peak serum concentration on life-threatening events after chronic theophylline intoxication. Arch Intern Med 1990;150:2045–8.

[89] Anderson CJ, Bardana EJ Jr. Asthma in the elderly: the importance of patient education. Compr Ther 1996;22:375–83.

[90] Allen SC, Jain M, Ragab S, et al. Acquisition and short-term retention of inhaler techniques require intact executive function in elderly subjects. Age Ageing 2003;32:299–302.

[91] Allen SC, Prior A. What determines whether an elderly patient can use a metered dose inhaler correctly? Br J Dis Chest 1986;80:45–9.

[92] Hayden ML. Asthma in the elderly: a diagnostic and management challenge. Adv Nurse Pract 2000;8:30–5.

[93] Stevens N. Inhaler devices for asthma and COPD: choice and technique. Prof Nurse 2003;18:641–5.

[94] Jarvis S, Ind PW, Shiner RJ. Inhaled therapy in elderly COPD patients: time for re-evaluation? Age Ageing 2007;36:213–8.

[95] Brennan VK, Osman LM, Graham H, et al. True device compliance: the need to consider both competence and contrivance. Respir Med 2005;99: 97–102.

[96] Daniels S, Meuleman J. Importance of assessment of metered-dose inhaler technique in the elderly. J Am Geriatr Soc 1994;42:82–4.

[97] Pounsford JC. Nebulisers for the elderly. Thorax 1997;52(Suppl 2):S53–5.

[98] Chapman KR, Love L, Brubaker H. A comparison of breath-actuated and conventional metered-dose inhaler inhalation techniques in elderly subjects. Chest 1993;104:1332–7.

[99] Donateo L, Gerardi R, Cantini L. A new spacer device for administration of inhaled salbutamol: use in elderly asthmatics. Adv Ther 1996;13:292–300.

[100] Kesten S, Elias M, Cartier A, et al. Patient handling of a multidose dry powder inhalation device for albuterol. Chest 1994;105:1077–81.

[101] Braman SS, Corrao WM, Kaemmerlen JT. The clinical outcome of asthma in the elderly: a 7-year

follow-up study. Ann N Y Acad Sci 1991;629: 449–50.

[102] Griswold SK, Nordstrom CR, Clark S, et al. Asthma exacerbations in North American adults: who are the "frequent fliers" in the emergency department? Chest 2005;127:1579–86.

[103] Diette GB, Krishnan JA, Dominici F, et al. Asthma in older patients: factors associated with hospitalization. Arch Intern Med 2002;162: 1123–32.

[104] Slavin RG, Haselkorn T, Lee JH, et al. Asthma in older adults: observations from the epidemiology and natural history of asthma. Outcomes and treatment regimens (TENOR) study. Ann Allergy Asthma Immunol 2006;96: 406–14.

ELSEVIER
SAUNDERS

CLINICS
IN CHEST
MEDICINE

Clin Chest Med 28 (2007) 703–715

Chronic Obstructive Pulmonary Disease in the Older Patient

Shoab A. Nazir, MD[a,b,*], Mohammad M. Al-Hamed, MD[a],
Marcia L. Erbland, MD[a,b]

[a]Division of Pulmonary and Critical Care Medicine, University of Arkansas for Medical Sciences,
4301 West Markham, Slot 555, Little Rock, AR 72205, USA
[b]Central Arkansas Veterans Health Care System, Little Rock, AR 72205, USA

Chronic obstructive pulmonary disease (COPD) is one of the most common chronic diseases in the world. It is a major cause of morbidity, mortality, and health care use, particularly in older adults. Although the definition of COPD has changed with time, an all-encompassing consensus definition is still lacking [1]. COPD includes a heterogeneous group of conditions characterized by expiratory airflow limitation. A key distinction from asthma is that the airflow limitation is not fully reversible, although COPD and asthma may frequently coexist [2].

The burden of COPD has been increasing for the last two decades, and it is projected to continue to increase for the next few [3,4]. In the year 2000, COPD became the fourth leading cause of death and is projected to be the fourth leading cause for disability worldwide by 2020 [5]. Worldwide it is the only leading cause of death with an increasing prevalence [6]. COPD is a leading cause of hospitalization in the United States and accounts for 19.9% of the total hospitalizations for patients aged 65 to 75 years and 18.2% of the total hospitalizations for patients aged 75 years and older [7].

The annual per-patient costs of COPD parallel those of other diseases, such as diabetes, arthritis, and cardiovascular disease [8]. The mean inpatient, outpatient, and pharmacy costs of patients aged 65 years or older who have COPD are more than twice those of age- and gender-matched control subjects who do not have COPD [9]. As the median age of the United States population increases, treatment of chronic conditions in older adults will have a significant impact on overall health care costs [10].

In the following sections, the authors review the diagnosis and management of COPD with a focus on special issues in older adults.

Risk factors

The major risk factor for the development of COPD is tobacco smoking, which accounts for 80% to 90% of the risk in the United States [11,12]. A highly significant quantitative relationship exists between pack-years of smoking and functional impairment [13]. In 2004 an estimated 20.9% (44.5 million) of United States adults were current smokers; of these, 81.3% (36.1 million) smoked every day and 18.7% (8.3 million) smoked some days [14]. Persons aged older than 65 years have the lowest prevalence (8.8%) of current cigarette smoking among all adults [14]. Data from all 50 states in the United States for 1996 through 2001 indicated that the median proportion of some-day smokers among current smokers decreased with age except in those aged 65 years and older, who had a rate of 20.3%, suggesting that older adults may smoke less heavily and less frequently [15].

Other risk factors for COPD include alpha-1 antitrypsin deficiency [16,17], occupational [18], environmental [19], and domestic air pollution, particularly in developing countries [20,21],

* Corresponding author. Division of Pulmonary and Critical Care Medicine, University of Arkansas for Medical Sciences, 4301 West Markham, Slot 555, Little Rock, AR 72205.
E-mail address: sanazir@uams.edu (S.A. Nazir).

0272-5231/07/$ - see front matter. Published by Elsevier Inc.
doi:10.1016/j.ccm.2007.07.003

chestmed.theclinics.com

mucous hypersecretion [22], and possibly airway hyper-responsiveness and asthma [23,24]. The prevalence of COPD is higher in men, but with the changing patterns in smoking habits, women may be at increased risk [25–27].

Diagnosis

The diagnosis is confirmed by the presence of mostly irreversible expiratory airflow limitation, also known as an obstructive defect, on spirometry. An obstructive defect is defined as a reduced post-bronchodilator forced expiratory volume in 1 second (FEV_1)/forced vital capacity (FVC) ratio. Most older subjects (approximately 80%) can perform reliable spirometry according to established standards [28–30]. Just what constitutes a reduced FEV_1/FVC ratio, however, has been the subject of some debate. The Global Initiative for Chronic Obstructive Lung Disease (GOLD) scientific committee has recommended assigning an FEV_1/FVC ratio of 0.7 as the lower limit of normal, or the cutoff value, in all subjects [2,31]. Other authorities recommend setting this cutoff at the fifth percentile of the normal distribution range of FEV_1/FVC ratios, rather than at a fixed value of 0.7 [32–36].

The criteria chosen to define airflow limitation on spirometry, and therefore to diagnose COPD, are especially important in older patients. The FEV_1/FVC ratio decreases with age, and this relative degree of airflow limitation is attributed to increased airway collapsibility in the normal aging lung [37,38]. Using a fixed FEV_1/FVC ratio to separate normal from "obstruction" creates a risk for over-diagnosis of COPD in older subjects [39–41]. Up to one fifth of current smokers and one seventh of never-smokers beyond the sixth decade may be misidentified as abnormal when a fixed cut-off is used [42]. Approximately one half of people greater than 80 years old would be misclassified as having COPD [40]. The debate is further complicated by data from the Cardiovascular Health Study, which showed that subjects aged 65 years or older who are identified as normal using the normal distribution cut-offs but who have an FEV_1/FVC ratio less than or equal to 0.7 are more likely to die and have COPD-related hospitalizations [43]. A clear consensus definition of pathologic airflow limitation and related diagnostic criteria for COPD in older patients is thus urgently needed.

On the other hand, under-diagnosis may also occur when the disease is mild. A population study applying the GOLD criteria found that only 5% of patients who had mild COPD were correctly diagnosed [44]. Older patients may be underdiagnosed because they are less likely to report mild symptoms [45,46]. Older subjects who have asthma may be misdiagnosed as having COPD, although the two conditions frequently coexist [47,48].

Prevalence

The estimation of the prevalence of COPD has been influenced by various factors, such as by the differences in the rates of disease occurrence, the definition used, and whether spirometry was used to confirm the diagnosis. Most well-designed studies have found a measured prevalence of between 4% and 10% of adults in Europe and North America [49]. Data from the Third National Health and Nutrition Examination Survey (NHANES III) estimated a prevalence of 6.8% across all age groups in the United States [50]. The prevalence of all classes of COPD increases with increasing age [45]. A Finnish population-based study found a prevalence of 12.5% in men and 3% in women of age greater than 80 years, and this increased among active smokers to 35% in men and 13% in women [51]. Using the GOLD criteria, 25% of the United States population aged 75 years or older have moderate COPD [7].

Management of stable chronic obstructive pulmonary disease

Smoking cessation

The most important intervention in the care of patients who have COPD is smoking cessation. Smoking cessation slows the smoking-induced accelerated rate of decline in lung function [52,53]. Older COPD patients are no exception; smoking cessation in older patients improves health and reduces mortality regardless of the severity of the pulmonary impairment [54,55]. Male smokers who quit at age 65 years stand to gain 2.0 years of life expectancy and female smokers who quit at age 65 years stand to gain 3.7 years [56].

Interventions to quit smoking, though not uniformly successful, significantly decrease mortality [57]. Useful interventions include physician counseling, behavioral therapy, and pharmacologic adjuncts. Effective first-line pharmacologic agents include nicotine replacement, bupropion, and varenicline. Nicotine [58], bupropion [59], and varenicline [60,61] seem to be effective, safe, and well-tolerated in the subgroups of subjects aged 65 to 75 years included in clinical trials. Unfortunately physicians are less likely to advise smoking cessation to older patients [62].

Pharmacologic management

After smoking cessation, pharmacologic treatment is focused on improving symptoms, exercise tolerance, and rates and severity of exacerbations. To date, none of the existing medications for COPD have been proven to modify the long-term decline in lung function.

Bronchodilators

Bronchodilators have long been the mainstay of symptom management in patients who have COPD, although they have not been shown to affect the rate of decline in lung function or survival [63,64]. The three main categories of bronchodilators are the β-agonists, the anticholinergics, and the methylxanthines. Current bronchodilator treatment emphasizes inhaled β-agonists, anticholinergics, or combinations of both. Short-acting bronchodilators increase exercise tolerance acutely and decrease dynamic hyperinflation, thereby decreasing the sensation of dyspnea [65,66]. Combination therapy with short-acting β-agonists and anticholinergics (ipratropium) may be better than monotherapy for improving spirometry and reducing the need for systemic steroids [67–69]. Long-acting β-agonists (LABA) improve lung function, health status, and frequency of exacerbations compared with placebo [70,71]. LABA improve lung function and possibly health status when compared with short-acting ipratropium [72], and combination therapy with these agents improves lung function and quality of life (QOL) more than either agent alone [73]. LABA and theophylline in combination may be more effective than either agent alone [74].

The long-acting anticholinergic agent tiotropium has shown to improve lung function, dyspnea, QOL, and frequency of exacerbations compared with placebo and with ipratropium [75,76]. Although no significant differences were found when tiotropium was compared with LABA in frequency of exacerbations or hospitalizations [77], tiotropium was shown to be superior in improving lung function [78,79].

Inhaled corticosteroids

Although anti-inflammatory inhaled corticosteroids (ICS) have a clear-cut role in the treatment of asthma, proof of benefit in patients who have COPD has been much harder to demonstrate or quantify. Use of ICS has been associated with some improvement in lung function, airway reactivity, frequency of exacerbations, and respiratory symptoms, but ICS do not affect the progressive decline in FEV_1 [80–83]. Higher rates of exacerbations were noted when ICS were withdrawn [84,85]. More data are needed on the incidence of adverse effects of ICS, particularly when used in a high-dose, prolonged maintenance approach that has been the objective of recent clinical trials. Although budesonide and fluticasone have not been shown to increase the risk for fractures or to decrease bone mineral density (BMD), BMD was significantly lower in those treated with triamcinolone for 3 years [80,82,86]. The long-term effects of ICS on BMD beyond 5 years are unknown. Recently the probability of having pneumonia has also been reported to be higher in those who were treated with ICS [87].

Combination therapy of inhaled corticosteroids and bronchodilators

Combination therapy with ICS and LABA has been associated with better lung function and symptom control, decreased frequency of exacerbations, and improved health status than either component alone, with greater benefit seen in those with more severe disease (FEV_1 <50% predicted) [87–91]. Thus far no survival benefit has been shown [87]. A recent trial showed that a combination of tiotropium plus fluticasone–salmeterol improved lung function and disease-specific QOL and reduced the number of hospitalizations for COPD exacerbation and all-cause hospitalizations compared with tiotropium plus placebo, without affecting the rates of COPD exacerbation [92]. The same study also showed that tiotropium plus salmeterol did not statistically improve lung function or hospitalization rates compared with tiotropium plus placebo, suggesting that these agents may work best in the presence of an ICS [92].

Aerosol formulations and delivery devices

Inhaled bronchodilators and corticosteroids can be delivered by way of metered dose inhaler (MDI), dry powder inhaler (DPI), or compressor nebulizer. The efficacy of inhaled medications depends on the amount of drug delivered to the airways. Drug deposition depends on several factors, including inhalation technique. In older patients, inhalation technique may be hindered by cognitive impairment and physical problems with vision, arthritis, and manual dexterity [93–96].

Although the MDI is most commonly prescribed, only 60% of older people have been reported to have adequate MDI technique subjectively, and the number decreases to 36% when objective criteria are used [97]. Most older patients are able to use MDI correctly when it is connected to large-volume spacer devices [98]. Up to 85% of older patients, however, do not use the spacer when prescribed [94].

As an alternative to the MDI, the breath-activated DPI requires less coordination, but a certain minimum negative peak inspiratory flow (PIF) is needed during inhalation for adequate drug delivery [99]. Older patients may not be able to generate sufficient PIF, because there is a significant negative correlation between age and the PIF, regardless of the severity of the underlying COPD [94].

For sicker, less capable patients, nebulizers are an option, but the benefits and limitations have not been adequately studied. Whichever device is prescribed, proper patient education on its use is critical, and assessment of inhalation technique should be part of subsequent visits to the physician [100].

Nonpharmacologic interventions

Long-term oxygen therapy

Two well-designed trials showed that, in COPD patients who have a resting Pao_2 of less than or equal to 55 mm Hg on room air, long-term oxygen therapy (LTOT) for at least 15 hours daily improves survival, exercise tolerance, sleep, and cognitive function [101,102]. Continuous long-term home oxygen therapy is therefore recommended for patients in this category. Although comparable benefits have not been demonstrated in patients who have mild to moderate hypoxemia (Pao_2 56–65 mm Hg) or nocturnal desaturation, some questions remain about the potential benefits of LTOT in these and other subgroups of patients [103,104]. The National Heart, Lung and Blood Institute (NHLBI) has targeted several unanswered questions about LTOT for future research [105].

Pulmonary rehabilitation

Patients who have advanced COPD complain of significant dyspnea and exercise intolerance. These symptoms have been attributed to ventilatory and gas exchange limitations, skeletal and respiratory muscle weakness, cardiac dysfunction,

and deconditioning [106,107]. Pulmonary rehabilitation improves dyspnea, exercise tolerance, and QOL, and these gains are maintained over an extended period of time [107–109]. It has also shown to improve anxiety and depression independent of the changes in dyspnea and QOL [110]. Although pulmonary rehabilitation does not have any significant effect on hospitalization rate or mortality, it has been shown to be cost-effective and benefits all stages of COPD [108,109,111]. Pulmonary rehabilitation can also be successfully undertaken from home [112]. Pulmonary rehabilitation is as successful in increasing effort tolerance in older patients as it is in younger patients [113]. Hence, age itself is not a limiting factor, and pulmonary rehabilitation should be offered to all patients who have COPD.

Immunizations

Older persons who have COPD are at high risk for complications from influenza. Immunization against influenza in this group is associated with a 52% reduction in hospitalizations for all episodes of influenza and pneumonia, a 70% reduction in deaths from all causes, and significant cost savings [114,115]. The role of pneumococcal vaccine in COPD is less clear. Although pneumococcal vaccine has shown to reduce mortality and hospitalization in the general older population, data for its effectiveness in patients who have COPD are sparse [116,117]. A recent Cochrane review found no evidence that pneumococcal vaccination in patients who have COPD had any significant impact on mortality or morbidity [118]. Large-scale randomized trials would be needed to address this issue.

Nutrition

A low body mass index (BMI) is widely prevalent in older patients, particularly in hospital or institutional settings, and is a key determinant of morbidity and mortality [119–124]. Malnutrition is a long-recognized complication of COPD; 20% to 30% of patients who have advanced COPD have a BMI of less than 20 [125–127]. A low BMI has been shown to be an independent predictor of mortality, regardless of the pulmonary status, even in those on long-term oxygen therapy [126–130]. Intervention to stop weight loss and to also reverse weight loss has been shown to be feasible in older patients [131]. Small studies have shown that nutritional supplementation in patients who have COPD improves respiratory muscle strength and endurance but not necessarily lung function [132–134]. In a prospective study, weight gain of greater than 2 kg over 8 weeks with either nutritional therapy alone or in combination with anabolic steroids was a significant predictor of survival [129]. A low fat-free mass (FFM) has been shown to be an independent predictor of mortality in patients who have COPD, even in patients who have a normal BMI [135–137]. This may explain why even a normal BMI in patients who have COPD has been shown to be associated with increased mortality [130]. A decline in FFM has also been shown to be associated with the frequency of COPD exacerbations and the use of corticosteroids [138]. The use of anabolic steroids in patients who have COPD has been shown to improve muscle strength, mass, and endurance, and the weight gained with their use is associated with increased survival [129,139,140]. Caution, however, has to be exercised, particularly in light of the adverse events associated with another anabolic hormone, growth hormone, noted in older patients [141]. Increased attention to nutrition in this vulnerable population may improve survival.

Role of comorbidities

Most patients who have COPD, particularly older adults, have additional clinically significant illnesses, or comorbidities, which are projected to have an increasing impact on QOL, health care costs, mortality risk, and actual cause of death [142–145]. Common comorbidities include cardiovascular diseases, lung cancer, and osteoporosis. In a cohort study of 270 patients discharged after a COPD exacerbation, the most common comorbidities were hypertension (28%), diabetes mellitus (14%), and ischemic heart disease (10%) [146]. In a small study of 27 older patients who had a mean age of 76 years, there was a significant correlation between increasing comorbidity and declining QOL and activities of daily living scores [147].

Among patients hospitalized with COPD exacerbation, individuals who have more comorbidities are more than five times more likely to die in hospital compared with patients who have COPD without comorbidities even after adjustment for a wide range of confounders, including age and sex [148]. Comorbidities are also predictive factors for all-cause and respiratory mortality in patients who have COPD treated with LTOT [130]. In evaluating the causes of death in patients who had chronic respiratory failure, Zielinski and colleagues [149] reported that acute-on-chronic respiratory failure caused death in only 38% of patients, whereas heart failure, pulmonary infection, pulmonary embolism, cardiac arrhythmia, lung cancer, and other malignancies were responsible for the remaining deaths. Furthermore, in the much larger Lung Health Study, deaths caused by respiratory causes other than lung cancer accounted for only 7.8% of the deaths, whereas lung cancer, cardiovascular disease, and non-lung organ cancers accounted for 33%, 22%, and 21%, respectively, highlighting the importance of comorbidities [57].

Cardiac dysfunction and cardiovascular diseases are emerging as major causes of death in patients who have COPD [145,146]. Pulmonary embolism nearly doubled the risk for dying within 1 year [150]. As the role of these other illnesses is further elucidated, future study design and patient management are likely to focus more on all-cause mortality and the role of adjunctive therapies for comorbid conditions.

Depression and anxiety

Depression and anxiety affect the functional status of older patients who have COPD [151]. Up to 42% of patients who have COPD across all age groups may be depressed [152,153]. Among older patients who have COPD, 42% to 46% have been reported to be depressed, and new onset of depression in these patients is a risk factor for the development of cognitive decline [154–156]. The rates of depression in community-dwelling patients who have COPD are comparable to the rates of depression in hospitalized older patients [157,158]. QOL measures correlate more with depression than spirometry or exercise tolerance [153,154,159]. Patients who report poor QOL caused by their COPD are more likely to be depressed and poorly adherent to treatment, and depressed patients are more likely to smoke [152,155].

Anxiety in patients who have COPD may be less prevalent, with reported prevalence ranging from 2% to 37% [152,153,155,160]. In older patients, anxiety is associated with the level of physical functioning and disability and is a major predictor for the frequency of hospital admission for the exacerbation of COPD [155,161].

Early detection and treatment of depression and anxiety may play a critical role in improving QOL for patients who have COPD. Smaller trials including patients from all age groups have attempted to address this issue using pharmacotherapy [162,163]. In one study from the United

Kingdom, use of the antidepressant paroxetine for at least 3 months was associated with significant improvement in depression and exercise tolerance as measured by the 6-minute walking test [164]. A small feasibility study, however, looking at the usefulness of antidepressants in older patients who had COPD and depression showed a high rate of refusal to take therapy (72%) [165]. Adding patient education to traditional pharmacotherapy for depression may improve adherence to depression and COPD treatments in older adults [166].

Quality of life

Factors that contribute to QOL in patients who have COPD are poorly understood. Studies looking at the relationship between FEV_1 and QOL have shown variable results. When studies used non–disease-specific measures of QOL, no relationship was noted between the percentage predicted of the FEV_1 and the QOL measures [167,168]. Others have shown that physiologic variables such as air flow limitation and diffusing capacity may have a correlation with QOL measures [169,170]. A disease-specific instrument is believed to give a more reasonable estimate of the QOL in a specific subpopulation [171]. In a larger study looking at 321 patients staged based on the American Thoracic Society criteria [33], patient scores on the St. George's Respiratory Questionnaire [172] were moderately to strongly associated with disease staging, and comorbid conditions influenced the deterioration of QOL across all stages [142].

Anxiety and depression in older adults seem to influence not only respiratory symptoms but also QOL [161,169,173]. QOL after a hospital discharge following a COPD exacerbation was poor, and in one study the frequency of exacerbations and the severity of dyspnea had the most significant effect on QOL [174].

Prognosis

Determining prognosis or remaining life expectancy in individual patients who have COPD is fraught with uncertainty. Across all age groups, age, smoking status, poor pulmonary function, and low BMI are important predictors of mortality [128,175–178]. Predictors of mortality in older outpatients who have COPD include FEV_1, the severity of physical disability, advancing age, and the use of long-term oxygen therapy, whereas

smoking status, depression and QOL scores, presence and number of comorbid diseases, and the frequency of hospitalization did not predict mortality [179]. Of note, in the same study, mortality was much higher in those on LTOT, which may define a subgroup of older patients who have a poor prognosis [179].

The frequency of COPD exacerbations, particularly those that result in hospitalization, correlates with increasing mortality and is an independent predictor of poor outcome [180]. In patients aged 65 years or older, mortality following an intensive care unit admission for COPD exacerbation may be as high as 30% at hospital discharge and 59% at 1 year [181]. The same study also showed that the hospital and longer-term mortality strongly correlated with the development of nonrespiratory organ system dysfunction and the severity of the lung disease, but not with the need for mechanical ventilation [181]. Following a hospital admission for COPD exacerbation, comorbidities, depression, marital status, and QOL have been shown to be strong predictors of mortality in older patients who have COPD [182].

Palliative care, end of life, and care-giver issues

Even with various mortality predictions, it can be difficult to identify when a patient who has COPD might be entering the terminal phase. In addition, much of the usual COPD treatment is symptom-related and of low toxicity. These factors limit the usefulness of sharp distinctions between active and palliative treatment in many patients during periods of relative stability. Usual care should address symptoms of pain, dyspnea, anxiety, and depression at all stages of disease. Approximately 20% to 25% of patients who have COPD experience severe pain, however, and many experience depression, anxiety, and breathlessness toward the end of their life [183–185]. Older patients who have severe COPD have worse QOL and emotional well-being than patients who have unresectable non-small cell lung cancer [186]. There is a definite role for symptom management by palliative care specialists, but management guidelines may not provide this emphasis [187,188].

In contrast to typical outpatient management, acute severe illness may offer major end-of-life choices, such as whether to forego intubation and mechanical ventilation or to limit its duration, whether to accept less invasive modes of treatment, or whether to forego hospitalization itself. Although patients who have advanced COPD are just as unwilling to remain on mechanical ventilation as patients who have lung cancer, they are provided with fewer palliative options than those who have cancer [183]. Patients need opportunities to discuss the benefits and burdens of these interventions versus a less invasive, comfort-based approach and they need adequate palliative care services to support the latter approach if preferred.

Older patients who have COPD should identify specific surrogate decision-makers, who should, along with other appropriate family members, be included in end-of-life discussions whenever possible. Patients and families are frequently unaware of the extent to which interventions such as mechanical ventilation may reduce the patient's own decision-making capacity and require a family member or other surrogate to act on the patient's behalf.

Caregivers suffer from excess strain in caring for these patients [189], and spouses may have levels of psychologic problems comparable to the patients themselves [190]. Attention to these issues over the entire course of the disease improves the lives of patients who have COPD.

Summary

The incidence and burden of COPD is high and continues to increase. With the aging of the general population, COPD will be an increasingly common problem in older adults. Most older patients can perform spirometry, which is needed for an accurate diagnosis. Consensus criteria are needed to define normal spirometry versus airflow limitation in older subjects. Older patients who have COPD benefit from all effective therapies available to treat COPD, including smoking cessation, immunization, home oxygen, and inhaled medications. The forms of inhaled medications prescribed for older patients must take into account their individual limitations with technique and the need for instruction. Older patients have more comorbidities that influence QOL, prognosis, and medical management. Many older patients who have COPD need guidance and support for end-of-life decisions and discussions, and adequate support services for a more palliative approach should be available if desired.

References

[1] Snider GL. Nosology for our day: its application to chronic obstructive pulmonary disease. Am J Respir Crit Care Med 2003;167(5):678–83.

[2] Pauwels RA, Buist AS, Calverley PM, et al. Global strategy for the diagnosis, management, and prevention of chronic obstructive pulmonary disease. NHLBI/WHO Global Initiative for Chronic Obstructive Lung Disease (GOLD) Workshop summary. Am J Respir Crit Care Med 2001;163(5): 1256–76.

[3] Lopez AD, Shibuya K, Rao C, et al. Chronic obstructive pulmonary disease: current burden and future projections. Eur Respir J 2006;27(2):397–412.

[4] Blanc PD, Balmes JR. Epidemiology and costs of COPD. Eur Respir J 2006;28(6):1290.

[5] Murray CJ, Lopez AD. Alternative projections of mortality and disability by cause 1990–2020: Global Burden of Disease Study. Lancet 1997; 349(9064):1498–504.

[6] Hurd SS. International efforts directed at attacking the problem of COPD. Chest 2000;117(5 Suppl 2): 336S–8S.

[7] Mannino DM. COPD: epidemiology, prevalence, morbidity and mortality, and disease heterogeneity. Chest 2002;121(5 Suppl):121S–6S.

[8] Miller JD, Foster T, Boulanger L, et al. Direct costs of COPD in the US, an analysis of Medical Expenditure Panel Survey (MEPS) data. COPD 2005; 2(3):311–8.

[9] Mapel DW, Hurley JS, Frost FJ, et al. Health care utilization in chronic obstructive pulmonary disease. A case-control study in a health maintenance organization. Arch Intern Med 2000;160(17): 2653–8.

[10] Garrett N, Martini EM. The boomers are coming: a total cost of care model of the impact of population aging on the cost of chronic conditions in the United States. Dis Manag 2007;10(2):51–60.

[11] Davis RM, Novotny TE. The epidemiology of cigarette smoking and its impact on chronic obstructive pulmonary disease. Am Rev Respir Dis 1989; 140(3 Pt 2):S82–4.

[12] Fletcher C, Peto R. The natural history of chronic airflow obstruction. Br Med J 1977;1(6077):1645–8.

[13] Burrows B, Knudson RJ, Cline MG, et al. Quantitative relationships between cigarette smoking and ventilatory function. Am Rev Respir Dis 1977; 115(2):195–205.

[14] Cigarette smoking among adults—United States, 2004. MMWR Morb Mortal Wkly Rep 2005; 54(44):1121–4.

[15] Prevalence of current cigarette smoking among adults and changes in prevalence of current and some day smoking—United States, 1996–2001. MMWR Morb Mortal Wkly Rep 2003;52(14): 303–4, 306–7.

[16] Eriksson S. Pulmonary emphysema and alpha1-antitrypsin deficiency. Acta Med Scand 1964;175: 197–205.

[17] Tobin MJ, Cook PJ, Hutchison DC. Alpha 1 antitrypsin deficiency: the clinical and physiological features of pulmonary emphysema in subjects

homozygous for Pi type Z. A survey by the British Thoracic Association. Br J Dis Chest 1983;77(1):14–27.

[18] Zock JP, Sunyer J, Kogevinas M, et al. Occupation, chronic bronchitis, and lung function in young adults. An international study. Am J Respir Crit Care Med 2001;163(7):1572–7.

[19] Tashkin DP, Clark VA, Coulson AH, et al. The UCLA population studies of chronic obstructive respiratory disease. VIII. Effects of smoking cessation on lung function: a prospective study of a free-living population. Am Rev Respir Dis 1984;130(5):707–15.

[20] Perez-Padilla R, Regalado J, Vedal S, et al. Exposure to biomass smoke and chronic airway disease in Mexican women. A case-control study. Am J Respir Crit Care Med 1996;154(3 Pt 1):701–6.

[21] Dennis RJ, Maldonado D, Norman S, et al. Woodsmoke exposure and risk for obstructive airways disease among women. Chest 1996;109(1):115–9.

[22] Vestbo J, Prescott E, Lange P. Association of chronic mucus hypersecretion with FEV1 decline and chronic obstructive pulmonary disease morbidity. Copenhagen City Heart Study Group. Am J Respir Crit Care Med 1996;153(5):1530–5.

[23] Tashkin DP, Altose MD, Connett JE, et al. Methacholine reactivity predicts changes in lung function over time in smokers with early chronic obstructive pulmonary disease. The Lung Health Study Research Group. Am J Respir Crit Care Med 1996;153(6 Pt 1):1802–11.

[24] Burrows B. Airways obstructive diseases: pathogenetic mechanisms and natural histories of the disorders. Med Clin North Am 1990;74(3):547–59.

[25] Connett JE, Murray RP, Buist AS, et al. Changes in smoking status affect women more than men: results of the Lung Health Study. Am J Epidemiol 2003;157(11):973–9.

[26] Chen Y, Horne SL, Dosman JA. Increased susceptibility to lung dysfunction in female smokers. Am Rev Respir Dis 1991;143(6):1224–30.

[27] de Torres JP, Campo A, Casanova C, et al. Gender and chronic obstructive pulmonary disease in high-risk smokers. Respiration 2006;73(3):306–10.

[28] De Filippi F, Tana F, Vanzati S, et al. Study of respiratory function in the elderly with different nutritional and cognitive status and functional ability assessed by plethysmographic and spirometric parameters. Arch Gerontol Geriatr 2003;37(1):33–43.

[29] Pezzoli L, Giardini G, Consonni S, et al. Quality of spirometric performance in older people. Age Ageing 2003;32(1):43–6.

[30] Sherman CB, Kern D, Richardson ER, et al. Cognitive function and spirometry performance in the elderly. Am Rev Respir Dis 1993;148(1):123–6.

[31] Celli BR, MacNee W. Standards for the diagnosis and treatment of patients with COPD: a summary of the ATS/ERS position paper. Eur Respir J 2004;23(6):932–46.

[32] Pellegrino R, Viegi G, Brusasco V, et al. Interpretative strategies for lung function tests. Eur Respir J 2005;26(5):948–68.

[33] Lung function testing: selection of reference values and interpretative strategies. American Thoracic Society. Am Rev Respir Dis 1991;144(5):1202–18.

[34] Crapo RO, Morris AH, Gardner RM. Reference spirometric values using techniques and equipment that meet ATS recommendations. Am Rev Respir Dis 1981;123(6):659–64.

[35] Hankinson JL, Odencrantz JR, Fedan KB. Spirometric reference values from a sample of the general U.S. population. Am J Respir Crit Care Med 1999;159(1):179–87.

[36] Knudson RJ, Lebowitz MD, Holberg CJ, et al. Changes in the normal maximal expiratory flow-volume curve with growth and aging. Am Rev Respir Dis 1983;127(6):725–34.

[37] Burrows B, Lebowitz MD, Camilli AE, et al. Longitudinal changes in forced expiratory volume in one second in adults. Methodologic considerations and findings in healthy nonsmokers. Am Rev Respir Dis 1986;133(6):974–80.

[38] Gelb AF, Zamel N. Effect of aging on lung mechanics in healthy nonsmokers. Chest 1975;68(4):538–41.

[39] Celli BR, Halbert RJ, Isonaka S, et al. Population impact of different definitions of airway obstruction. Eur Respir J 2003;22(2):268–73.

[40] Hardie JA, Buist AS, Vollmer WM, et al. Risk of over-diagnosis of COPD in asymptomatic elderly never-smokers. Eur Respir J 2002;20(5):1117–22.

[41] Medbo A, Melbye H. Lung function testing in the elderly—can we still use FEV(1)/FVC < 70% as a criterion of COPD? Respir Med 2007;10(6):1097–105.

[42] Hansen JE, Sun XG, Wasserman K. Spirometric criteria for airway obstruction: use percentage of FEV1/FVC ratio below the fifth percentile, not < 70%. Chest 2007;131(2):349–55.

[43] Mannino DM, Sonia Buist A, Vollmer WM. Chronic obstructive pulmonary disease in the older adult: what defines abnormal lung function? Thorax 2007;62(3):237–41.

[44] Lindberg A, Bjerg-Backlund A, Ronmark E, et al. Prevalence and underdiagnosis of COPD by disease severity and the attributable fraction of smoking report from the Obstructive Lung Disease in Northern Sweden Studies. Respir Med 2006;100(2):264–72.

[45] Lundback B, Gulsvik A, Albers M, et al. Epidemiological aspects and early detection of chronic obstructive airway diseases in the elderly. Eur Respir J Suppl 2003;40:3s–9s.

[46] Lindstrom M, Jonsson E, Larsson K, et al. Underdiagnosis of chronic obstructive pulmonary disease in Northern Sweden. Int J Tuberc Lung Dis 2002;6(1):76–84.

[47] Sciurba FC. Physiologic similarities and differences between COPD and asthma. Chest 2004;126(2 Suppl):117S–24S [discussion: 159S–161S].

[48] Bellia V, Battaglia S, Catalano F, et al. Aging and disability affect misdiagnosis of COPD in elderly asthmatics: the SARA study. Chest 2003;123(4):1066–72.

[49] Halbert RJ, Isonaka S, George D, et al. Interpreting COPD prevalence estimates: what is the true burden of disease? Chest 2003;123(5):1684–92.

[50] Mannino DM, Gagnon RC, Petty TL, et al. Obstructive lung disease and low lung function in adults in the United States: data from the National Health and Nutrition Examination Survey, 1988–1994. Arch Intern Med 2000;160(11):1683–9.

[51] Isoaho R, Puolijoki H, Huhti E, et al. Prevalence of chronic obstructive pulmonary disease in elderly Finns. Respir Med 1994;88(8):571–80.

[52] Burchfiel CM, Marcus EB, Curb JD, et al. Effects of smoking and smoking cessation on longitudinal decline in pulmonary function. Am J Respir Crit Care Med 1995;151(6):1778–85.

[53] Pelkonen M, Notkola IL, Tukiainen H, et al. Smoking cessation, decline in pulmonary function and total mortality: a 30-year follow up study among the Finnish cohorts of the Seven Countries Study. Thorax 2001;56(9):703–7.

[54] Higgins MW, Enright PL, Kronmal RA, et al. Smoking and lung function in elderly men and women. The Cardiovascular Health Study. JAMA 1993;269(21):2741–8.

[55] Vollset SE, Tverdal A, Gjessing HK. Smoking and deaths between 40 and 70 years of age in women and men. Ann Intern Med 2006;144(6):381–9.

[56] Taylor DH Jr, Hasselblad V, Henley SJ, et al. Benefits of smoking cessation for longevity. Am J Public Health 2002;92(6):990–6.

[57] Anthonisen NR, Skeans MA, Wise RA, et al. The effects of a smoking cessation intervention on 14.5-year mortality: a randomized clinical trial. Ann Intern Med 2005;142(4):233–9.

[58] Tait RJ, Hulse GK, Waterreus A, et al. Effectiveness of a smoking cessation intervention in older adults. Addiction 2007;102(1):148–55.

[59] Hurt RD, Sachs DP, Glover ED, et al. A comparison of sustained-release bupropion and placebo for smoking cessation. N Engl J Med 1997;337(17):1195–202.

[60] Gonzales D, Rennard SI, Nides M, et al. Varenicline, an alpha4beta2 nicotinic acetylcholine receptor partial agonist, vs sustained-release bupropion and placebo for smoking cessation: a randomized controlled trial. JAMA 2006;296(1):47–55.

[61] Jorenby DE, Hays JT, Rigotti NA, et al. Efficacy of varenicline, an alpha4beta2 nicotinic acetylcholine receptor partial agonist, vs placebo or sustained-release bupropion for smoking cessation: a randomized controlled trial. JAMA 2006;296(1):56–63.

[62] Maguire CP, Ryan J, Kelly A, et al. Do patient age and medical condition influence medical advice to stop smoking? Age Ageing 2000;29(3):264–6.

[63] Anthonisen NR, Connett JE, Kiley JP, et al. Effects of smoking intervention and the use of an inhaled anticholinergic bronchodilator on the rate of decline of FEV1. The Lung Health Study. JAMA 1994;272(19):1497–505.

[64] Anthonisen NR, Connett JE, Enright PL, et al. Hospitalizations and mortality in the Lung Health Study. Am J Respir Crit Care Med 2002;166(3):333–9.

[65] Belman MJ, Botnick WC, Shin JW. Inhaled bronchodilators reduce dynamic hyperinflation during exercise in patients with chronic obstructive pulmonary disease. Am J Respir Crit Care Med 1996;153(3):967–75.

[66] O'Donnell DE, Lam M, Webb KA. Spirometric correlates of improvement in exercise performance after anticholinergic therapy in chronic obstructive pulmonary disease. Am J Respir Crit Care Med 1999;160(2):542–9.

[67] In chronic obstructive pulmonary disease, a combination of ipratropium and albuterol is more effective than either agent alone. An 85-day multicenter trial. COMBIVENT Inhalation Aerosol Study Group. Chest 1994;105(5):1411–9.

[68] Appleton S, Jones T, Poole P, et al. Ipratropium bromide versus short acting beta-2 agonists for stable chronic obstructive pulmonary disease. Cochrane Database Syst Rev 2006;2:CD001387.

[69] Routine nebulized ipratropium and albuterol together are better than either alone in COPD. The COMBIVENT Inhalation Solution Study Group. Chest 1997;112(6):1514–21.

[70] Appleton S, Poole P, Smith B, et al. Long-acting beta2-agonists for poorly reversible chronic obstructive pulmonary disease. Cochrane Database Syst Rev 2006;3 CD001104.

[71] Jones PW, Bosh TK. Quality of life changes in COPD patients treated with salmeterol. Am J Respir Crit Care Med 1997;155(4):1283–9.

[72] Dahl R, Greefhorst LA, Nowak D, et al. Inhaled formoterol dry powder versus ipratropium bromide in chronic obstructive pulmonary disease. Am J Respir Crit Care Med 2001;164(5):778–84.

[73] Appleton S, Jones T, Poole P, et al. Ipratropium bromide versus long-acting beta-2 agonists for stable chronic obstructive pulmonary disease. Cochrane Database Syst Rev 2006;3:CD006101.

[74] ZuWallack RL, Mahler DA, Reilly D, et al. Salmeterol plus theophylline combination therapy in the treatment of COPD. Chest 2001;119(6):1661–70.

[75] Casaburi R, Mahler DA, Jones PW, et al. A long-term evaluation of once-daily inhaled tiotropium in chronic obstructive pulmonary disease. Eur Respir J 2002;19(2):217–24.

[76] Vincken W, van Noord JA, Greefhorst AP, et al. Improved health outcomes in patients with COPD during 1 yr's treatment with tiotropium. Eur Respir J 2002;19(2):209–16.

[77] Barr RG, Bourbeau J, Camargo CA, et al. Tiotropium for stable chronic obstructive pulmonary disease: a meta-analysis. Thorax 2006;61(10):854–62.

[78] Brusasco V, Hodder R, Miravitlles M, et al. Health outcomes following treatment for six months with once daily tiotropium compared with twice daily salmeterol in patients with COPD. Thorax 2003; 58(5):399–404.

[79] Donohue JF, van Noord JA, Bateman ED, et al. A 6-month, placebo-controlled study comparing lung function and health status changes in COPD patients treated with tiotropium or salmeterol. Chest 2002;122(1):47–55.

[80] Effect of inhaled triamcinolone on the decline in pulmonary function in chronic obstructive pulmonary disease. N Engl J Med 2000;343(26):1902–9.

[81] Burge PS, Calverley PM, Jones PW, et al. Randomised, double blind, placebo controlled study of fluticasone propionate in patients with moderate to severe chronic obstructive pulmonary disease: the ISOLDE trial. BMJ 2000;320(7245):1297–303.

[82] Pauwels RA, Lofdahl CG, Laitinen LA, et al. Long-term treatment with inhaled budesonide in persons with mild chronic obstructive pulmonary disease who continue smoking. European Respiratory Society Study on chronic obstructive pulmonary disease. N Engl J Med 1999;340(25):1948–53.

[83] Vestbo J, Sorensen T, Lange P, et al. Long-term effect of inhaled budesonide in mild and moderate chronic obstructive pulmonary disease: a randomised controlled trial. Lancet 1999;353(9167): 1819–23.

[84] Jarad NA, Wedzicha JA, Burge PS, et al. An observational study of inhaled corticosteroid withdrawal in stable chronic obstructive pulmonary disease. ISOLDE Study Group. Respir Med 1999;93(3): 161–6.

[85] van der Valk P, Monninkhof E, van der Palen J, et al. Effect of discontinuation of inhaled corticosteroids in patients with chronic obstructive pulmonary disease: the COPE study. Am J Respir Crit Care Med 2002;166(10):1358–63.

[86] Johnell O, Pauwels R, Lofdahl CG, et al. Bone mineral density in patients with chronic obstructive pulmonary disease treated with budesonide Turbuhaler. Eur Respir J 2002;19(6):1058–63.

[87] Calverley PM, Anderson JA, Celli B, et al. Salmeterol and fluticasone propionate and survival in chronic obstructive pulmonary disease. N Engl J Med 2007;356(8):775–89.

[88] Calverley P, Pauwels R, Vestbo J, et al. Combined salmeterol and fluticasone in the treatment of chronic obstructive pulmonary disease: a randomised controlled trial. Lancet 2003;361(9356): 449–56.

[89] Calverley PM, Boonsawat W, Cseke Z, et al. Maintenance therapy with budesonide and formoterol in chronic obstructive pulmonary disease. Eur Respir J 2003;22(6):912–9.

[90] Mahler DA, Wire P, Horstman D, et al. Effectiveness of fluticasone propionate and salmeterol combination delivered via the Diskus device in the treatment of chronic obstructive pulmonary disease. Am J Respir Crit Care Med 2002;166(8): 1084–91.

[91] Szafranski W, Cukier A, Ramirez A, et al. Efficacy and safety of budesonide/formoterol in the management of chronic obstructive pulmonary disease. Eur Respir J 2003;21(1):74–81.

[92] Aaron SD, Vandemheen KL, Fergusson D, et al. Tiotropium in combination with placebo, salmeterol, or fluticasone-salmeterol for treatment of chronic obstructive pulmonary disease: a randomized trial. Ann Intern Med 2007;146(8):545–55.

[93] Diggory P, Fernandez C, Humphrey A, et al. Comparison of elderly people's technique in using two dry powder inhalers to deliver zanamivir: randomised controlled trial. BMJ 2001;322(7286):577–9.

[94] Jarvis S, Ind PW, Shiner RJ. Inhaled therapy in elderly COPD patients; time for re-evaluation? Age Ageing 2007;36(2):213–8.

[95] Allen SC. Competence thresholds for the use of inhalers in people with dementia. Age Ageing 1997; 26(2):83–6.

[96] Allen SC, Ragab S. Ability to learn inhaler technique in relation to cognitive scores and tests of praxis in old age. Postgrad Med J 2002;78(915):37–9.

[97] Chapman KR, Love L, Brubaker H. A comparison of breath-actuated and conventional metered-dose inhaler inhalation techniques in elderly subjects. Chest 1993;104(5):1332–7.

[98] Ho SF, O'Mahoney MS, Steward JA, et al. Inhaler technique in older people in the community. Age Ageing 2004;33(2):185–8.

[99] Jones V, Fernandez C, Diggory P. A comparison of large volume spacer, breath-activated and dry powder inhalers in older people. Age Ageing 1999; 28(5):481–4.

[100] Dolovich MB, Ahrens RC, Hess DR, et al. Device selection and outcomes of aerosol therapy: evidence-based guidelines: American College of Chest Physicians/American College of Asthma, Allergy, and Immunology. Chest 2005;127(1):335–71.

[101] Continuous or nocturnal oxygen therapy in hypoxemic chronic obstructive lung disease: a clinical trial. Nocturnal Oxygen Therapy Trial Group. Ann Intern Med 1980;93(3):391–8.

[102] Long term domiciliary oxygen therapy in chronic hypoxic cor pulmonale complicating chronic bronchitis and emphysema. Report of the Medical Research Council Working Party. Lancet 1981; 1(8222):681–6.

[103] Gorecka D, Gorzelak K, Sliwinski P, et al. Effect of long-term oxygen therapy on survival in patients with chronic obstructive pulmonary disease with moderate hypoxaemia. Thorax 1997;52(8):674–9.

[104] Chaouat A, Weitzenblum E, Kessler R, et al. A randomized trial of nocturnal oxygen therapy in

chronic obstructive pulmonary disease patients. Eur Respir J 1999;14(5):1002–8.

[105] Croxton TL, Bailey WC. Long-term oxygen treatment in chronic obstructive pulmonary disease: recommendations for future research: an NHLBI workshop report. Am J Respir Crit Care Med 2006;174(4):373–8.

[106] Pulmonary rehabilitation—1999. American Thoracic Society. Am J Respir Crit Care Med 1999; 159(5 Pt 1):1666–82.

[107] Nici L, Donner C, Wouters E, et al. American Thoracic Society/European Respiratory Society statement on pulmonary rehabilitation. Am J Respir Crit Care Med 2006;173(12):1390–413.

[108] Guell R, Casan P, Belda J, et al. Long-term effects of outpatient rehabilitation of COPD: a randomized trial. Chest 2000;117(4):976–83.

[109] Troosters T, Gosselink R, Decramer M. Short- and long-term effects of outpatient rehabilitation in patients with chronic obstructive pulmonary disease: a randomized trial. Am J Med 2000;109(3):207–12.

[110] Paz-Diaz H, Montes de Oca M, Lopez JM, et al. Pulmonary rehabilitation improves depression, anxiety, dyspnea and health status in patients with COPD. Am J Phys Med Rehabil 2007;86(1): 30–6.

[111] Takigawa N, Tada A, Soda R, et al. Comprehensive pulmonary rehabilitation according to severity of COPD. Respir Med 2007;101(2):326–32.

[112] Wijkstra PJ, Ten Vergert EM, van Altena R, et al. Long term benefits of rehabilitation at home on quality of life and exercise tolerance in patients with chronic obstructive pulmonary disease. Thorax 1995;50(8):824–8.

[113] Couser JI Jr, Guthmann R, Hamadeh MA, et al. Pulmonary rehabilitation improves exercise capacity in older elderly patients with COPD. Chest 1995;107(3):730–4.

[114] Hak E, van Essen GA, Buskens E, et al. Is immunising all patients with chronic lung disease in the community against influenza cost effective? Evidence from a general practice-based clinical prospective cohort study in Utrecht, The Netherlands. J Epidemiol Community Health 1998;52(2):120–5.

[115] Nichol KL, Margolis KL, Wuorenma J, et al. The efficacy and cost effectiveness of vaccination against influenza among elderly persons living in the community. N Engl J Med 1994;331(12): 778–84.

[116] Jackson LA, Neuzil KM, Yu O, et al. Effectiveness of pneumococcal polysaccharide vaccine in older adults. N Engl J Med 2003;348(18):1747–55.

[117] Vila-Corcoles A, Ochoa-Gondar O, Hospital I, et al. Protective effects of the 23-valent pneumococcal polysaccharide vaccine in the elderly population: the EVAN-65 study. Clin Infect Dis 2006; 43(7):860–8.

[118] Granger R, Walters J, Poole PJ, et al. Injectable vaccines for preventing pneumococcal infection in patients with chronic obstructive pulmonary disease. Cochrane Database Syst Rev 2006;4: CD001390.

[119] Keller HH. Malnutrition in institutionalized elderly: how and why? J Am Geriatr Soc 1993; 41(11):1212–8.

[120] Lipski PS, Torrance A, Kelly PJ, et al. A study of nutritional deficits of long-stay geriatric patients. Age Ageing 1993;22(4):244–55.

[121] Bienia R, Ratcliff S, Barbour GL, et al. Malnutrition in the hospitalized geriatric patient. J Am Geriatr Soc 1982;30(7):433–6.

[122] Constans T, Bacq Y, Brechot JF, et al. Protein-energy malnutrition in elderly medical patients. J Am Geriatr Soc 1992;40(3):263–8.

[123] Payette H, Coulombe C, Boutier V, et al. Weight loss and mortality among free-living frail elders: a prospective study. J Gerontol A Biol Sci Med Sci 1999;54(9):M440–5.

[124] Sullivan DH, Sun S, Walls RC. Protein-energy undernutrition among elderly hospitalized patients: a prospective study. JAMA 1999;281(21):2013–9.

[125] Vandenbergh E, Van de Woestijne KP, Gyselen A. Weight changes in the terminal stages of chronic obstructive pulmonary disease. Relation to respiratory function and prognosis. Am Rev Respir Dis 1967;95(4):556–66.

[126] Chailleux E, Laaban JP, Veale D. Prognostic value of nutritional depletion in patients with COPD treated by long-term oxygen therapy: data from the ANTADIR observatory. Chest 2003;123(5):1460–6.

[127] Gray-Donald K, Gibbons L, Shapiro SH, et al. Nutritional status and mortality in chronic obstructive pulmonary disease. Am J Respir Crit Care Med 1996;153(3):961–6.

[128] Landbo C, Prescott E, Lange P, et al. Prognostic value of nutritional status in chronic obstructive pulmonary disease. Am J Respir Crit Care Med 1999;160(6):1856–61.

[129] Schols AM, Slangen J, Volovics L, et al. Weight loss is a reversible factor in the prognosis of chronic obstructive pulmonary disease. Am J Respir Crit Care Med 1998;157(6 Pt 1):1791–7.

[130] Marti S, Munoz X, Rios J, et al. Body weight and comorbidity predict mortality in COPD patients treated with oxygen therapy. Eur Respir J 2006; 27(4):689–96.

[131] Payette H, Boutier V, Coulombe C, et al. Benefits of nutritional supplementation in free-living, frail, undernourished elderly people: a prospective randomized community trial. J Am Diet Assoc 2002; 102(8):1088–95.

[132] Efthimiou J, Fleming J, Gomes C, et al. The effect of supplementary oral nutrition in poorly nourished patients with chronic obstructive pulmonary disease. Am Rev Respir Dis 1988; 137(5):1075–82.

[133] Rogers RM, Donahoe M, Costantino J. Physiologic effects of oral supplemental feeding in

malnourished patients with chronic obstructive pulmonary disease. A randomized control study. Am Rev Respir Dis 1992;146(6):1511–7.

[134] Whittaker JS, Ryan CF, Buckley PA, et al. The effects of refeeding on peripheral and respiratory muscle function in malnourished chronic obstructive pulmonary disease patients. Am Rev Respir Dis 1990;142(2):283–8.

[135] Schols AM, Broekhuizen R, Weling-Scheepers CA, et al. Body composition and mortality in chronic obstructive pulmonary disease. Am J Clin Nutr 2005;82(1):53–9.

[136] Slinde F, Gronberg A, Engstrom CP, et al. Body composition by bioelectrical impedance predicts mortality in chronic obstructive pulmonary disease patients. Respir Med 2005;99(8):1004–9.

[137] Vestbo J, Prescott E, Almdal T, et al. Body mass, fat-free body mass, and prognosis in patients with chronic obstructive pulmonary disease from a random population sample: findings from the Copenhagen City Heart Study. Am J Respir Crit Care Med 2006;173(1):79–83.

[138] Hopkinson NS, Tennant RC, Dayer MJ, et al. A prospective study of decline in fat free mass and skeletal muscle strength in chronic obstructive pulmonary disease. Respir Res 2007;8:25–32.

[139] Creutzberg EC, Wouters EF, Mostert R, et al. A role for anabolic steroids in the rehabilitation of patients with COPD? A double-blind, placebo-controlled, randomized trial. Chest 2003;124(5):1733–42.

[140] Schols AM, Soeters PB, Mostert R, et al. Physiologic effects of nutritional support and anabolic steroids in patients with chronic obstructive pulmonary disease. A placebo-controlled randomized trial. Am J Respir Crit Care Med 1995;152(4 Pt 1):1268–74.

[141] Liu H, Bravata DM, Olkin I, et al. Systematic review: the safety and efficacy of growth hormone in the healthy elderly. Ann Intern Med 2007;146(2):104–15.

[142] Ferrer M, Alonso J, Morera J, et al. Chronic obstructive pulmonary disease stage and health-related quality of life. The Quality of Life of Chronic Obstructive Pulmonary Disease Study Group. Ann Intern Med 1997;127(12):1072–9.

[143] Stewart AL, Greenfield S, Hays RD, et al. Functional status and well-being of patients with chronic conditions. Results from the Medical Outcomes Study. JAMA 1989;262(7):907–13.

[144] Schellevis FG, van der Velden J, van de Lisdonk E, et al. Comorbidity of chronic diseases in general practice. J Clin Epidemiol 1993;46(5):469–73.

[145] Fuso L, Incalzi RA, Pistelli R, et al. Predicting mortality of patients hospitalized for acutely exacerbated chronic obstructive pulmonary disease. Am J Med 1995;98(3):272–7.

[146] Antonelli Incalzi R, Fuso L, De Rosa M, et al. Comorbidity contributes to predict mortality of patients with chronic obstructive pulmonary disease. Eur Respir J 1997;10(12):2794–800.

[147] Yeo J, Karimova G, Bansal S. Co-morbidity in older patients with COPD—its impact on health service utilisation and quality of life, a community study. Age Ageing 2006;35(1):33–7.

[148] Patil SP, Krishnan JA, Lechtzin N, et al. In-hospital mortality following acute exacerbations of chronic obstructive pulmonary disease. Arch Intern Med 2003;163(10):1180–6.

[149] Zielinski J, MacNee W, Wedzicha J, et al. Causes of death in patients with COPD and chronic respiratory failure. Monaldi Arch Chest Dis 1997;52(1):43–7.

[150] Carson JL, Terrin ML, Duff A, et al. Pulmonary embolism and mortality in patients with COPD. Chest 1996;110(5):1212–9.

[151] Kim HF, Kunik ME, Molinari VA, et al. Functional impairment in COPD patients: the impact of anxiety and depression. Psychosomatics 2000;41(6):465–71.

[152] Bosley CM, Corden ZM, Rees PJ, et al. Psychological factors associated with use of home nebulized therapy for COPD. Eur Respir J 1996;9(11):2346–50.

[153] Light RW, Merrill EJ, Despars JA, et al. Prevalence of depression and anxiety in patients with COPD. Relationship to functional capacity. Chest 1985;87(1):35–8.

[154] Yohannes AM, Roomi J, Baldwin RC, et al. Depression in elderly outpatients with disabling chronic obstructive pulmonary disease. Age Ageing 1998;27(2):155–60.

[155] Yohannes AM, Baldwin RC, Connolly MJ. Depression and anxiety in elderly outpatients with chronic obstructive pulmonary disease: prevalence, and validation of the BASDEC screening questionnaire. Int J Geriatr Psychiatry 2000;15(12):1090–6.

[156] Incalzi RA, Chiappini F, Fuso L, et al. Predicting cognitive decline in patients with hypoxaemic COPD. Respir Med 1998;92(3):527–33.

[157] Koenig HG, George LK, Peterson BL, et al. Depression in medically ill hospitalized older adults: prevalence, characteristics, and course of symptoms according to six diagnostic schemes. Am J Psychiatry 1997;154(10):1376–83.

[158] McCusker J, Cole M, Dufouil C, et al. The prevalence and correlates of major and minor depression in older medical inpatients. J Am Geriatr Soc 2005;53(8):1344–53.

[159] Engstrom CP, Persson LO, Larsson S, et al. Functional status and well being in chronic obstructive pulmonary disease with regard to clinical parameters and smoking: a descriptive and comparative study. Thorax 1996;51(8):825–30.

[160] Yellowlees PM, Alpers JH, Bowden JJ, et al. Psychiatric morbidity in patients with chronic airflow obstruction. Med J Aust 1987;146(6):305–7.

[161] Cully JA, Graham DP, Stanley MA, et al. Quality of life in patients with chronic obstructive pulmonary disease and comorbid anxiety or depression. Psychosomatics 2006;47(4):312–9.

[162] Argyropoulou P, Patakas D, Koukou A, et al. Buspirone effect on breathlessness and exercise performance in patients with chronic obstructive pulmonary disease. Respiration 1993;60(4): 216–20.

[163] Borson S, McDonald GJ, Gayle T, et al. Improvement in mood, physical symptoms, and function with nortriptyline for depression in patients with chronic obstructive pulmonary disease. Psychosomatics 1992;33(2):190–201.

[164] Eiser N, Harte R, Spiros K, et al. Effect of treating depression on quality-of-life and exercise tolerance in severe COPD. COPD 2005;2(2):233–41.

[165] Yohannes AM, Connolly MJ, Baldwin RC. A feasibility study of antidepressant drug therapy in depressed elderly patients with chronic obstructive pulmonary disease. Int J Geriatr Psychiatry 2001; 16(5):451–4.

[166] Sirey JA, Raue PJ, Alexopoulos GS. An intervention to improve depression care in older adults with COPD. Int J Geriatr Psychiatry 2007;22(2): 154–9.

[167] Prigatano GP, Wright EC, Levin D. Quality of life and its predictors in patients with mild hypoxemia and chronic obstructive pulmonary disease. Arch Intern Med 1984;144(8):1613–9.

[168] McSweeny AJ, Grant I, Heaton RK, et al. Life quality of patients with chronic obstructive pulmonary disease. Arch Intern Med 1982;142(3): 473–8.

[169] Peruzza S, Sergi G, Vianello A, et al. Chronic obstructive pulmonary disease (COPD) in elderly subjects: impact on functional status and quality of life. Respir Med 2003;97(6):612–7.

[170] Tsukino M, Nishimura K, Ikeda A, et al. Physiologic factors that determine the health-related quality of life in patients with COPD. Chest 1996; 110(4):896–903.

[171] Jones PW. Issues concerning health-related quality of life in COPD. Chest 1995;107(5 Suppl): 187S–93S.

[172] Jones PW, Quirk FH, Baveystock CM. The St George's respiratory questionnaire. Respir Med 1991;85(Suppl B):25–31 [discussion: 27–33].

[173] Okubadejo AA, Jones PW, Wedzicha JA. Quality of life in patients with chronic obstructive pulmonary disease and severe hypoxaemia. Thorax 1996;51(1):44–7.

[174] Wang Q, Bourbeau J. Outcomes and health-related quality of life following hospitalization for an acute exacerbation of COPD. Respirology 2005;10(3): 334–40.

[175] Anthonisen NR, Wright EC, Hodgkin JE. Prognosis in chronic obstructive pulmonary disease. Am Rev Respir Dis 1986;133(1):14–20.

[176] Kanner RE, Renzetti AD Jr, Stanish WM, et al. Predictors of survival in subjects with chronic airflow limitation. Am J Med 1983;74(2):249–55.

[177] Postma DS, Gimeno F, van der Weele LT, et al. Assessment of ventilatory variables in survival prediction of patients with chronic airflow obstruction: the importance of reversibility. Eur J Respir Dis 1985;67(5):360–8.

[178] Burrows B, Earle RH. Prediction of survival in patients with chronic airway obstruction. Am Rev Respir Dis 1969;99(6):865–71.

[179] Yohannes AM, Baldwin RC, Connolly M. Mortality predictors in disabling chronic obstructive pulmonary disease in old age. Age Ageing 2002; 31(2):137–40.

[180] Soler-Cataluna JJ, Martinez-Garcia MA, Roman Sanchez P, et al. Severe acute exacerbations and mortality in patients with chronic obstructive pulmonary disease. Thorax 2005;60(11):925–31.

[181] Seneff MG, Wagner DP, Wagner RP, et al. Hospital and 1-year survival of patients admitted to intensive care units with acute exacerbation of chronic obstructive pulmonary disease. JAMA 1995;274(23):1852–7.

[182] Almagro P, Calbo E, Ochoa de Echaguen A, et al. Mortality after hospitalization for COPD. Chest 2002;121(5):1441–8.

[183] Claessens MT, Lynn J, Zhong Z, et al. Dying with lung cancer or chronic obstructive pulmonary disease: insights from SUPPORT. Study to Understand Prognoses and Preferences for Outcomes and Risks of Treatments. J Am Geriatr Soc 2000; 48(5 Suppl):S146–53.

[184] Lynn J, Ely EW, Zhong Z, et al. Living and dying with chronic obstructive pulmonary disease. J Am Geriatr Soc 2000;48(5 Suppl):S91–S100.

[185] Elkington H, White P, Addington-Hall J, et al. The last year of life of COPD: a qualitative study of symptoms and services. Respir Med 2004;98(5): 439–45.

[186] Gore JM, Brophy CJ, Greenstone MA. How well do we care for patients with end stage chronic obstructive pulmonary disease (COPD)? A comparison of palliative care and quality of life in COPD and lung cancer. Thorax 2000;55(12):1000–6.

[187] Mast KR, Salama M, Silverman GK, et al. End-of-life content in treatment guidelines for life-limiting diseases. J Palliat Med 2004;7(6):754–73.

[188] Shee CD. Palliation in chronic respiratory disease. Palliat Med 1995;9(1):3–12.

[189] Seamark DA, Blake SD, Seamark CJ, et al. Living with severe chronic obstructive pulmonary disease (COPD): perceptions of patients and their carers. An interpretative phenomenological analysis. Palliat Med 2004;18(7):619–25.

[190] Kara M, Mirici A. Loneliness, depression, and social support of Turkish patients with chronic obstructive pulmonary disease and their spouses. J Nurs Scholarsh 2004;36(4):331–6.

ELSEVIER
SAUNDERS

Clin Chest Med 28 (2007) 717–733

CLINICS
IN CHEST
MEDICINE

Pulmonary Hypertension in Older Adults

John R. McArdle, MD[a,*], Terence K. Trow, MD[a,b],
Kathryn Lerz, APRN[a,b]

[a]Division of Internal Medicine, Section of Pulmonary and Critical Care Medicine, Yale University School of Medicine,
333 Cedar Street, LCI 105D, P.O. Box 208057, New Haven, CT 06520-8057, USA
[b]Pulmonary Hypertension Center, Yale University School of Medicine, 333 Cedar Street, LCI 105D,
P.O. Box 208057, New Haven, CT 06520-8057, USA

Pulmonary hypertension (PH) is a frequently encountered problem in older patients. There is some suggestion in the literature that the prevalence of PH and mortality from PH in this cohort may be increasing [1–4]. Although diseases resulting in systolic and diastolic dysfunction with accompanying pulmonary venous hypertension (PVH) account for a large percentage of PH in this population, PH associated with other respiratory diseases, such as chronic obstructive pulmonary disease (COPD), interstitial lung disease (ILD), and sleep apnea, and PH associated with connective tissue disease, pulmonary emboli, tumor emboli, or pulmonary hypertension complicating cancer therapies is also encountered by the practicing clinician. True idiopathic pulmonary arterial hypertension (IPAH) can also be seen and requires careful exclusion in older patients. Institution of therapies must be tempered with an appreciation of individual comorbidities and functional limitations that may affect patients' ability to comply and benefit from the complex treatments available for pulmonary arterial hypertension (PAH). This article reviews the existing data on the various forms of PH presenting in older patients and on appropriate therapy in this challenging population.

Prevalence and mortality

Accurate data on the prevalence and incidence of PH in older patients is scarce and is often confounded by inaccurate diagnosis, selection bias, and retrospective study design [5]. Because right heart catheterization is necessary to formally diagnose and classify PH [6,7], large unselected prospective studies are not likely to be done. Rich and colleagues [5] attempted to examine the prevalence of PH in the adult population using chest roentgenogram (CXR) criteria in a population of 10,000 subjects entered into the Second National Health and Nutrition Examination Survey. They concluded that the overall prevalence was too low to project within reasonable confidence limits. They estimated the prevalence of PH in men above the age of 64 to be 28.2% [5]. When nonagenarians living at high altitudes were assessed using radiographic criteria alone in a small cohort of 28 patients, up to 59% demonstrated abnormal enlargement of the pulmonary arteries in posterior-anterior and lateral radiographs [8]. The applicability of these findings to nonagenarians in general is likely limited because this cohort represented a highly selected population living at high altitudes. These CXR studies are limited by the subjective nature of interpreting CXRs and interobserver variability and by the limited sensitivity and specificity of CXR in the diagnosis of PH when compared with catheterization data [7,9].

More recently, the Centers for Disease Control and Prevention's Survey of the United States population observed increasing rates of hospitalizations for PH over the past 20 years, noting that 30% of the patients dying with PH were 75 years of age or older (Fig. 1) [3]. In addition, age-specific death rates for PH increased among men 65 years of age or older, whites 75 years of age or older, and blacks 65 years of age or older

* Corresponding author.
E-mail address: john.mcardle@yale.edu
(J.R. McArdle).

0272-5231/07/$ - see front matter © 2007 Elsevier Inc. All rights reserved.
doi:10.1016/j.ccm.2007.08.006

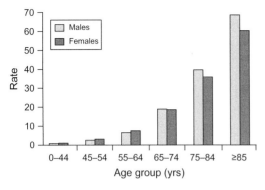

Fig. 1. Age-specific death rates among decedents with pulmonary hypertension as any contributing cause of death by sex and age group in the United States, 2000 to 2002. (*From* Hyduk A, Croft JB, Ayala C, et al. Pulmonary hypertension surveillance: United States 1980–2002. MMWR Surveill Summ 2005;54(5):1–28.)

(Fig. 2). The annual number of hospitalizations for PH tripled among Medicare enrollees 65 years of age and older from 1999 to 2002. The proportion of patients dying with PH who were 75 years of age or older increased from 1980 to 2002: 30.6% of all patients dying with PH from 2000 to 2002 were 75 to 84 years of age, and 18.1% were 85 years of age or older, compared with 23.7% and 6.5%, respectively, from 1980 to 1984. Although these statistics may reflect increased physician awareness and changes in diagnosis and reporting, the size of the database makes the observed trends reliable [4]. Further research is needed to answer the many questions that remain regarding the special features of unexplained PH in older patients [2]. Al-Shaer

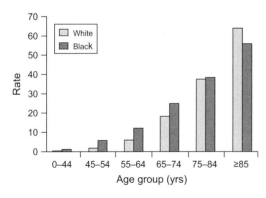

Fig. 2. Age-specific death rates among decedents with pulmonary hypertension as any contributing cause of death, by race and age group in the United States, 2000 to 2002. (*From* Hyduk A, Croft JB, Ayala C, et al. Pulmonary hypertension surveillance: United States 1980–2002. MMWR Surveill Summ 2005;54(5):1–28.)

and colleagues [10] have suggested that normal aging may result in global vascular dysfunction due to attenuation in endothelial nitric oxide (NO) synthase activity that may subject older adults to increased vulnerability to develop PH. Others have suggested similar age-related impairment of NO release and impaired endothelium dependent relaxation by acetylcholine in older patients [11,12]. In addition, spontaneous endothelial injury, possibly as a result of oxygen-derived free radicals and defective endothelial repair mechanisms, increases in older patients [13].

Classifying pulmonary hypertension in the older adults

In 2003, the World Health Organization (WHO) convened to a panel of world experts to develop a classification schema of PH to aid clinicians in their approach to patients who have elevated pulmonary artery pressures [14]. Although a large percentage of older adults have WHO group 2 (PVH) secondary to valvular heart disease, systolic heart failure, or diastolic heart failure, precise data on the breakdown of WHO-classified PH disease in older adults must be gleaned indirectly from existing reports.

WHO group I forms of pulmonary hypertension

Idiopathic pulmonary hypertension

Although IPAH has historically been reported most frequently in adults in the third and fourth decades of life [14–17], its diagnosis in older adults has been increasingly noted [2,18–20]. In the National Institutes of Health study of "primary" pulmonary hypertension, 9% of the registry was older than 60 years of age [17]. More recently, Humbert and colleagues [19] studied 674 adult patients from PH centers throughout France and found 25% of all cases presenting after the age of 60, with first diagnosis as late at 80 years of age. Nine percent of their population was older than 70 years at the time of diagnosis (Fig. 3). Shapiro and colleagues [2] recently reported that 24% of 197 patients retrospectively evaluated at the Mayo Clinic who had unexplained PH (IPAH) were 65 years or older and that the percentage of older patients was greater in the period from 1996 to 2003 than in earlier periods (1987–1995). They also observed that the mean age of patients who met clinical and hemodynamic criteria for IPAH was 48 years, which was greater than 10 years older than in a series

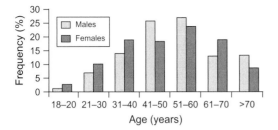

Fig. 3. Distribution of pulmonary hypertension by age based on sex. (*From* Humbert M, Sitbon O, Chaouat A, et al. Pulmonary arterial hypertension in France: results from a national registry. Am J Resp Crit Care Med 2006;173:1023–30; with permission. Copyright © 2006, American Thoracic Society.)

previously reported from the same institution from 1955 to 1977 [21]. Older patients had higher pulmonary capillary wedge pressures (PCWP) than did younger patients and more frequently failed to meet hemodynamic criteria of IPAH. This subset also had worse survival than the younger patients. The authors suggested that enhanced left ventricular interdependence along with increases in left ventricular free wall stiffness unique to the aging heart may result in elevated filling pressures in older patients who otherwise seem to have isolated pulmonary arteriopathy, raising the question as to whether new criteria should be adopted for PCWP cutoffs in the diagnosis of PAH in older adults [2]. These investigators did not include exercise provocation as a routine part of their algorithm in older patients, and as such the contribution of diastolic impairments could not be assessed. Taken together, these reports suggest that IPAH does not spare older adults and may be increasing in prevalence. A careful evaluation that includes right, and often left, heart catheterization is imperative in assessing older patients who have echocardiographically determined elevations of pulmonary systolic pressure.

Other forms of PAH encountered in older adults include connective tissue disease–associated PAH (CTAPAH), PAH associated with congenital heart disease (CHD), and portopulmonary-associated PAH (PPHTN). A less likely form of PAH seen in older adults is HIV-associated PAH, although this may change with the longer survival seen in the era of highly active antiretroviral therapy. Little data exist for anorexigen-induced PAH in older patients, although surveillance reports from France [22] and the United States [23] document cases of patients over the age of

60 with this form of PAH. Another WHO class I form of PAH rarely encountered in older adults is pulmonary veno-occlusive disease. This form of PH mimics IPAH in presentation and is usually diagnosed postmortem. Rarely, pulmonary capillary hemagiomatosis has been described in older patients [24].

Connective tissue associated pulmonary arterial hypertension

The prevalence of CTAPAH in those older than 60 years is unknown. However, a retrospective study of patients who had scleroderma found that increasing age at presentation was associated with a risk of PAH that was twice as high as those with younger age at onset of scleroderma [25]. When patients older than 60 years of age who had scleroderma were assessed, 56.7% developed PAH (Table 1) [25]. When age was viewed as a continuous variable, there was a 22% increase in risk for PAH development for every 10 years of age at disease onset [25]. This was not confounded by longer duration of disease nor by degree of restrictive lung disease as reflected by forced vital capacity. After adjusting for relevant confounders, the risk of PAH was more than twofold greater for patients diagnosed with scleroderma when they were older than 60 years compared with a diagnosis before age 60 [25]. Chang and colleagues [26] have also recently suggested that older age is a risk factor for PAH disease progression in systemic sclerosis. In another retrospective cross-sectional study of 619 patients who had scleroderma, the same investigators found that the presence of restrictive lung disease along with PAH was associated with

Table 1
Frequency of pulmonary arterial hypertension by decade of age at onset of scleroderma

Decade of life (years)	Patients, no.	Frequency of PAH, no. (%)
First (age <10)	4	1 (25.0)
Second (10–19)	40	9 (22.5)
Third (20–29)	108	38 (35.2)
Fourth (30–39)	164	57 (34.8)
Fifth (40–49)	188	70 (37.2)
Sixth (50–59)	123	54 (43.9)
Seventh (60–69)	60	34 (56.7)
Eighth (70–79)	22	11 (50)
Overall	709	274 (38.7)

From Schachna L, Wigley FM, Chang B, et al. Age and risk of pulmonary arterial hypertension in scleroderma. Chest 2003;124:2098–104; with permission.

a mortality risk ratio of 2.9 when compared with isolated restrictive lung disease alone [27]. Whether the age association accounts for the observed poor prognosis of scleroderma-associated PAH in general is unknown [28–30].

Congenital heart disease–associated pulmonary arterial hypertension

The presence of PAH in association with CHD defects persisting to adulthood is well recognized [7,31,32]. It is less clear why only some patients with similarly sized defects develop an arteriopathy resulting in PH. Theories include congestive arteriopathy on the basis of intercurrent left-sided heart disease [33], shear-stress injury from excessive blood flow over a long period of time, and hypoxia from right-to-left shunting as triggers in genetically predisposed persons [31,34]. Although the molecular biology of PAH development in CHD is unclear, evidence exists for overexuberant generation of endothelin-1 [35,36]. To this end, the literature suggests that anywhere from 6% to 15% of unrepaired atrial septal defects (ASDs) progress to PAH over time [34,37–40], with sinus venosus types more commonly progressing to PAH [40]. Much of this natural history data predate the era of surgical and, more recently, percutaneous closure of such defects early in life. In contrast, ventricular septal defects (VSDs) have been reported to progress to PAH in approximately 50% of cases [34], although this depends to some degree on the size of the defect [34,41]. Paradoxically, the murmur of VSDs is less easily detected on examination despite the larger the size of the defect [7,42,43].

Although the presence of persistent unrepaired septal defects has been associated with shorter life expectancy [37], many case reports exist of patients living into their 90s with such defects [44,45]. Great controversy exists about the advisability of closure in older patients [46]. Although many proponents for closure in patients not displaying Eisenmenger's physiology exist in the literature [39,47–57], these studies are limited by study size and design and differ greatly in populations enrolled, the number of subjects who have significant pulmonary hypertension, and the primary outcomes examined. Other researchers have concluded that outcome in adults who have ASDs was not improved by surgical closure [58–62]. Murphy and colleagues [60] followed a cohort of 123 patients who underwent surgical closure of ASDs and concluded that survival was significantly less in those older than 25 years.

Konstantinides and colleagues [52], while concluding that all-cause mortality was reduced by a surgical approach, caution that the incidence of new atrial arrhythmias and potentially new cerebrovascular insults required close postsurgical follow-up. The only prospective, randomized trial of 521 patients over the age of 40 showed no clear survival advantage for surgery versus medical management but showed statistically significant improvements in a composite end point that included death, pulmonary embolism, major arrhythmic events, embolic cerebral events, and recurrent pulmonary infections [63]. Many of these studies suggest that the most important factor in poor outcomes was the degree of PH at the time of surgery [31,39,47,52,53,56,57,60], although the definition of significant PH varied substantially in these studies, with mean pulmonary artery pressures from 40 mm Hg to 58 mm Hg [47,60], a systolic pulmonary artery pressure of greater than 70 [63], or a pulmonary vascular resistance cut-off of 5 to 15 Wood Units [39,56,57]. The implication of these therapies is unclear for older patients who have long-standing disease who may have difficulty tolerating and complying with infused prostanoid therapy.

Portopulmonary-associated pulmonary arterial hypertension

Although portopulmonary-associated PAH is occasionally encountered in older adults, this form of PAH is rarely an issue in persons of advanced age primarily because its onset is typically in the fifth decade and within 4 to 7 years of the diagnosis of portal hypertension [64]. Most patients die of complications of their disease before the age of 65. Kawut and colleagues [65] show substantially worse survival rates for patients who have PPHTN when compared with patients who have IPAH even after adjustment for age and ethnicity. In the pretransplant era, Robalino and Moodie [66] reported a mean and median survival for PPHTN of 15 and 6 months, respectively. Although response to therapy with prostanoid infusion can significantly lower mean pulmonary artery pressures and PVR, a minority of patients improve enough to undergo orthotopic liver transplantation [67].

WHO group II: pulmonary hypertension associated with left heart disease

Elevation of the pulmonary venous pressure due to impaired function of the left heart remains a common cause of elevated pulmonary artery pressure. Diseases of the mitral and aortic valves and abnormalities of systolic and diastolic function occur with increasing frequency with age, making the assessment of left heart pathology particularly important in patients with PH who are of advanced age. PVH should be considered especially likely in those with PH in the setting of left atrial (LA) enlargement, left ventricular hypertrophy (LVH), a history of atrial fibrillation or obesity [68]. This article focuses on several major contributors to pulmonary venous hypertension, with the exception of constrictive pericardial disease and infiltrative disorders.

Diastolic dysfunction

Congestive heart failure (CHF) occurs in the absence of overt systolic dysfunction in a close to half of patients hospitalized for CHF [69]. The terms "diastolic dysfunction" or "heart failure with normal ejection fraction" have been used to describe this syndrome, which is less well characterized in terms of pathophysiology and therapeutic alternatives when compared with systolic dysfunction [70,71].

Normal diastole is comprised of isovolumic relaxation time (IVRT), early diastolic filling, and the atrial phase of diastolic filling. IVRT is the time between aortic valve closure and mitral valve (MV) opening, is influenced by heart rate and afterload, and is proportional to the rate of ventricular relaxation [72]. In a healthy person, diastolic filling of the left ventricle occurs predominantly during early diastole (ie, during the period of ventricular relaxation), whereas the atrial phase of diastolic filling tends to account for a lesser amount of diastolic filling of the left ventricle [72]. Abnormalities in diastolic function may include impairments in ventricular relaxation, decreased ventricular compliance, or both [73]. Risk factors for abnormalities in the normal pattern of diastolic filling include advanced age, female gender, hypertension, coronary artery disease, and diabetes [74].

Characteristics of diastolic function are frequently detectable by echocardiography but require careful attention on the part of the echocardiographer. Alterations in E/A ratio and deceleration time (Fig. 4) can provide insight into abnormalities of diastolic function, but pseudonormalization of early diastolic filling occurs as left atrial pressure rises in moderate and severe diastolic dysfunction [72]. IVRT, the time between the end of flow in the left ventricular (LV) outflow tract to the beginning of LV diastolic inflow, is

lengthened in patients who have impaired relaxation and can be measured by simultaneous acquisition of velocities in the LV outflow and inflow tract [68]. The use of pulmonary venous flow characteristics and tissue Doppler analysis of the velocity of diastolic relaxation can improve the echocardiographic evaluation of diastolic function but may not be performed routinely at all centers [72].

PH can occur due to elevated left atrial pressures with resultant engorgement of the pulmonary veins in patients with diastolic dysfunction. Right heart catheterization in this setting generally reveals PH with an elevated PCWP and may also reveal a prominent V wave due to decreased left atrial compliance even in the absence of significant mitral regurgitation (MR) [75]. Although passive congestion is expected to result in PH with a normal pulmonary vascular resistance (PVR), a subset of patients who have CHF due to systolic, diastolic, or valvular abnormalities have an elevated PVR in the absence of a clear alternative explanation [76]. Such patients may continue to have elevated pulmonary artery pressures even after medical therapy has rendered a normal PCWP or after surgical correction of valvular lesions has been performed. Elevated endothelin-1 levels have been noted in patients who have chronic congestive heart failure, as have impaired NO-dependent relaxation, suggesting that endothelial dysfunction and possibly vasoconstriction and smooth muscle proliferation may occur [77].

Pulmonary arterial hypertension (WHO group I) may lead to abnormalities of LV diastolic function [68]. Pressure and volume overload in the right ventricle results in a leftward displacement of the intraventricular septum. This displacement results in flattening of the septum and impairment of septal motion from left to right during diastole. This may result in abnormalities of diastolic filling and a decrease in E/A ratio, mimicking LV diastolic dysfunction [78–81]. Decreases in LV compliance are also possible in this setting, although expansion of the LV free wall into the pericardial space may minimize changes in compliance in this setting [81]. Care must be taken to avoid the pitfall of ascribing elevated pulmonary pressures to LV diastolic dysfunction in this setting so that appropriate therapies are not withheld. Right heart catheterization remains the diagnostic test of choice unless overt pulmonary edema makes the correct diagnosis obvious.

The treatment of PH associated with diastolic dysfunction is not well characterized. Control of

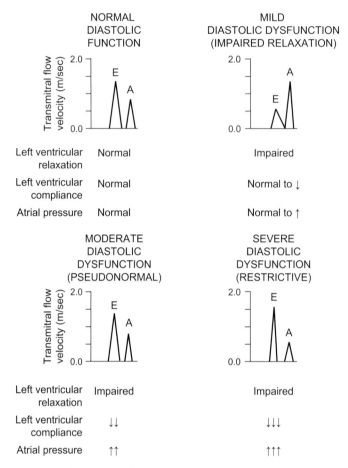

Fig. 4. Normal diastole is notable for an E/A ratio >1 in the setting of normal atrial pressure. Mild diastolic dysfunction is notable for reduced early diastolic filling of the left ventricle (LV) and pronounced increase in velocity associated with atrial contraction. In moderate and severe diastolic dysfunction, elevations in left atrial pressure normalize or elevate the E wave velocity (pseudo normalization). The former is attenuated with preload reducing maneuvers (Valsalva maneuver), whereas the latter is not (restrictive pattern). E, early phase of diastolic filling; A, atrial phase of diastolic filling. (*From* Aurigemma GP, Gaasch WH. Clinical practice: diastolic heart failure. N Engl J Med 2004;351: 1097–105; with permission. Copyright © 2004, Massachusetts Medical Society.)

volume status with judicious diuresis is considered one of the mainstays of therapy, although abnormal LV compliance predisposes such patients to pronounced underfilling if LA pressure is dropped too sharply, with resultant renal insufficiency and hypotension [82]. Beta blockers or calcium channel blockers may be used to control heart rate, allowing prolonged ventricular relaxation and preventing the deleterious effects of tachycardia on early diastolic filling [82]. Candesartan and valsartan have been investigated as therapies in patients who had heart failure with preserved ejection fraction, given that neurohumoral activation is felt to contribute to left ventricular hypertrophy and fibrosis [83,84]. In the CHARM study, 3023

patients who had CHF, NYHA Class II-IV symptoms, and LV ejection fraction (LVEF) >40% were randomized to the angiotensin receptor blocker candesartan or placebo. Although there was no significant difference in survival between the two groups at a median follow-up of 36.6 months, candesartan demonstrated a significant decrease in admissions for heart failure [84]. A similar study investigated the angiotensin receptor blocker valsartan as compared with placebo in patients who had hypertension and diastolic dysfunction. Both groups received additional antihypertensives not targeting the renin-angiotensin system to achieve similar levels of blood pressure control. Both groups had similar improvements in echocardiographic parameters, suggesting that control of systemic hypertension, as opposed to the effects on neurohumoral activation, may underlie the observed benefits [83].

The use of specific pulmonary vasodilators in patients who have diastolic heart failure has not been evaluated in a prospective fashion, and their use cannot be routinely recommended due to an absence of clinical data. Moreover, pulmonary vasodilation in the setting of elevated left atrial pressures and impaired atrial and ventricular compliance runs the risk of precipitating pulmonary edema [85,86].

Systolic dysfunction

PH may occur due to passive venous congestion in patients who have left ventricular systolic dysfunction. Abramson and colleagues [87], in long-term follow-up of 108 patients who had dilated cardiomyopathy (ischemic or idiopathic), demonstrated that patients who had PH as assessed by echocardiography (tricuspid regurgitant jet velocity >2.5 m/s) had markedly increased mortality as compared with patients who did not have PH (57% versus 17% at 28 months); furthermore, there was a threefold increase in the percentage of patients hospitalized for CHF.

Despite the association of systolic dysfunction with pulmonary hypertension, there is not a clear association between LVEF and the presence or absence of PH [75,88,89]. When evaluated noninvasively, PH in patients who have had dilated cardiomyopathy is independently associated with parameters of diastolic function, such as deceleration time [75,88,89], functional MR [89], and the peak velocities of forward pulmonary venous flow during systole [75,88]. The correlation with diastolic filling parameters suggests that patients who have diastolic dysfunction in the setting of systolic dysfunction are at greatest risk for developing PH. On interval follow-up of 100 patients who had systolic dysfunction before and after optimization of treatment, Dini and colleagues [88] found that improvements in PH were apparent only in subjects who had favorable changes in mitral inflow patterns on echocardiography, from restrictive or pseudo-normal pattern to the less severe impaired relaxation pattern of diastolic dysfunction. The association of impaired diastolic function with PH in patients who have impaired systolic function suggests that the excess mortality seen by Abrahamson and colleagues [87] may relate to the coexistence of systolic and diastolic abnormalities in the same patient.

The mainstay of therapy for PH associated with systolic dysfunction is optimization of therapy for the patient's underlying cardiomyopathy, the discussion of which is beyond the scope of this article. The use of traditional PAH therapies in patients who have systolic dysfunction has been met with disappointing results. The Flolan International Randomized Survival Trial evaluated the effects of epoprostenol versus standard care on survival in 471 patients who had decreased ejection fraction and advanced symptomatic heart failure [85]. Secondary endpoints included CHF symptoms, 6-minute walk distance, quality of life measures, and clinical events. The trial was terminated early due to a trend toward excess mortality in the epoprostenol group despite improvements in symptoms and hemodynamic parameters [85].

Bosentan has been studied in two randomized, placebo-controlled trials in patients who had systolic dysfunction and advanced heart failure symptoms. The ENABLE trial enrolled 1613 patients who had advanced CHF and LVEF <35% and randomized them to usual care plus placebo or bosentan with the primary endpoint being a composite of all-cause mortality and hospitalization for CHF. The primary endpoint in this study was not met [90]. The REACH-1 study enrolled 370 patients who had severe symptomatic heart failure with depressed ejection fraction [91]. Patients were randomized to placebo versus slow or rapid titration of bosentan to a dose of 500 mg daily. Patients receiving bosentan were more likely to have heart failure during the first month of treatment but a decreased risk of heart failure in the fourth, fifth, and sixth months of therapy. Treatment with bosentan was terminated early due to safety concerns, so no conclusion about the possible late benefits could be drawn [91].

Sildenafil has not been studied in an ongoing prospective fashion in patients who have CHF and depressed ejection fraction. Bocchi and colleagues [92] performed a prospective, randomized, crossover, single-dose trial of sildenafil in patients who had erectile dysfunction and heart failure. Sildenafil improved maximal exercise capacity as measured by cardiopulmonary exercise test in this population [92]. In an acute hemodynamic study, oral sildenafil, inhaled NO, or both were given to 11 patients who had LV systolic dysfunction and PH. Sildenafil decreased mean pulmonary artery pressure, PCWP, PVR, and systemic vascular resistance while increasing cardiac output [93]. The effects were more pronounced when combined with NO [93]. Although neither of these studies rises to a level of evidence allowing a recommendation of sildenafil in patients who have LV systolic dysfunction, they provide grounds for hypothesis generation.

Mitral valve disease

Mitral stenosis (MS) is a slowly progressive process that results in gradual leaflet thickening, commissural and chordal fusion, and calcification [94]. Impaired pulmonary venous outflow may lead to severe pulmonary congestion, PH, exercise intolerance, and death. Given the slow progression of this disorder (typically over decades), a substantial number of patients who have severe MS are older [94]. The presence of PH in patients who have MS is associated with decreased survival and worsened exercise tolerance [95]. The most common method for evaluating the severity of MS echocardiographically is the pressure half-time method, which relies on the relationship between pressure decay and orifice size of the stenotic valve [96]. Transesophageal echocardiography may be required for optimal evaluation of the hemodynamic characteristics in patients who have MS [94]. There exists substantial variability between the measured MV area (MVA) and the degree of PH in patients who have MS [97]. Ha and colleagues [97] performed right heart and transseptal catheterization in 113 patients who had rheumatic MS, all of whom were in sinus rhythm. Of this group, the presence of a large atrial V wave in the absence of concomitant MR was significantly associated with the presence of PH, as was an elevated mean mitral gradient. The V wave is a reflection of changes in atrial pressure brought on by atrial filling during ventricular systole. In the absence of MR, a large V wave is reflective of impaired atrial compliance [97]. Schwammenthal and colleagues [96] found an association between low atrioventricular compliance and the development of PH with rest and exercise. The authors conclude that MVA may be overestimated in patients who have low atrial compliance due to changes in the pressure half-time brought on by altered atrial distensibility.

Given the relationship between PH and worsened outcome in MS, its presence is a consideration when determining the therapeutic approach, irrespective of the presence of symptoms. Patients who do not have symptoms but have pulmonary artery systolic pressure (PASP) >50 mm Hg are considered to have a Class I indication for percutaneous intervention when MVA is <1.5 cm^2 according to the American College of Cardiology/American Heart Association 2006 practice guidelines [94]. Exercise echocardiography may unmask severe PH with exercise, considered a marker of more severe disease and an indication for intervention whether MVA is <1.5 cm^2 (Class I indication) or >1.5 cm^2 (Class IIb indication) [94,98]. A variety of procedures is available to treat MS. Valve replacement is generally reserved for symptomatic patients who have heavily calcified valves and restricted leaflet mobility. In patients who have less severely calcified, more pliable valves and in the absence of significant concomitant MR, percutaneous mitral balloon valvotomy is the most commonly performed procedure [94,99]. Fawzy and colleagues [100] has presented his experience with percutaneous mitral balloon valvotomy in 559 patients who had severe MS (Fig. 5). He demonstrated substantial improvements in PH, with normalization of PH over 6 to 12 months even in patients who had PASP >80 mm Hg at baseline.

MR is a common finding in adult patients [94]. There are a variety of underlying causes for MR,

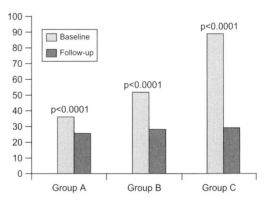

Fig. 5. Impact of mitral valvotomy in patients who have mitral stenosis and pulmonary hypertension. Baseline and 12-month follow-up pulmonary artery systolic pressure (PASP) in patients undergoing balloon valvotomy. Group A (n = 345) had mild pulmonary hypertension (PH) at baseline (defined as PASP <50 mm Hg), Group B (n = 183) had moderate PH at baseline (PASP 50–79 mm Hg), and Group C (n = 31) had severe PH at baseline (PASP >80 mm Hg). Postoperative PASP was similar in all three groups and significantly reduced from baseline. (*From* Fawzy ME. Percutaneous mitral balloon valvotomy. Catheterization Cardiovasc Inter 2007;69:313–21; with permission. Copyright © 2007. Reprinted with permission of Wiley-Liss, Inc., a subsidary of John Wiley & Sons, Inc.)

including myxomatous degeneration, rheumatic valvular disease, ischemia, rupture of chorda tendinae, and infectious endocarditis, many of which are more likely to be present with advancing age [94,101]. The Framingham Heart Study notes that the prevalence of MR increases 1.3-fold with each decade of life [101]. Significant MR leads to increased preload given the regurgitation of a substantial volume of blood into the left atrium during ventricular systole and decreased afterload due to the ejection of blood into the lower pressure left atrium and pulmonary veins. The presence of decreased LV afterload and increased LV preload can lead to an overestimation of the adequacy of LV systolic function.

Pulmonary hypertension complicating MR is associated with increased symptoms and shortened survival and is a factor favoring surgical rather than medical therapy in asymptomatic patients who have MR [94,102]. Advanced age (> 75 years) is associated with a higher mortality; overall operative mortality is 14% for MV replacement in this population. MV repair reduces these risks and should be preferred in this population if feasible [94]. Preoperative PH in patients who have MR generally improves postoperatively [103,104], although its presence is associated with worsened LV systolic function postoperatively [105]. Severe PH and marked elevations in PVR define a high-risk group with substantial surgical mortality, although patients who survive surgery generally have significant reductions in PH over time [103,104,106]. Salzberg and colleagues [107] reported a series of 14 patients who had severe MR undergoing MV surgery (repair or replacement) treated preoperatively with nesiritide, resulting in reductions of pulmonary artery pressures, PCWP, and central venous pressure before surgery. The surgical mortality in this group was 0%, raising the possibility that nesiritide may help optimize the PH patient who has severe MR for surgery.

There are little data to guide the appropriate therapy in patients who have persistent severe PH with elevated PVR post mitral valvotomy, commisurotomy, repair or replacement for MS, or MR. For patients who have no evidence of CHF or elevated PCWP with exercise provocation, specific pulmonary vasodilator therapy may be warranted.

Aortic stenosis

PH most frequently complicates aortic stenosis in the presence of coexisting MV disease or depressed LV systolic function [108]. Aragam and colleagues [109] evaluated operative outcome in 74 men undergoing aortic valve replacement (AVR). Patients were divided into groups based on preoperative systolic PA pressure. Normal (≤ 30 mm Hg), mild (31–49 mm Hg), and severe (≥ 50 mm Hg) groups were evaluated separately. Overall, 58% of patients had PH using these definitions, and 22% had severe elevations in PA systolic pressure. The degree of PH did not correlate well with aortic valve area or with LVEF; rather, the closest correlation was with LV end diastolic pressure. Operative mortality did not differ between the three groups and was 5% overall [109]. Malouf and colleagues [110] reported outcomes of 47 patients who had severe AS, a mean age of 78 years, and severe PH. Thirty-seven patients underwent AVR, and 10 were managed medically. Those who underwent AVR had a lower LVEF (39% versus 56%); furthermore, there was a higher proportion of patients who had NYHA Class III or IV symptoms and a lower percentage of patients who had systemic hypertension before surgery. Although perioperative mortality was high (16%), PASP was significantly reduced, functional class improved, and long-term follow-up of a median of 460 days revealed 29% mortality in patients undergoing AVR as compared with 80% in patients managed medically [110]. These data suggest that PH may increase the risk of AVR, but the results seem to be favorable when compared with conservative management.

WHO group III: pulmonary hypertension associated with disorders of the respiratory system or hypoxemia

Many older patients have PH associated with disorders of respiration or hypoxemia. These include COPD, sleep apnea, chronic exposure to high altitude, kyphoscoliosis, and ILD. Although many reports link the presence of PH in these settings to worse survival [111–115], it is unclear whether PH is an independent predictor of survival or a reflection of underlying disease severity. In a population of patients who had COPD and ILD (mean age, 52 years) who were carefully assessed by echocardiography and concomitant right heart catheterization, echocardiography proved inaccurate: 48% of patients were misclassified as having PH [116]. Given the preponderance of valvular heart disease, systolic heart failure, and diastolic dysfunction in older patients, caution about relying on echocardiography must be emphasized even more. Treatment of patients who have these forms of associated PH is controversial. Anecdotal suggestions of successful acute treatment in older patients who have IPF without worsened ventilation-perfusion matching exist in the literature [117–119]. No randomized controlled trials of PH-specific therapy in COPD-associated PH have been performed, making evidence-based recommendations in this large cohort of older patients impossible.

The prevalence of sleep apnea in older adults is generally believed to be increased [120–125]. Little data exist addressing specifically the incidence or prevalence of PH associated with sleep-disordered breathing in older adults or its impact on mortality. This represents an area for future study. When overall rates of PH in obstructive sleep apnea are examined, PH is present in 17% to 20% of patients who have obstructive sleep apnea and is usually of mild to moderate severity, with mean PAP usually less than 30 mm Hg [126]. It is more likely to occur in the setting of more severe apnea index and hypoxemia and in patients who have other comorbidities, such as COPD, ILD, or obesity-hypoventilation syndrome [126].

WHO group IV: pulmonary hypertension due to chronic thrombotic or embolic disease

The incidence of chronic thromboembolic pulmonary hypertension (CTEPH) after recognized or occult acute pulmonary embolism is is reported to be 0.1% to as high as 3.8% [127–130], usually diagnosed within the first 2 years of the acute event [129]. Although precise data regarding incidence or prevalence rates in older patients are lacking, this is clearly a form of PH encountered in older patients [130]. In the most recent studies of CTEPH development, the mean age of the populations studied was older than 60 years [127–129]. Risk factors that have been proposed for the development of CTEPH include abnormal fibrinolysis due to genetic defects in fibrin side chain sialation [131,132] and prior splenectomy [133], which may predispose the pulmonary vascular bed to senescent red cells and surface phosphatidylserine with activation of the coagulation process [134,135]. It is crucial to consider the possibility of CTEPH in old and young patients because it is the only surgically curable form of PH. Although some reports suggest that patient age is a preoperative risk factor for in hospital mortality postpulmonary thromboendartectomy

(PEA) [136], advanced age alone should not be considered an absolute contraindication for PEA [137]. In patients who are not operative candidates for PEA, the role of medical therapy is uncertain, although small, uncontrolled series suggesting short-term benefits from prostanoids, sildenafil, and bosentan exist in the literature [138].

Other forms of emboli can rarely cause PH in older patients and need to enter into the differential diagnosis of CTEPH. Pulmonary artery sarcomas, which can present identically to CTEPH, are rare tumors of the pulmonary vascular bed, and distinction preoperatively alters the surgical approach [139]. Tumor emboli to the proximal pulmonary vascular bed [140] or distal to the pulmonary arteriolar bed leading to PH have been reported in a number of case reports in the literature in older patients [141–143]. These presentations of PH are rarely diagnosed premortem [144]. Another rare form of PH from vascular luminal occlusion is schistosomiasis in endemic areas [14].

Miscellaneous causes of pulmonary hypertension in older adults

Although a comprehensive list of all the rare associations of PH that exist in the literature is beyond the scope of this article, a number of associations encountered in older adults are worth noting. These include vascular involvement from diffuse amyloidosis [145], PH arising from chemotherapy with attendant microangiopathic hemolytic anemia and pulmonary veno-occlusive disease [146], and PH developing in patients who have agnogenic myeloid metaplasia or other forms of myeloid fibrosis [147–150]. In some presentations of the latter, it seems that extramedullary hematopoiesis may be occurring in the lungs of some of these patients and that low-dose radiation therapy may help mitigate the concomitant PH [151,152]. Finally, high-output states acquired through surgically created arterio-venous fistulae may present with significant PH [153,154]. These unusual presentations of PH underscore the need for keeping an open mind and a broad differential when approaching the older patient who has unexplained dyspnea or echocardiographically determined PH.

Special considerations in treating the older patient who has pulmonary hypertension

Once the diagnosis of PAH has been confirmed, a cautious assessment and thorough discussion between the patient and the physician should occur. The physician should keep in mind the patient's comorbidities, concomitant medications, sensory limitations, cognitive abilities, safety, financial resources, and emotional support.

With PAH on the rise in this population [2–4], treatment with the six current FDA-approved therapies (bosentan, sildenafil, ambrisentan, iloprost, treprostinil, and epoprostenol) presents interesting challenges to the clinician and the patient. Until recently, many clinical drug trials for PH did not include healthy volunteers or patients whose age was over 75 years [155]. Only sildenafil was studied in healthy volunteers over the age of 65 years, but even that study did not include a sufficient number of volunteers to determine whether older patients have a different response than their younger counterparts [156,157]. It was noted that these healthy older volunteers had a reduced clearance of sildenafil, with a 40% greater increase in free plasma concentrations than in younger volunteers [156,157]. The potential age-related pharmacokinetic changes of the other PAH medications is unknown.

The easiest therapies to use, for all ages, are the oral agents bosentan, sildenafil, and ambrisentan. Once this therapeutic approach is chosen, the clinician should carefully review the patient's list of medications. Drug–drug interactions with potentially harmful side effects (eg, sildenafil and nitrates [156,157] and bosentan and glyburide [158]) have been identified when oral therapy is prescribed in conjunction with certain medications. If feasible, choosing the oral agent that does not interact with the other medications is advised; however, if a certain agent must be selected, it is imperative that the patient understand the changes that might be required in his or her medication list.

The other available therapies, the prostacyclin analogs, are the most complex and present special challenges for the older patient who has PAH. These therapies are delivered via ambulatory infusion pumps through central lines, subcutaneously under the skin, or via a special inhalation device. These medications must be meticulously prepared and infused to avoid potential life-threatening side effects. Special attention to sterility is imperative to minimize the risk of line sepsis. A care partner should be educated in the use and preparation of these medications in the event that the older patient becomes unable. The clinician should recognize the challenge that these medications pose on this population. Many older patients have impaired vision, thus making it difficult to read the vials of medications or the amount to draw up in a syringe or to program the infusion pump.

Patients who have arthritic hands, malformations from rheumatoid arthritis, or difficulty with hand grasp and mobility related to scleroderma may have logistical problems complying with these complex medical regimes. All of these factors must be taken into account before deciding the advisability of PAH-specific therapy in any patient.

Summary

PH is a disorder with multiple underlying etiologies. As the age of the United States population and awareness of this disease increase, PH will likely continue to be a more frequent diagnosis. Although left-sided heart disease is more prevalent with advancing age and is likely causative in many of the older patients referred for PH evaluation, all WHO Groups are represented in older adults, and their evaluation should be as rigorous and thoughtful as that in younger patients who have PH.

Careful consideration should be given to percutaneous or even surgical interventions to address structural cardiac lesions (whether congenital or acquired) because significant regression of the PH may be seen with correction of the underlying cause. Patients should be carefully evaluated for diastolic cardiac dysfunction, and full advantage should be taken of the capabilities provided by echocardiography, including measurement of IVRT, tissue Doppler assessment of relaxation, and morphology of E and A waves. Diastolic dysfunction in isolation or in combination with systolic or valvular disease is an important contributor to PH in older patients.

Although some data exist on the use of pulmonary vasodilator therapy in older patients, these agents should be considered only in carefully selected patients after a thorough evaluation of the underlying mechanism for their PH. Special considerations in older patients relate to the ability to operate the infusion pumps, the ability to care for indwelling catheters, and the presence of medical comorbidities.

References

[1] Lilienfeld DE, Rubin LJ. Mortality from primary pulmonary hypertension in the United States, 1979–1996. Chest 2000;117(3):796–800.

[2] Shapiro BP, McGoon MD, Redfield MM. Unexplained pulmonary hypertension in elderly patients. Chest 2007;131(1):94–100.

[3] Hyduk A, Croft JB, Ayala C, et al. Pulmonary hypertension surveillance: United States, 1980–2002. MMWR Surveill Summ 2005;54(5):1–28.

[4] Rich S. How do we explain unexplained pulmonary hypertension in the elderly? Chest 2007;131(1):5–6.

[5] Rich S, Chomka E, Hasara L, et al. The prevalence of pulmonary hypertension in the United States: adult population estimates obtained from measurements of chest roentgenograms from the NHANES II Survey. Chest 1989;96(2):236–41.

[6] McGoon M, Gutterman D, Steen V, et al. Screening, early detection, and diagnosis of pulmonary arterial hypertension: ACCP evidence-based clinical practice guidelines. Chest 2004;126(1 Suppl): 14S–34S.

[7] Trow TK, McArdle JR. Diagnosis of pulmonary arterial hypertension. Clin Chest Med 2007;28(1): 59–73, viii.

[8] Crausman RS, Lewin JM. Pulmonary arterial hypertension in nonagenarians. J Am Geriatr Soc 1995;43(10):1177.

[9] Algeo S, Morrison D, Ovitt T, et al. Noninvasive detection of pulmonary hypertension. Clin Cardiol 1984;7(3):148–56.

[10] Al-Shaer MH, Choueiri NE, Correia ML, et al. Effects of aging and atherosclerosis on endothelial and vascular smooth muscle function in humans. Int J Cardiol 2006;109(2):201–6.

[11] Marin J, Rodriguez-Martinez MA. Age-related changes in vascular responses. Exp Gerontol 1999;34(4):503–12.

[12] Moreau P, d'Uscio LV, Luscher TF. Structure and reactivity of small arteries in aging. Cardiovasc Res 1998;37(1):247–53.

[13] Ames BN, Shigenaga MK, Hagen TM. Oxidants, antioxidants, and the degenerative diseases of aging. Proc Natl Acad Sci U S A 1993;90(17):7915–22.

[14] Simonneau G, Galie N, Rubin LJ, et al. Clinical classification of pulmonary hypertension. J Am Coll Cardiol 2004;43(12 Suppl S):5S–12S.

[15] Appelbaum L, Yigla M, Bendayan D, et al. Primary pulmonary hypertension in Israel: a national survey. Chest 2001;119(6):1801–6.

[16] Dantzker DR. Primary pulmonary hypertension: the American experience. Chest 1994;105(2 Suppl):26S–8S.

[17] Rich S, Dantzker DR, Ayres SM, et al. Primary pulmonary hypertension: a national prospective study. Ann Intern Med 1987;107(2):216–23.

[18] Braman SS, Eby E, Kuhn C, et al. Primary pulmonary hypertension in the elderly. Arch Intern Med 1991;151(12):2433–8.

[19] Humbert M, Sitbon O, Chaouat A, et al. Pulmonary arterial hypertension in France: results from a national registry. Am J Respir Crit Care Med 2006;173(9):1023–30.

[20] Phipps B, Wong B, Chang CH, et al. Unexplained severe pulmonary hypertension in the older age group. Chest 1983;84(4):399–402.

[21] Fuster V, Steele PM, Edwards WD, et al. Primary pulmonary hypertension: natural history and the importance of thrombosis. Circulation 1984;70(4): 580–7.

[22] Simonneau G, Fartoukh M, Sitbon O, et al. Primary pulmonary hypertension associated with the use of fenfluramine derivatives. Chest 1998;114(3 Suppl):195S–9S.

[23] Rich S, Rubin L, Walker AM, et al. Anorexigens and pulmonary hypertension in the United States: results from the surveillance of North American pulmonary hypertension. Chest 2000;117(3):870–4.

[24] Cioffi U, De Simone M, Pavoni G, et al. Pulmonary capillary hemangiomatosis in an asymptomatic elderly patient. Int Surg 1999;84(2):168–70.

[25] Schachna L, Wigley FM, Chang B, et al. Age and risk of pulmonary arterial hypertension in scleroderma. Chest 2003;124(6):2098–104.

[26] Chang B, Schachna L, White B, et al. Natural history of mild-moderate pulmonary hypertension and the risk factors for severe pulmonary hypertension in scleroderma. J Rheumatol 2006;33(2): 269–74.

[27] Chang B, Wigley FM, White B, et al. Scleroderma patients with combined pulmonary hypertension and interstitial lung disease. J Rheumatol 2003; 30(11):2398–405.

[28] Kawut SM, Taichman DB, Archer-Chicko CL, et al. Hemodynamics and survival in patients with pulmonary arterial hypertension related to systemic sclerosis. Chest 2003;123(2):344–50.

[29] Koh ET, Lee P, Gladman DD, et al. Pulmonary hypertension in systemic sclerosis: an analysis of 17 patients. Br J Rheumatol 1996;35(10):989–93.

[30] MacGregor AJ, Canavan R, Knight C, et al. Pulmonary hypertension in systemic sclerosis: risk factors for progression and consequences for survival. Rheumatology (Oxford) 2001;40(4): 453–9.

[31] Webb G, Gatzoulis MA. Atrial septal defects in the adult: recent progress and overview. Circulation 2006;114(15):1645–53.

[32] Barst RJ, McGoon M, Torbicki A, et al. Diagnosis and differential assessment of pulmonary arterial hypertension. J Am Coll Cardiol 2004;43(12 Suppl S):40S–7S.

[33] Sanders C, Bittner V, Nath PH, et al. Atrial septal defect in older adults: atypical radiographic appearances. Radiology 1988;167(1):123–7.

[34] Vongpatanasin W, Brickner ME, Hillis LD, et al. The Eisenmenger syndrome in adults. Ann Intern Med 1998;128(9):745–55.

[35] Cacoub P, Dorent R, Maistre G, et al. Endothelin-1 in primary pulmonary hypertension and the Eisenmenger syndrome. Am J Cardiol 1993;71(5): 448–50.

[36] Yoshibayashi M, Nishioka K, Nakao K, et al. Plasma endothelin concentrations in patients with pulmonary hypertension associated with congenital heart defects: evidence for increased production of endothelin in pulmonary circulation. Circulation 1991;84(6):2280–5.

[37] Campbell M. Natural history of atrial septal defect. Br Heart J 1970;32(6):820–6.

[38] Craig RJ, Selzer A. Natural history and prognosis of atrial septal defect. Circulation 1968;37(5):805–15.

[39] Steele PM, Fuster V, Cohen M, et al. Isolated atrial septal defect with pulmonary vascular obstructive disease: long-term follow-up and prediction of outcome after surgical correction. Circulation 1987;76(5):1037–42.

[40] Vogel M, Berger F, Kramer A, et al. Incidence of secondary pulmonary hypertension in adults with atrial septal or sinus venosus defects. Heart 1999; 82(1):30–3.

[41] Kidd L, Driscoll DJ, Gersony WM, et al. Second natural history study of congenital heart defects: results of treatment of patients with ventricular septal defects. Circulation 1993;87(2 Suppl):I38–51.

[42] Leatham A, Segal B. Auscultatory and phonocardiographic signs of ventricular septal defect with left to-right shunt. Circulation 1962;25:318–27.

[43] Newburger JW, Rosenthal A, Williams RG, et al. Noninvasive tests in the initial evaluation of heart murmurs in children. N Engl J Med 1983;308(2): 61–4.

[44] Landi F, Cipriani L, Cocchi A, et al. Ostium secundum atrial septal defect in the elderly. J Am Geriatr Soc 1991;39(1):60–3.

[45] Tikoff G, Wilson JF. Atrial septal defect in a nonagenarian. Chest 1970;58(6):628–30.

[46] Borow KM, Karp R. Atrial septal defect: lessons from the past, directions for the future. N Engl J Med 1990;323(24):1698–700.

[47] Breyer RH, Monson DO, Ruggie NT, et al. Atrial septal defect: repair in patients over thirty-five years of age. J Cardiovasc Surg (Torino) 1979; 20(6):583–6.

[48] de Lezo JS, Medina A, Romero M, et al. Effectiveness of percutaneous device occlusion for atrial septal defect in adult patients with pulmonary hypertension. Am Heart J 2002;144(5):877–80.

[49] Hairston P, Parker EF, Arrants JE, et al. The adult atrial septal defect: results of surgical repair. Ann Surg 1974;179(5):799–804.

[50] Horvath KA, Burke RP, Collins JJ Jr, et al. Surgical treatment of adult atrial septal defect: early and long-term results. J Am Coll Cardiol 1992;20(5): 1156–9.

[51] John Sutton MG, Tajik AJ, McGoon DC. Atrial septal defect in patients ages 60 years or older: operative results and long-term postoperative follow-up. Circulation 1981;64(2):402–9.

[52] Konstantinides S, Geibel A, Olschewski M, et al. A comparison of surgical and medical therapy for atrial septal defect in adults. N Engl J Med 1995; 333(8):469–73.

[53] Mattila S, Merikallio E, Tala P. ASD in patients over 40 years of age. Scand J Thorac Cardiovasc Surg 1979;13(1):21–4.

[54] Miyaji K, Furuse A, Tanaka O, et al. Surgical repair for atrial septal defect in patients over 70 years of age. Jpn Heart J 1997;38(5):677–84.

[55] Nasrallah AT, Hall RJ, Garcia E, et al. Surgical repair of atrial septal defect in patients over 60 years of age: long-term results. Circulation 1976; 53(2):329–31.

[56] Paolillo V, Dawkins KD, Miller GA. Atrial septal defect in patients over the age of 50. Int J Cardiol 1985;9(2):139–47.

[57] Reed WA, Dunn MI. Long-term results of repair of atrial septal defects. Am J Surg 1971;121(6):724–7.

[58] Cohn LH, Morrow AG, Braunwald E. Operative treatment of atrial septal defect: clinical and haemodynamic assessments in 175 patients. Br Heart J 1967;29(5):725–34.

[59] Magilligan DJ Jr, Lam CR, Lewis JW Jr, et al. Late results of atrial septal defect repair in adults. Arch Surg 1978;113(11):1245–7.

[60] Murphy JG, Gersh BJ, McGoon MD, et al. Long-term outcome after surgical repair of isolated atrial septal defect: follow-up at 27 to 32 years. N Engl J Med 1990;323(24):1645–50.

[61] Shah D, Azhar M, Oakley CM, et al. Natural history of secundum atrial septal defect in adults after medical or surgical treatment: a historical prospective study. Br Heart J 1994;71(3):224–7 [discussion: 228].

[62] Ward C. Secundum atrial septal defect: routine surgical treatment is not of proven benefit. Br Heart J 1994;71(3):219–23.

[63] Attie F, Rosas M, Granados N, et al. Surgical treatment for secundum atrial septal defects in patients >40 years old: a randomized clinical trial. J Am Coll Cardiol 2001;38(7):2035–42.

[64] Golbin JM, Krowka MJ. Portopulmonary hypertension. Clin Chest Med 2007;28(1):203–18, ix.

[65] Kawut SM, Taichman DB, Ahya VN, et al. Hemodynamics and survival of patients with portopulmonary hypertension. Liver Transpl 2005;11(9): 1107–11.

[66] Robalino BD, Moodie DS. Association between primary pulmonary hypertension and portal hypertension: analysis of its pathophysiology and clinical, laboratory and hemodynamic manifestations. J Am Coll Cardiol 1991;17(2):492–8.

[67] Fix OK, Bass NM, De Marco T, et al. Long-term follow-up of portopulmonary hypertension: effect of treatment with epoprostenol. Liver Transpl 2007;13(6):875–85.

[68] Shapiro BP, Nishimura RA, McGoon MD, et al. Diagnostic dilemmas: diastolic heart failure causing pulmonary hypertension and pulmonary hypertension causing diastolic dysfunction. Advances in Pulmonary Hypertension 2006;5:13–20.

[69] Owan TE, Hodge DO, Herges RM, et al. Trends in prevalence and outcome of heart failure with preserved ejection fraction. N Engl J Med 2006; 355(3):251–9.

[70] Vasan RS, Levy D. Defining diastolic heart failure: a call for standardized diagnostic criteria. Circulation 2000;101(17):2118–21.

[71] Zile MR, Gaasch WH, Carroll JD, et al. Heart failure with a normal ejection fraction: is measurement of diastolic function necessary to make the diagnosis of diastolic heart failure? Circulation 2001;104(7):779–82.

[72] Garcia MJ, Thomas JD, Klein AL. New Doppler echocardiographic applications for the study of diastolic function. J Am Coll Cardiol 1998;32(4): 865–75.

[73] Zile MR, Baicu CF, Gaasch WH. Diastolic heart failure: abnormalities in active relaxation and passive stiffness of the left ventricle. N Engl J Med 2004;350(19):1953–9.

[74] Owan TE, Redfield MM. Epidemiology of diastolic heart failure. Prog Cardiovasc Dis 2005;47(5): 320–32.

[75] Capomolla S, Febo O, Guazzotti G, et al. Invasive and non-invasive determinants of pulmonary hypertension in patients with chronic heart failure. J Heart Lung Transplant 2000;19(5):426–38.

[76] Benza RL, Tallaj JA. Pulmonary hypertension out of proportion to left heart disease. Advances in Pulmonary Hypertension 2006;5:21–9.

[77] Moraes DL, Colucci WS, Givertz MM. Secondary pulmonary hypertension in chronic heart failure: the role of the endothelium in pathophysiology and management. Circulation 2000;102(14): 1718–23.

[78] Louie EK, Rich S, Brundage BH. Doppler echocardiographic assessment of impaired left ventricular filling in patients with right ventricular pressure overload due to primary pulmonary hypertension. J Am Coll Cardiol 1986;8(6):1298–306.

[79] Stojnic BB, Brecker SJ, Xiao HB, et al. Left ventricular filling characteristics in pulmonary hypertension: a new mode of ventricular interaction. Br Heart J 1992;68(1):16–20.

[80] Tutar E, Kaya A, Gulec S, et al. Echocardiographic evaluation of left ventricular diastolic function in chronic cor pulmonale. Am J Cardiol 1999;83(9): 1414–7.

[81] Little WC, Badke FR, O'Rourke RA. Effect of right ventricular pressure on the end-diastolic left ventricular pressure-volume relationship before and after chronic right ventricular pressure overload in dogs without pericardia. Circ Res 1984; 54(6):719–30.

[82] Aurigemma GP, Gaasch WH. Clinical practice: diastolic heart failure. N Engl J Med 2004; 351(11):1097–105.

[83] Solomon SD, Janardhanan R, Verma A, et al. Effect of angiotensin receptor blockade and antihypertensive drugs on diastolic function in patients with hypertension and diastolic dysfunction: a randomised trial. Lancet 2007;369(9579): 2079–87.

[84] Yusuf S, Pfeffer MA, Swedberg K, et al. Effects of candesartan in patients with chronic heart failure and preserved left-ventricular ejection fraction: the CHARM-Preserved Trial. Lancet 2003; 362(9386):777–81.

[85] Califf RM, Adams KF, McKenna WJ, et al. A randomized controlled trial of epoprostenol therapy for severe congestive heart failure: the Flolan International Randomized Survival Trial (FIRST). Am Heart J 1997;134(1):44–54.

[86] Farber HW, Graven KK, Kokolski G, et al. Pulmonary edema during acute infusion of epoprostenol in a patient with pulmonary hypertension and limited scleroderma. J Rheumatol 1999;26(5): 1195–6.

[87] Abramson SV, Burke JF, Kelly JJ Jr, et al. Pulmonary hypertension predicts mortality and morbidity in patients with dilated cardiomyopathy. Ann Intern Med 1992;116(11):888–95.

[88] Dini FL, Nuti R, Barsotti L, et al. Doppler-derived mitral and pulmonary venous flow variables are predictors of pulmonary hypertension in dilated cardiomyopathy. Echocardiography 2002;19(6): 457–65.

[89] Enriquez-Sarano M, Rossi A, Seward JB, et al. Determinants of pulmonary hypertension in left ventricular dysfunction. J Am Coll Cardiol 1997; 29(1):153–9.

[90] Teerlink JR. Recent heart failure trials of neurohormonal modulation (OVERTURE and ENABLE): approaching the asymptote of efficacy? J Card Fail 2002;8(3):124–7.

[91] Packer M, McMurray J, Massie BM, et al. Clinical effects of endothelin receptor antagonism with bosentan in patients with severe chronic heart failure: results of a pilot study. J Card Fail 2005; 11(1):12–20.

[92] Bocchi EA, Guimaraes G, Mocelin A, et al. Sildenafil effects on exercise, neurohormonal activation, and erectile dysfunction in congestive heart failure: a double-blind, placebo-controlled, randomized study followed by a prospective treatment for erectile dysfunction. Circulation 2002;106(9):1097–103.

[93] Lepore JJ, Maroo A, Bigatello LM, et al. Hemodynamic effects of sildenafil in patients with congestive heart failure and pulmonary hypertension: combined administration with inhaled nitric oxide. Chest 2005;127(5):1647–53.

[94] Bonow RO, Carabello BA, Kanu C, et al. ACC/ AHA 2006 guidelines for the management of patients with valvular heart disease: a report of the American College of Cardiology/American Heart Association Task Force on Practice Guidelines (writing committee to revise the 1998 Guidelines for the Management of Patients With Valvular

Heart Disease). Developed in collaboration with the Society of Cardiovascular Anesthesiologists. Endorsed by the Society for Cardiovascular Angiography and Interventions and the Society of Thoracic Surgeons. Circulation 2006;114(5):e84–231.

[95] Walston A, Peter RH, Morris JJ, et al. Clinical implications of pulmonary hypertension in mitral stenosis. Am J Cardiol 1973;32(5):650–5.

[96] Schwammenthal E, Vered Z, Agranat O, et al. Impact of atrioventricular compliance on pulmonary artery pressure in mitral stenosis: an exercise echocardiographic study. Circulation 2000; 102(19):2378–84.

[97] Ha JW, Chung N, Jang Y, et al. Is the left atrial v. wave the determinant of peak pulmonary artery pressure in patients with pure mitral stenosis? Am J Cardiol 2000;85(8):986–91.

[98] Okay T, Deligonul U, Sancaktar O, et al. Contribution of mitral valve reserve capacity to sustained symptomatic improvement after balloon valvulotomy in mitral stenosis: implications for restenosis. J Am Coll Cardiol 1993;22(6):1691–6.

[99] Fawzy ME. Percutaneous mitral balloon valvotomy. Catheter Cardiovasc Interv 2007;69(2):313–21.

[100] Fawzy ME, Hassan W, Stefadouros M, et al. Prevalence and fate of severe pulmonary hypertension in 559 consecutive patients with severe rheumatic mitral stenosis undergoing mitral balloon valvotomy. J Heart Valve Dis 2004;13(6): 942–7 [discussion: 947–8].

[101] Singh JP, Evans JC, Levy D, et al. Prevalence and clinical determinants of mitral, tricuspid, and aortic regurgitation (the Framingham Heart Study). Am J Cardiol 1999;83(6):897–902.

[102] Ward C, Hancock BW. Extreme pulmonary hypertension caused by mitral valve disease: natural history and results of surgery. Br Heart J 1975; 37(1):74–8.

[103] Cesnjevar RA, Feyrer R, Walther F, et al. High-risk mitral valve replacement in severe pulmonary hypertension: 30 years experience. Eur J Cardiothorac Surg 1998;13(4):344–51 [discussion: 351–2].

[104] Foltz BD, Hessel EA 2nd, Ivey TD. The early course of pulmonary artery hypertension in patients undergoing mitral valve replacement with cardioplegic arrest. J Thorac Cardiovasc Surg 1984;88(2):238–47.

[105] Yang H, Davidson WR Jr, Chambers CE, et al. Preoperative pulmonary hypertension is associated with postoperative left ventricular dysfunction in chronic organic mitral regurgitation: an echocardiographic and hemodynamic study. J Am Soc Echocardiogr 2006;19(8):1051–5.

[106] Cevese PG, Gallucci V, Valfre C, et al. Pulmonary hypertension in mitral valve surgery. J Cardiovasc Surg (Torino) 1980;21(1):7–10.

[107] Salzberg SP, Filsoufi F, Anyanwu A, et al. High-risk mitral valve surgery: perioperative hemodynamic optimization with nesiritide (BNP). Ann Thorac Surg 2005;80(2):502–6.

[108] Silver K, Aurigemma G, Krendel S, et al. Pulmonary artery hypertension in severe aortic stenosis: incidence and mechanism. Am Heart J 1993; 125(1):146–50.

[109] Aragam JR, Folland ED, Lapsley D, et al. Cause and impact of pulmonary hypertension in isolated aortic stenosis on operative mortality for aortic valve replacement in men. Am J Cardiol 1992; 69(16):1365–7.

[110] Malouf JF, Enriquez-Sarano M, Pellikka PA, et al. Severe pulmonary hypertension in patients with severe aortic valve stenosis: clinical profile and prognostic implications. J Am Coll Cardiol 2002; 40(4):789–95.

[111] Chaouat A, Bugnet AS, Kadaoui N, et al. Severe pulmonary hypertension and chronic obstructive pulmonary disease. Am J Respir Crit Care Med 2005;172(2):189–94.

[112] Fell CD, Martinez FJ. The impact of pulmonary arterial hypertension on idiopathic pulmonary fibrosis. Chest 2007;131(3):641–3.

[113] Hamada K, Nagai S, Tanaka S, et al. Significance of pulmonary arterial pressure and diffusion capacity of the lung as prognosticator in patients with idiopathic pulmonary fibrosis. Chest 2007;131(3): 650–6.

[114] Lettieri CJ, Nathan SD, Barnett SD, et al. Prevalence and outcomes of pulmonary arterial hypertension in advanced idiopathic pulmonary fibrosis. Chest 2006;129(3):746–52.

[115] Oswald-Mammosser M, Weitzenblum E, Quoix E, et al. Prognostic factors in COPD patients receiving long-term oxygen therapy: importance of pulmonary artery pressure. Chest 1995;107(5):1193–8.

[116] Arcasoy SM, Christie JD, Ferrari VA, et al. Echocardiographic assessment of pulmonary hypertension in patients with advanced lung disease. Am J Respir Crit Care Med 2003;167(5):735–40.

[117] Ghofrani HA, Wiedemann R, Rose F, et al. Sildenafil for treatment of lung fibrosis and pulmonary hypertension: a randomised controlled trial. Lancet 2002;360(9337):895–900.

[118] Olschewski H, Ghofrani HA, Walmrath D, et al. Inhaled prostacyclin and iloprost in severe pulmonary hypertension secondary to lung fibrosis. Am J Respir Crit Care Med 1999;160(2):600–7.

[119] Shapiro S. Management of pulmonary hypertension resulting from interstitial lung disease. Curr Opin Pulm Med 2003;9(5):426–30.

[120] Bixler EO, Vgontzas AN, Ten Have T, et al. Effects of age on sleep apnea in men: I. Prevalence and severity. Am J Respir Crit Care Med 1998;157(1): 144–8.

[121] Fleury B. Sleep apnea syndrome in the elderly. Sleep 1992;15(6 Suppl):S39–41.

[122] Hoch CC, Reynolds CF 3rd, Monk TH, et al. Comparison of sleep-disordered breathing among

healthy elderly in the seventh, eighth, and ninth decades of life. Sleep 1990;13(6):502–11.

[123] Launois SH, Pepin JL, Levy P. Sleep apnea in the elderly: a specific entity? Sleep Med Rev 2007; 11(2):87–97.

[124] Tishler PV, Larkin EK, Schluchter MD, et al. Incidence of sleep-disordered breathing in an urban adult population: the relative importance of risk factors in the development of sleep-disordered breathing. JAMA 2003;289(17):2230–7.

[125] Zamarron C, Gude F, Otero Y, et al. Prevalence of sleep disordered breathing and sleep apnea in 50- to 70-year-old individuals: a survey. Respiration 1999;66(4):317–22.

[126] Atwood CW Jr, McCrory D, Garcia JG, et al. Pulmonary artery hypertension and sleep-disordered breathing: ACCP evidence-based clinical practice guidelines. Chest 2004;126(1 Suppl):72S–7S.

[127] Becattini C, Agnelli G, Pesavento R, et al. Incidence of chronic thromboembolic pulmonary hypertension after a first episode of pulmonary embolism. Chest 2006;130(1):172–5.

[128] Miniati M, Monti S, Bottai M, et al. Survival and restoration of pulmonary perfusion in a long-term follow-up of patients after acute pulmonary embolism. Medicine (Baltimore) 2006;85(5):253–62.

[129] Pengo V, Lensing AW, Prins MH, et al. Incidence of chronic thromboembolic pulmonary hypertension after pulmonary embolism. N Engl J Med 2004;350(22):2257–64.

[130] Tapson VF, Humbert M. Incidence and prevalence of chronic thromboembolic pulmonary hypertension: from acute to chronic pulmonary embolism. Proc Am Thorac Soc 2006;3(7):564–7.

[131] Morris TA, Marsh JJ, Chiles PG, et al. Fibrin derived from patients with chronic thromboembolic pulmonary hypertension is resistant to lysis. Am J Respir Crit Care Med 2006;173(11):1270–5.

[132] Morris TA, Marsh JJ, Chiles PG, et al. Abnormally sialylated fibrinogen gamma-chains in a patient with chronic thromboembolic pulmonary hypertension. Thromb Res 2007;119(2):257–9.

[133] Bonderman D, Jakowitsch J, Adlbrecht C, et al. Medical conditions increasing the risk of chronic thromboembolic pulmonary hypertension. Thromb Haemost 2005;93(3):512–6.

[134] Kuypers FA, Yuan J, Lewis RA, et al. Membrane phospholipid asymmetry in human thalassemia. Blood 1998;91(8):3044–51.

[135] Lang I, Kerr K. Risk factors for chronic thromboembolic pulmonary hypertension. Proc Am Thorac Soc 2006;3(7):568–70.

[136] Tscholl D, Langer F, Wendler O, et al. Pulmonary thromboendarterectomy: risk factors for early survival and hemodynamic improvement. Eur J Cardiothorac Surg 2001;19(6):771–6.

[137] Kim NH. Assessment of operability in chronic thromboembolic pulmonary hypertension. Proc Am Thorac Soc 2006;3(7):584–8.

[138] Peacock A, Simonneau G, Rubin L. Controversies, uncertainties and future research on the treatment of chronic thromboembolic pulmonary hypertension. Proc Am Thorac Soc 2006;3(7):608–14.

[139] Widera E, Sulica R. Pulmonary artery sarcoma misdiagnosed as chronic thromboembolic pulmonary hypertension. Mt Sinai J Med 2005;72(6): 360–4.

[140] Wilson MK, Granger EK, Preda VA. Pulmonary hypertension due to isolated metastatic squamous cell carcinoma thromboemboli. Heart Lung Circ 2006;15(2):143–5.

[141] Malani AK, Gupta C, Kutty AV, et al. Pulmonary tumor thrombotic microangiopathy from metastatic gallbladder carcinoma: an unusual cause of severe pulmonary hypertension. Dig Dis Sci 2007; 52(2):555–7.

[142] Nakamura H, Adachi H, Sudoh A, et al. Subacute cor pulmonale due to tumor embolism. Intern Med 2004;43(5):420–2.

[143] Stucki A, Kruse A, Iff S, et al. A rare cause of fatal right heart failure. Eur J Intern Med 2006;17(1): 68–70.

[144] Roberts KE, Hamele-Bena D, Saqi A, et al. Pulmonary tumor embolism: a review of the literature. Am J Med 2003;115(3):228–32.

[145] Shiue ST, McNally DP. Pulmonary hypertension from prominent vascular involvement in diffuse amyloidosis. Arch Intern Med 1988;148(3):687–9.

[146] Waldhorn RE, Tsou E, Smith FP, et al. Pulmonary veno-occlusive disease associated with microangiopathic hemolytic anemia and chemotherapy of gastric adenocarcinoma. Med Pediatr Oncol 1984; 12(6):394–6.

[147] Coates GG, Eisenberg B, Dail DH. Tc-99m sulfur colloid demonstration of diffuse pulmonary interstitial extramedullary hematopoiesis in a patient with myelofibrosis: a case report and review of the literature. Clin Nucl Med 1994;19(12): 1079–84.

[148] Garcia-Manero G, Schuster SJ, Patrick H, et al. Pulmonary hypertension in patients with myelofibrosis secondary to myeloproliferative diseases. Am J Hematol 1999;60(2):130–5.

[149] Marvin KS, Spellberg RD. Pulmonary hypertension secondary to thrombocytosis in a patient with myeloid metaplasia. Chest 1993;103(2): 642–4.

[150] Rumi E, Passamonti F, Boveri E, et al. Dyspnea secondary to pulmonary hematopoiesis as presenting symptom of myelofibrosis with myeloid metaplasia. Am J Hematol 2006;81(2):124–7.

[151] Steensma DP, Hook CC, Stafford SL, et al. Low-dose, single-fraction, whole-lung radiotherapy for pulmonary hypertension associated with myelofibrosis with myeloid metaplasia. Br J Haematol 2002;118(3):813–6.

[152] Weinschenker P, Kutner JM, Salvajoli JV, et al. Whole-pulmonary low-dose radiation therapy in

agnogenic myeloid metaplasia with diffuse lung involvement. Am J Hematol 2002;69(4):277–80.

[153] Bhatia S, Morrison JF, Bower TC, et al. Pulmonary hypertension in the setting of acquired systemic arteriovenous fistulas. Mayo Clin Proc 2003; 78(7):908–12.

[154] Tayyareci G, Dayi SU, Akgoz H, et al. A rare case of pulmonary hypertension as a result of arteriovenous fistula after cardiac surgery. Int Heart J 2005; 46(3):551–6.

[155] Petrone K, Katz P. Approaches to appropriate drug prescribing for the older adult. Prim Care 2005;32(3):755–75.

[156] Muirhead GJ, Wilner K, Colburn W, et al. The effects of age and renal and hepatic impairment on the pharmacokinetics of sildenafil. Br J Clin Pharmacol 2002;53(Suppl 1):21S–30S.

[157] Zusman RM, Morales A, Glasser DB, et al. Overall cardiovascular profile of sildenafil citrate. Am J Cardiol 1999;83(5A):35C–44C.

[158] van Giersbergen PL, Treiber A, Clozel M, et al. In vivo and in vitro studies exploring the pharmacokinetic interaction between bosentan, a dual endothelin receptor antagonist, and glyburide. Clin Pharmacol Ther 2002;71(4): 253–62.

ELSEVIER
SAUNDERS

Clin Chest Med 28 (2007) 735–749

CLINICS
IN CHEST
MEDICINE

Treatment of Lung Cancer in Older Patients

Lynn T. Tanoue, MD[a],*, Scott Gettinger, MD[b]

[a]Section of Pulmonary and Critical Care Medicine, Yale School of Medicine, 333 Cedar St., New Haven, CT 06520, USA
[b]Section of Medical Oncology, Yale School of Medicine, 333 Cedar St., New Haven, CT 06520, USA

Lung cancer is the most common cause of cancer death in men and women in this country. In 2007, an estimated 160,390 deaths will be attributable to cancer of the lung and bronchus [1]. Eighty percent of these deaths occur in patients over the age of 60, with approximately 20% occurring in patients over the age of 80 [1]. Lung cancer, like most solid tumors, predominantly affects older persons. Cigarette smoking remains the major risk factor, with risk influenced by smoking intensity and duration [2,3]. Cessation of smoking abrogates risk over time, even in persons who have smoked into the sixth decade of life [4]. Other recognized risk factors include a family history of lung cancer, exposures to occupational carcinogens (eg, asbestos, radon, polycyclic aromatic hydrocarbons), domestic exposure to radon, exposure to environmental tobacco smoke, air pollution, and underlying lung disease, including chronic airflow obstruction and fibrosing pulmonary disorders [5,6]. Age, per se, is not considered a risk factor; however, because most lung cancers occur in older persons, age inevitably is a factor that may influence treatment choices.

The definition of "older" is vague at best. Chronologic age is easily definable, biologic age less so. Webster's defines "elderly" as "approaching old age, past middle age" [7]. From a practical perspective, an age of 65 years is often used as a threshold for defining "older" because it defines eligibility for Medicare and Social Security benefits, which may be linked to the age of retirement from active occupation. The age cut-off for

medical research in older persons varies, however, with arbitrary thresholds set typically between the ages of 60 and 80. What is generally agreed upon is that chronologic age does not define health status. Decisions related to therapeutic options for older patients who have lung cancer, or in reality, any disease, should be influenced by an assessment of overall health and function rather than by the number of years of life. Unfortunately, bias exists among physicians that older persons who have cancer have shorter life expectancy, have more comorbid medical conditions, and are less likely to tolerate invasive diagnostic evaluation or aggressive treatments, such as surgery or chemotherapy [8,9]. Such bias may influence physicians not to confirm a diagnosis of cancer, pursue clinical staging, or refer an older patient for further treatment evaluation [9–12]. The attainment of older age itself is a predictor of longevity, however. In 2004 in the United States, the life expectancy at birth for men and women combined was 77.8 years [13]. Among persons who had reached the age of 65, life expectancy was an additional 18.7 years (ie, 83.7 years); among persons who had attained the age of 75, life expectancy was an additional 11.9 years (ie, 86.9 years) [13]. It is true that comorbid medical conditions are more common in older patients, as are age-related reductions in organ function. Concerns about an older person's ability to tolerate surgical resection or their risk for chemotherapy-related toxicities are legitimate. Considerations for these specific risks in an individual patient should determine whether to exclude older persons from such treatments, however, not absolute age.

In all patients, but perhaps particularly in older persons, objective assessments of global health and functional status should be used

* Corresponding author.
E-mail address: lynn.tanoue@yale.edu
(L.T. Tanoue).

0272-5231/07/$ - see front matter © 2007 Elsevier Inc. All rights reserved.
doi:10.1016/j.ccm.2007.08.003

routinely in determining suitability of individual patients for evaluation and treatment. In oncology practice, this is typically defined by what is termed "performance status," which is an assessment of how disease affects activities and abilities of daily living. Measurements of performance status are widely used to evaluate cancer progression and determine appropriate treatment and prognosis [14]. Performance status metrics incorporate elements of physical activity, ability to perform work and self-care, and mobility in an assessment of function rather than disease status. The Eastern Cooperative Oncology Group (ECOG) performance status measurement is one such tool and is typically used as part of the determination of a patient's ability to tolerate treatment and assess eligibility for clinical trials of cancer treatment interventions (Table 1) [15]. In all patients, but particularly in a geriatric population, assessments of cognition, nutrition, and social environment should be performed, because dementia, poor nutritional status, and the absence of social support are all associated with decreased survival [16–20]. In patients of any age, poor performance status, impaired cognition, poor nutritional status, and poor social support may define individuals as poor candidates for aggressive therapeutic or even diagnostic interventions. If the presence of a lung cancer is clearly not the life-limiting factor, then an aggressive approach to treatment of that cancer may be inappropriate. Conversely, the approach to older patients who have good overall health and good performance status should be the same as for younger persons and not arbitrarily limited by age.

Non–small-cell lung cancer

More than 80% of all lung cancers are non–small-cell lung cancers (NSCLC). The major histologic groups that comprise this category include squamous cell, large cell, and adenocarcinomas. Until recently, treatments for all three histologies have been grouped together under the NSCLC classification. Newer therapies, however, have focused increasingly on targeting to histology and tumor protein expression or gene mutational analysis [21–24]. This shift in treatment paradigm is likely to burgeon in the future with development of more targeted agents and an increasing understanding of lung cancer biology. The major determinants of survival for NSCLC are performance status, histology, and stage, with better performance status, adenocarcinoma histology, and

Table 1
Eastern Cooperative Oncology Group performance status

ECOG performance status[a]	
Grade	ECOG
0	Fully active, able to carry on all predisease performance without restriction
1	Restricted in physically strenuous activity but ambulatory and able to carry out work of a light or sedentary nature (eg, light house work, office work)
2	Ambulatory and capable of all self-care but unable to carry out any work activities, up and about more than 50% of waking hours
3	Capable of only limited sel-care, confined to bed or chair more than 50% of waking hours
4	Completely disabled; cannot carry on any self-care Totally confined to bed or chair
5	Dead

[a] Robert Comis, MD, Group Chair.
From Oken MM, Creech RH, Tormey DC, et al. Toxicity and response criteria of the Eastern Cooperative Oncology Group. Am J Clin Oncol 1982;5(6): 654. Courtesy of the Eastern Cooperative Oncology Group, Robert Comis, MD, Group CHair.

earlier stage all correlating with better outcome. Determination of clinical stage (ie, the assessment of the extent of NSCLC by means other than complete surgical resection) typically defines optimal treatment recommendations for NSCLC and provides an estimate of survival (Fig. 1 and Table 2) [25,26]. A general guide to current recommendations for treatment modalities according to NSCLC stage is presented in Table 3.

Surgical treatment for early-stage non–small-cell lung cancer

Surgery is the treatment of choice for patients who have stages I and II NSCLC without medical contraindication to operation and is a consideration in selected patients who have stage IIIA NSCLC (see Table 3). Patients who have stage I

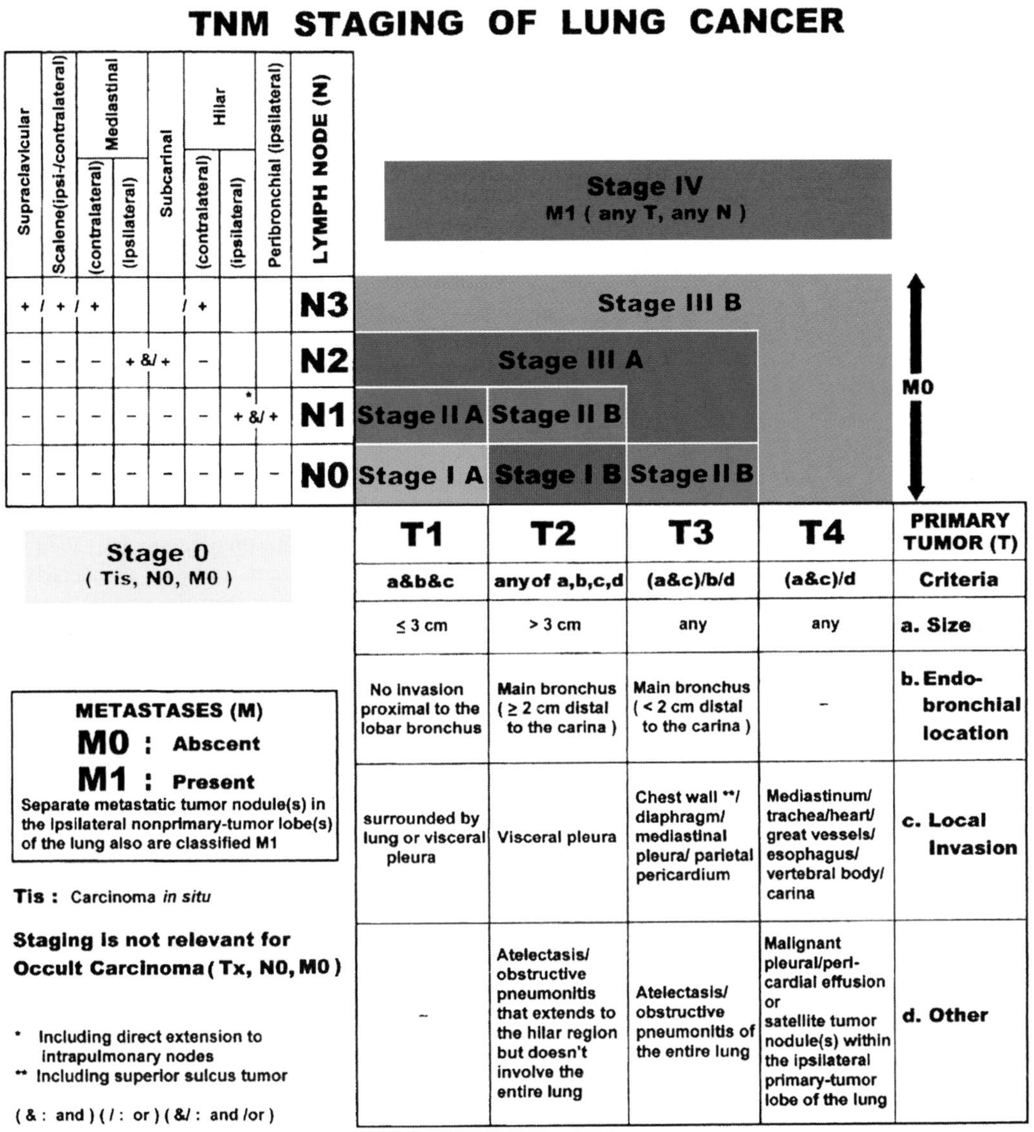

TNM STAGING OF LUNG CANCER

Stage IV M1 (any T, any N)

Supraclavicular	Scalene (ipsi-/contralateral)	Mediastinal (contralateral)	Mediastinal (ipsilateral)	Subcarinal	Hilar (contralateral)	Hilar (ipsilateral)	Peribronchial (ipsilateral)	LYMPH NODE (N)	
+	/	+	/		/	+		**N3**	Stage III B
−	−	−	+ &/	+	−			**N2**	Stage III A
−	−	−	−	−	−	+ &/	+	**N1**	Stage II A / Stage II B
−	−	−	−	−	−	−	−	**N0**	Stage I A / Stage I B / Stage II B

MO

Stage 0 (Tis, N0, M0)

	T1	T2	T3	T4	PRIMARY TUMOR (T)
Criteria	a&b&c	any of a,b,c,d	(a&c)/b/d	(a&c)/d	**Criteria**
a. Size	≤ 3 cm	> 3 cm	any	any	**a. Size**
b. Endobronchial location	No invasion proximal to the lobar bronchus	Main bronchus (≥ 2 cm distal to the carina)	Main bronchus (< 2 cm distal to the carina)	−	**b. Endobronchial location**
c. Local Invasion	surrounded by lung or visceral pleura	Visceral pleura	Chest wall **/ diaphragm/ mediastinal pleura/ parietal pericardium	Mediastinum/ trachea/heart/ great vessels/ esophagus/ vertebral body/ carina	**c. Local Invasion**
d. Other	−	Atelectasis/ obstructive pneumonitis that extends to the hilar region but doesn't involve the entire lung	Atelectasis/ obstructive pneumonitis of the entire lung	Malignant pleural/peri-cardial effusion or satellite tumor nodule(s) within the ipsilateral primary-tumor lobe of the lung	**d. Other**

METASTASES (M)

M0 : Absent

M1 : Present
Separate metastatic tumor nodule(s) in the ipsilateral nonprimary-tumor lobe(s) of the lung also are classified M1

Tis : Carcinoma *in situ*

Staging is not relevant for Occult Carcinoma (Tx, N0, M0)

* Including direct extension to intrapulmonary nodes
** Including superior sulcus tumor

(& : and) (/ : or) (&/ : and /or)

Fig. 1. TNM staging of lung cancer. (*From* Lababede O, Meziane MA, Rice TW. TNM staging of lung cancer: a quick reference chart. Chest 1999;115(1):1495; with permission.)

NSCLC confirmed at surgical resection have an overall 5-year survival rate of 67% [25]. The subset of stage IA patients who have very small (<1 cm diameter) tumors have a 5-year survival rate in excess of 90% [27,28]. Recent clinical trials suggested that adjuvant chemotherapy may improve survival in patients who have resected stages IB and II disease [29–31]. Although there is current debate regarding the natural history of very small stage I NSCLC in persons identified by screening with CT scanning, historically cure without surgery in patients who have early stage NSCLC is unlikely [28,32–36]. The selection of patients suitable for surgical resection is largely determined by the presence of comorbidities, primarily cardiovascular disease, and by predicted postoperative pulmonary function. Widely practiced algorithms for patient selection do not include age as a criterion for surgery [37,38]. The American College of Chest Physicians' evidence-based guidelines on

Table 2
Non–small-cell lung cancer survival at 2 and 5 years based on clinical staging at diagnosis

| Clinical stage | Percent surviving | |
| | Years after treatment | |
	2 years (%)	5 years (%)
IA	79	61
IB	54	38
IIA	49	34
IIB	41	24
IIIA	25	13
IIIB	13	5
IV	6	1

Data from Mountain CF. Revisions in the International System for Staging Lung Cancer. Chest 1997;111(6):1710–7.

the diagnosis and management of lung cancer summary recommendations for the physiologic evaluation of patients who have lung cancer being considered for resectional surgery specifically state, "Patients with lung cancer should not be denied lung resection surgery on the grounds of age alone" [37].

Concern relating to the possibility of increased perioperative morbidity undoubtedly factors into treatment decisions for older patients who have early-stage NSCLC. In an analysis of the Surveillance, Epidemiology, and End Results (SEER) database analysis by Mery and colleagues [39], 30% of patients over the age of 75 with early-stage NSCLC did not receive curative surgery, compared with 8% of patients under the age of 65. The reasons for withholding surgery could not be determined, but medical comorbidities,

functional status, physician discretion, and patient and family preference all likely factor into such decisions. Other studies have demonstrated that surgery and other therapies are less commonly offered to older patients [40,41]. Although current cancer clinical treatment trials tend not to use age as a criterion for eligibility, older patients have been underrepresented in such trials, and so efficacy and toxicity of newer therapies in older populations are often poorly understood [42]. Diagnostic evaluations also tend to be more limited and less invasive in older patients [12,43]. Because staging by clinical as opposed to pathologic information tends to understage patients, a more limited and less accurate approach may contribute to the observation that older persons have a higher incidence of early-stage lung cancer than younger patients [39,41,44–46]. If older persons tend to be understaged, then that may factor into their observed worse long-term survival. Conversely, if the staging is accurate, then the smaller percentage of older patients who receive curative surgery for early-stage disease becomes even more of an issue.

A comprehensive patient evaluation is critical to making decisions related to surgery in any patient who has lung cancer, particularly in older patients. In all patients, cancer staging and physiologic assessment should be augmented by an assessment of medical appropriateness for surgery. For patients who have lung cancer, the latter includes measurement of performance status. In an older population, a more focused functional evaluation also may be indicated. Dementia is an independent predictor of decreased survival in older adults [18,19]. A report by

Table 3
Treatment of non–small-cell lung cancer by stage

Stage	Surgery	Adjuvant chemotherapy	Concurrent chemotherapy and radiation therapy with curative intent	Palliative chemotherapy
IA	X			
IB	X	?		
IIA/B incidental IIIA	X	X		
IIIA, N2	?		X	
IIIB (without supraclavicular or scalene nodal involvement, and without pleural involvement)[a]			X	
IV/IIIB wet (malignant pleural involvement)				X

[a] IIIB with contralateral supraclavicular/scalene involvement is approached with palliative chemotherapy. Although somewhat controversial, ipsilateral supraclavicular/scalene involvement generally also precludes definitive therapy with combination CRT.

Fukuse and colleagues [20], which evaluated 120 patients over the age of 60 undergoing thoracic surgery for lung cancer, identified disability in performing activities of daily living (P = .041) and dementia (P = .0065) as factors strongly correlating with the development of postoperative complications, whereas age, per se, was not. In this study, ability to perform activities of daily living was measured by the Barthel Index of function [47,48] and dementia by the Mini Mental State Examination [49,50]. Many other instruments are available for evaluating functional or cognitive impairment, the choice of which depends on physician preference, available time, and patient population [51]. The use of such metrics in a comprehensive geriatric assessment should be incorporated into the evaluation of older patients being considered for lung cancer surgery to identify patients at higher risk for complications and patients for whom surgery is appropriate [52,53].

Debate exists as to whether older age is associated with an increase in the incidence of perioperative complications and mortality. Several studies have reported worse short- and long-term survival in older compared with younger patients undergoing surgical resection for lung cancer [54–57]. The Lung Cancer Study Group reported that 30-day mortality rate from surgical treatment for lung cancer was directly influenced by age [56]. In this multicenter study that included more than 2000 resections for lung cancer, the surgical mortality rate in patients aged 60 years or younger was 1.3% compared with 4.1% in patients aged 60 to 69 years and 7.1% in patients over age 70 (P < .01). In another large study from the Netherlands that evaluated more than 2300 patients undergoing pulmonary resection for NSCLC, 5-year survival rate in patients under the age of 65 was 44% compared with 38% in patients over the age of 65 (P < .0001) [54]. In their SEER analysis, Mery and colleagues [39] confirmed that age was an independent predictor of long-term survival. Median survival times for patients younger than 65, 65 to 74, and 75 years and older were 71, 47, and 28 months, respectively (P < .0001). None of these studies controlled for factors such as the presence of comorbid medical conditions, limitations of pulmonary reserve, or impairment in functional status, however, all of which might be anticipated to be more prevalent in older persons and might be expected to contribute to perioperative complications. In contrast, other studies taking these and other factors into consideration have reported

no differences in operative mortality between older and younger patients [44,58–61]. In a retrospective study of 534 patients in Japan undergoing surgery for NSCLC, older (≥ 76 years) patients who had good performance status (ECOG performance status 0-2) and no medical comorbidities had similar perioperative mortality and long-term survival compared with younger patients [61]. In this study, a smaller percentage of older patients compared with younger patients actually underwent surgery (36.1% versus 51.0%), related to a higher prevalence of poor performance status and greater comorbidity in the older group. Similarly, in a nested case-control study of 726 patients matched for $FEV_1\%$ of predicted, ECOG performance status, stage, type of tumor, and type of pulmonary resection, Cerfolio and Bryant [44] found no differences in short-term morbidity and mortality between older (≥ 70 years) and younger (< 70 years) patients. These studies demonstrated that consideration of patient factors other than the tumor itself—specifically inclusion of assessments of functional status and comorbidities—can identify fit older patients for whom the outcomes of surgery for early-stage NSCLC are equal to their younger counterparts.

Factors other than age may influence the extent of surgery or the choice of a treatment other than resection. In their SEER analysis, Mery and colleagues [39] reported that among patients older than 70 years, there was no difference in survival between patients who underwent a standard lobectomy compared with patients who had limited resection (median survival 42 versus 44 months; P = .47) for early-stage NSCLC. This finding should raise consideration for a limited surgical procedure in older persons for whom the physiologic stresses of lobectomy may be problematic.

Based on the available evidence, it seems clear that careful selection of older patients for surgery can minimize perioperative mortality and provide good long-term survival. In all persons, but particularly in older adults, preoperative medical evaluation should include an assessment of performance status and function and the usual physiologic measurements. This type of comprehensive approach, as opposed to absolute age, should guide decisions relating to operability.

*Radiotherapy as an alternative treatment
for early-stage non–small-cell lung cancer*

Unfortunately, the likelihood of medical comorbidities, lessened pulmonary reserve, and higher prevalence of cognitive and functional disabilities render many older patients who have early-stage NSCLC inoperable. For these patients, conventional single-modality radiotherapy (RT) has been the primary definitive treatment option [62–64]. Typically treatment is given as an uninterrupted course of radiotherapy, usually 60 Gy in 30 fractions over 6 weeks [65]. In selected medically inoperable patients who have early-stage NSCLC, Haffty and colleagues [62] reported a 5-year survival rate of 45% compared with 12% in patients undergoing no treatment. Numerous other retrospective reports demonstrated long-term disease-free and overall survival rates that were modestly superior to that expected with no treatment, but both local and distant failure continue to be significant issues. Conventional RT remains a viable treatment option for patients who have early-stage disease and should be considered in older persons who, by medical criteria or personal choice, are not suitable for surgery.

A body of recent evidence suggests that new radiation therapy modalities may be potential treatment alternatives for medically inoperable patients who have early-stage NSCLC. Radiofrequency ablation is one such strategy being investigated for primary and metastatic pulmonary lesions. Radiofrequency ablation typically is performed percutaneously under CT or ultrasound guidance, with placement of an electrode directly in the tumor. Current between this electrode and one on the skin produces localized heating and coagulation necrosis in tissue within a certain distance of the electrode. Radiofrequency ablation is most effective in patients who have smaller tumors (<3 cm). Initial studies have evaluated radiofrequency ablation for pain management and treatment of medically inoperable tumors. In general, results have been reported in terms of local control, with sparse information about long-term survival. Complications reported with radiofrequency ablation include pneumothorax in 30% to 40% and pleural effusion in 10% to 20% of patients [66–68]. Stereotactic body radiation therapy is another novel cancer treatment strategy that incorporates image guidance to safely deliver ultra-high radiation doses in a few fractions. Stereotactic body radiation therapy plays an established role in treatment of intracranial neoplasms, both primary and metastatic [69]. Stereotactic body radiation therapy is being investigated as a possible treatment option for extracranial sites, including the lung. Because the thorax is constantly moving with respiration, stereotactic body radiation therapy of pulmonary lesions requires either gating of treatment to the respiratory cycle or immobilization of the chest and abdominal walls. Toxicities have been relatively few, with the most common being radiation-associated pneumonitis and esophagitis. Early studies have reported 2- to 3-year survival rates after stereotactic body radiation therapy ranging from 32% to 88% [70–72]. Because the technology is relatively new, long-term survival data are not yet available.

Medical treatment of non–small-cell lung cancer

Most patients who have NSCLC present with advanced disease, for which chemotherapy is the mainstay of therapy (see Table 3). A growing body of evidence also supports adjunctive chemotherapy in the treatment of patients who have earlier stage disease. Treating older lung cancer patients with chemotherapy is challenging. Older persons often have significant comorbidities and age-related declines in organ function and bone marrow reserve. Coexisting medical conditions frequently require other medications that may interfere with chemotherapy, which leads to decreased efficacy and/or increased toxicity. Cognitive, social, and financial issues also can be particularly limiting in this population. Despite these challenges, retrospective and prospective trials suggest that fit older patients derive as much benefit from chemotherapy as their younger counterparts. Increasingly, efforts are being focused on creating and validating instruments to distinguish biologic from chronologic age to aid in determining who should receive therapy and which therapy they should be prescribed.

Chemotherapy has been clearly shown to improve survival in patients who have stages II, III, and IV NSCLC. Clinical data relating to chemotherapy as adjunctive treatment for stage I disease are less convincing, although there may be a role in select patients. For example, the subset of patients with stage IB NSCLC with a tumor size 4 cm or larger may benefit from adjuvant chemotherapy after surgical resection [73]. The role of chemotherapy in older patients has been established firmly in advanced disease; however, there are no completed elderly-specific phase III trials in early-stage or locally advanced NSCLC. Recommendations in these settings are confined to retrospective analyses; it should be noted that the relatively sparse inclusion of older patients in lung cancer clinical trials limits the interpretation of these analyses.

Adjuvant chemotherapy for early-stage non–small-cell lung cancer

Three recent clinical trials have established the benefits of cisplatin-based adjuvant chemotherapy [30,31,74]. Two of these trials used only modern cisplatin regimens and together reported an 8.6% to 15% absolute 5-year survival advantage over surgery alone in patients who had stage IB, II, or IIIA NSCLC [30,31]. Treatment was generally well tolerated, with the main toxicity being significant neutropenia. The pooled treatment-related death rate from all three trials was 1.1% (16 deaths/1450 patients).

Information concerning older adults in adjuvant clinical trials is scarce, with a dedicated subset analysis available for only one trial. The National Cancer Institute of Canada BR.10 trial randomized patients who had completely resected stage IB ($n = 91$) and stage II ($n = 109$) NSCLC to four cycles of cisplatin/vinorelbine doublet chemotherapy or observation [30]. With median follow-up of 62 months, 5-year survival rate with chemotherapy was 69% versus 54% (hazard ratio 0.69, 95% CI 0.52–0.91; $P = .04$). Subset analysis did not show a significant survival advantage in stage IB patients. There was a 0.8% treatment-related death rate. Of the 155 patients on the BR.10 trial over 65 years of age, there was an absolute improvement in 5-year survival rate of 10% with chemotherapy (5-year survival rate 68% versus 58%, hazard ratio 0.61, 95% CI 0.38–0.98; $P = .04$) [75]. There were no significant differences between age groups in toxicities, hospitalizations, or treatment-related deaths, which may be partly accounted for by the observations that significantly less chemotherapy was delivered to older compared with younger patients and fewer older patients completed all four cycles of therapy. Further analysis of patients aged 75 years or older did not demonstrate the same benefit from adjuvant chemotherapy; however, the small size of this subset (23 patients) limits interpretation of these results.

A recently presented meta-analysis also addressed the safety and efficacy of cisplatin-based chemotherapy in older patients [76]. The Lung Adjuvant Cisplatin Evaluation project analyzed individual patient data from five large phase III trials in an effort to identify trial characteristics associated with benefit from cisplatin-based adjuvant chemotherapy [76]. Patients were pooled and divided into three age groups: younger than age 65 years ($n = 3269$), 65 to 69 years ($n = 901$), and 70 years or older ($n = 414$). Patients aged 70 years or older received less cisplatin than younger patients, but there were no significant differences in overall survival or toxicities. Hazard ratios for death for the three age groups in order of increasing age were 0.86 (95% CI 0.78–0.95), 1.10 (95% CI 0.85–1.21), and 0.9 (95% CI 0.7–1.160).

In the absence of other clinical trial data, recommendations concerning adjuvant chemotherapy in older patients cannot be definitive. In fit older patients who can tolerate cisplatin chemotherapy, however, it is reasonable to treat with the same chemotherapy protocol used for younger patients. Retrospective analyses of other adjuvant trials are anticipated and may provide more clarity for treating older patients who have early-stage NSCLC. However, retrospective analyses suffer from selection bias and must be interpreted with caution. Although elderly-specific randomized adjuvant trials are clearly warranted, they may never be undertaken secondary to concerns about accrual.

Chemotherapy for locally advanced non–small-cell lung cancer

The treatment of locally advanced NSCLC has evolved substantively over the last several years. Phase III clinical trials have established that chemotherapy adds to the survival benefit seen with definitive radiotherapy [77,78] and that chemotherapy concurrent with radiation is superior to sequential therapy [79,80]. The role of surgery in stage IIIA disease with ipsilateral mediastinal lymph node involvement remains unclear and is being evaluated further in ongoing clinical trials.

The addition of chemotherapy to thoracic irradiation (RT) is associated with increased toxicity, which is particularly concerning in older persons. Retrospective analyses of older populations in four cooperative group trials evaluating concurrent chemoradiotherapy (CRT) are available. The Radiation Therapy Oncology Group (RTOG) 94-10 trial randomized patients to sequential chemotherapy (cisplatin/vinblastine) with once-daily RT, concurrent chemotherapy (cisplatin/vinblastine) with once-daily RT, or concurrent chemotherapy (cisplatin/etoposide) with hyperfractionated RT (two fractions per day) [80,81]. Of the 595 patients enrolled, 104 were aged 70 years or older. In this older cohort, improved survival was demonstrated with concurrent therapy, albeit with more severe neutropenia and esophagitis. Median survival was 22.4 months with concurrent daily RT and 16.4 months with concurrent twice-daily RT versus 10.8 months with sequential therapy ($P = .069$). The Cancer and Leukemia Group B reported their experience with older patients in a subset analysis of a phase III trial investigating sequential CRT (cisplatin/vinblastine) versus induction chemotherapy (cisplatin/vinblastine) followed by concurrent CRT with carboplatin [82]. An increase in the frequency of neutropenia and renal toxicity was observed in older patients; however, there was no difference in response rate or survival by age. The North Central Cancer Treatment Group conducted a trial of concurrent CRT (cisplatin/etoposide) with conventional daily radiation or hyperfractioned RT, including 63 patients who were aged 70 years or older [83]. Again there was more severe neutropenia in older patients and more pneumonitis (1% in younger patients compared with 6% in older patients, $P = .02$). Despite these acute toxicities, there was no significant difference in disease progression or survival based on age. Finally, the Hoosier Oncology Group recently presented a subset analysis of older patients from a phase III trial that evaluated the benefit of consolidation chemotherapy (docetaxel) after standard concurrent CRT (cisplatin/etoposide) [84]. In this study, 52 patients aged 70 years or older experienced more frequent significant neutropenia and esophagitis, but there was no difference in median survival compared with younger patients.

To our knowledge, only one elderly-specific phase III trial has evaluated definitive concurrent CRT. In a study from Japan, patients aged 70 years or older were randomized to either definitive daily RT alone or concurrent carboplatin chemotherapy with the same RT schedule [85]. This trial was terminated prematurely after four deaths related to therapy were reported, three on the concurrent arm. Subsequent analysis found significant protocol violations, including radiation field noncompliance in two of the four patients who succumbed to treatment-related toxicities. Of the 46 patients enrolled, the median survival was 18.5 months in patients who received concurrent therapy, compared with 14.3 months in patients who underwent radiation alone. This difference was not statistically significant.

Taken together, the available data suggest that fit older patients may benefit as much as their younger counterparts from concurrent CRT strategies in locally advanced NSCLC. However, this approach comes with increases in acute toxicities, primarily neutropenia and esophagitis. Careful monitoring with supportive measures is required if such an aggressive approach is considered. Alternative treatment options currently being evaluated for locally advanced disease include concurrent therapy with attenuated doses of cisplatin-based chemotherapy, non–platinum-containing chemotherapy, and targeted therapies.

Chemotherapy for advanced non–small-cell lung cancer

The current treatment standard for patients who have advanced NSCLC (stages IIIB with malignant effusion and stage IV) is combination chemotherapy with a platinum-based doublet [86]. Addition of bevacizumab, an inhibitor of vascular endothelial growth factor, is also recommended for some patients who have advanced NSCLC of nonsquamous histology [22]. These regimens can be difficult to tolerate, even for younger patients, but comprise first-line therapy for patients who have advanced disease.

The role of modern platinum-based doublet chemotherapy, specifically in an older population that has advanced NSCLC, is less clear, with clinical trial data only available from retrospective analyses of phase III trials. Two such trials compared platinum-based doublet therapy with single-agent therapy. The Cancer and Leukemia Group B 9730 trial randomized patients to either paclitaxel or the combination of paclitaxel with carboplatin [87]. In a subset analysis of 155 patients aged 70 years or older, median survival with combination therapy was 8 months versus 5.8 months with paclitaxel alone; however, this result was not statistically significant (hazard ratio 0.84, 95% CI 0.61–1.16; $P = .29$). Data concerning toxicity, specifically in the older cohort, are not available, but both regimens were generally tolerated well, with less than 10% incidence of neutropenic fever and two treatment-related deaths. A similarly designed trial conducted by the Swedish Lung Cancer Study Group also reported a trend toward improvement in median survival with combination chemotherapy (carboplatin/gemcitabine) versus gemcitabine alone (11 months versus 9.4 months; hazard ratio 0.74, 95% CI 0.51–1.1, $P = .12$) [88]. Although there was more severe hematologic toxicity with therapy in older patients compared with younger ones, it did not lead to an increased incidence of neutropenic fever, hospitalizations, or death.

Subset analyses of several randomized trials that compared modern platinum-based doublet chemotherapy together have suggested similar efficacy in older patients, with slightly more hematologic toxicity. The largest of these trials randomized 1155 patients to four different doublet regimens [86]. There was no significant difference in survival between the four chemotherapy arms. In a retrospective age-specific analysis of this study, 227 patients were identified as aged 70 years or older. Median survival in this subset was 8.2 months, compared with 8.1 months in patients younger than 70 years [89]. One-year survival rates were 35% ($\geq$70 years) and 33% ($<$70 years). Toxicities were similar in both cohorts. In the small subset of patients aged 80 years and older ($n = 9$) enrolled in the trial, only one patient was able to complete more than three cycles of therapy, and no responses to chemotherapy were observed.

Recently, the addition of the anti-angiogenesis agent, bevacizumab, to carboplatin/paclitaxel chemotherapy has been shown to improve median survival in patients who have advanced NSCLC [22]. Patients who had squamous cell histology were not eligible for this trial, because an earlier trial noted an increased incidence of fatal hemoptysis in this population. Those patients who had pre-existing hemoptysis, a need for coagulation, or brain metastases were excluded also. A retrospective analysis of 224 patients aged 70 years or older found a trend toward improved response rate (20% versus 17%, $P = .067$) and median progression-free survival (5.9 months versus 4.9 months, $P = .063$) with the addition of bevacizumab, but no improvement in median survival (11.3 months with bevacizumab versus 12.1 months without, $P = .4$) [90]. Severe treatment-related toxicity was more common with bevacizumab (87% versus 61%, $P < .001$), with seven treatment-related deaths associated with the addition of bevacizumab compared with two in patients receiving chemotherapy alone.

As an alternative to platinum-based doublet chemotherapy, a series of elderly-specific phase III trials over the last 10 years has evaluated the benefits of single-agent chemotherapy in advanced NSCLC. The landmark Elderly Lung Cancer Vinorelbine Italian Study Group trial initially established that monotherapy with vinorelbine was superior to best supportive care, with improved survival and quality of life [91,92]. One hundred fifty-four patients aged 70 years or older were randomized to either weekly vinorelbine or best supportive care. Median survival was increased from 4.8 months to 6.4 months with chemotherapy ($P < .05$), with 1-year survival rate of 32% versus 14% with best supportive care.

Chemotherapy was also associated with overall improvement in quality of life. The subsequent Multicenter Italian Lung Cancer in the Elderly Study evaluated the use of either weekly vinorelbine or gemcitabine or the combination of both agents in 698 patients aged 70 or older [93]. There was no statistically significant difference in survival or quality of life among the three arms; however, there was substantially more toxicity with combination chemotherapy. Median survival ranged from 6.4 to 8.3 months between the three arms, with 1-year survival rates of 28% to 38%. More recently, the West Japan Thoracic Oncology Group compared docetaxel to vinorelbine in 180 patients aged 70 years or older and reported a trend toward improved median survival with docetaxel (14.3 months versus 9.9 months, $P = .138$) with 1-year survival rate of 58.6% versus 36.7% in the vinorelbine arm [94]. Response rates were significantly higher with docetaxel (22.7% versus 9.9%, $P = .019$), as was median progression-free survival (5.5 months versus 3.1 months; $P < .001$). Despite increased hematologic toxicities, patients who received docetaxel reported overall improvement in disease-related symptoms.

Based on these retrospective analyses, it is reasonable to consider first-line therapy with platinum-based doublet chemotherapy in fit older patients who have advanced NSCLC. The increased risk of significant neutropenia in such patients may be lessened with the use of myeloid growth factors. Alternatively, single-agent therapy, such as vinorelbine or docetaxel, should be considered. The safety and efficacy of bevacizumab with chemotherapy in older persons needs to be evaluated further. Particular caution must be exercised when considering treatment of fit patients aged 80 years or older, because data relating to safety and outcomes are sparse.

Small-cell lung cancer

Limited-stage small-cell lung cancer

Limited-stage small-cell lung cancer (SCLC) is defined as disease confined to the ipsilateral hemithorax (but may include contralateral mediastinal lymph node involvement) in the absence of a malignant effusion that can be encompassed within a single radiation port [95]. Chemotherapy is the cornerstone of treatment for limited-stage SCLC (Table 4). The addition of thoracic radiotherapy to chemotherapy has been associated with improvements in local control and survival, with

Table 4
Treatment of small-cell lung cancer by stage

Small-cell lung cancer				
Stage	Surgery	Adjuvant chemotherapy	Concurrent chemotherapy and radiation therapy with curative intent	Palliative chemotherapy
Limited stage[a]			X	
Extensive stage[a]				X

[a] Prophylactic cranial irradiation should be offered to responders with either limited- or extensive-stage SCLC.

a meta-analysis of 13 randomized clinical trials reporting a 5.4% overall survival advantage at 3 years compared with chemotherapy alone [96]. Generally, thoracic irradiation is recommended early, to be initiated concurrently with either the first or second cycle of chemotherapy.

Limited clinical data exist concerning feasibility and benefit of CRT, particularly with standard cisplatin-based regimens, in older patients who have SCLC. Two retrospective analyses of cisplatin-based CRT trials in older patients are available. The landmark Intergroup 0096 trial compared the use of twice-daily RT with concurrent chemotherapy (cisplatin/etoposide) to conventional once-daily RT with the same chemotherapy [97]. Five-year survival rate with twice-daily RT was 26% versus 16% for conventional dosing of RT ($P = .04$). Although acute toxicity was greater with twice-daily RT, particularly esophagitis (27% versus 11%, $P < .001$), there was no significant difference in treatment-related deaths. A subsequent retrospective analysis of the 50 patients aged 70 years or older reported that severe hematologic toxicities (61% versus 84%, $P < .01$) and fatal toxicity (1% versus 10%, $P < .01$) were more frequent in older patients. Overall 5-year survival rate in older patients was 16% compared with 22% in younger patients ($P = .05$), with no significant differences in 5-year event-free survival, time to local failure, response, or duration of response [98]. Unlike the Intergroup 0096 trial, a North Central Cancer Treatment Group trial that compared once-daily versus split-course, twice-daily radiotherapy with the cisplatin/etoposide platform failed to show a survival advantage with twice-daily RT [99]. This finding was likely because RT was delayed until the fourth cycle of chemotherapy and was only given in a continuous fashion on the once-daily regimen. Five-year survival rate was found to be 21% with once-daily RT versus 22% with split-course, twice-daily administration ($P = .68$). A retrospective analysis of the 56 patients aged

70 years or older reported 5-year survival rate of 17% compared with 22% in younger patients ($P = .14$) [100]. There were no significant differences in severe or fatal toxicities other than increased incidence of pneumonitis in older patients (6% versus 0% in younger patients).

Although these analyses are subject to selection bias and suffer from small sample size, they suggest that standard curative concurrent CRT regimens should be considered in fit older patients who have limited-stage SCLC. For less fit patients of any age, alternative treatment with sequential therapy or attenuated doses of concurrent chemotherapy should be considered.

Extensive-stage small-cell lung cancer

Extensive-stage SCLC is defined as disease not meeting criteria for limited-stage disease (ie, distant metastatic disease, malignant effusion, or locally advanced disease that cannot be encompassed within a reasonable radiation port) [95]. The standard of current treatment for extensive-stage SCLC is platinum-based chemotherapy doublet. A small number of elderly-specific prospective trials have evaluated the use of chemotherapy in extensive-stage SCLC. Considering that the goal of therapy in this population is not curative, carboplatin is often substituted for cisplatin, because it appears similar in efficacy but is better tolerated. Split dosing of cisplatin (eg, over 3 days rather than 1) has been another strategy to reduce toxicity. Generally, these approaches result in high response rates with significant clinical benefit. The Japan Clinical Oncology Group conducted a phase III trial of combination chemotherapy with carboplatin and etoposide versus split-dose cisplatin and etoposide in older or poor risk patients ($n = 220$) with extensive-stage SCLC [101]. Both regimens were tolerated well, with approximately two thirds of patients receiving the full four cycles of therapy.

There was more severe thrombocytopenia with carboplatin and etoposide and equally high rates of severe neutropenia in both arms (95% with carboplatin and etoposide; 90% with split-dose cisplatin and etoposide), but only 6% of patients experienced serious infections and there were no significant bleeding episodes. Response rates were 73% in both arms with no significant difference in median survival (10.6 months with carboplatin and etoposide; 9.9 months with split-dose cisplatin and etoposide, $P = .54$).

Another approach in older patients has been to use single-agent therapy, usually oral etoposide, or attenuated doses of doublet chemotherapy. Although this may be appropriate in significantly compromised patients, it should not be routinely practiced in fit older patients. This was demonstrated in a randomized phase II trial of low-dose versus standard-dose cisplatin/etoposide chemotherapy with growth factor support [102]. Response rate and 1-year survival rate in patients receiving full-dose chemotherapy were 69% and 39%, respectively, compared with a 39% response rate and an 18% 1-year survival with low-dose therapy. Both regimens were well tolerated, but patients who received full-dose chemotherapy experienced more severe myelotoxicity (12% versus 0%).

Prophylactic cranial irradiation

Prophylactic cranial irradiation (PCI) has an established role in SCLC patients who have demonstrated a good response to chemotherapy or chemoradiation. Not only does such therapy reduce the incidence of brain metastases but it also leads to improved survival. This benefit was initially shown in a meta-analysis of seven randomized trials that enrolled 987 patients who had complete response to induction therapy [103]. Patients randomized to PCI versus observation experienced a decreased incidence of brain metastases (relative risk 0.46, 95% CI 0.38–0.57; $P < .001$) and a 5.4% absolute improvement in the rate of 3-year survival (relative risk 0.84, 95% CI 0.73–0.97; $P = .01$). More recently, a randomized trial of PCI versus observation demonstrated benefit of PCI in 286 patients who had extensive-stage disease and responded to first line chemotherapy [104]. At 1 year, symptomatic brain metastases developed in 15% of patients who received PCI compared with 40% in the observation arm ($P < .001$). One-year survival rate was 27% with PCI versus 13% without PCI (hazard ratio 0.68, 95% CI 0.52–0.88; $P = .003$). PCI was tolerated well; however, less than 10% of patients survived 2 years, when late cognitive deficits might be expected to manifest.

The survival benefit noted with PCI does not seem to be influenced by age. PCI should be used cautiously in older adults, however, because the potential for late neurocognitive dysfunction is of special concern in these patients. Pre-existing neuropsychological impairment and patient support systems must be considered, particularly with limited-stage disease, in which up to 20% of patients may experience long-term survival. Still, available data indicate that the risk of neurocognitive decline with modern PCI schedules seems to be minimal, and such therapy should not be denied to selected fit older patients who experience a good response to chemotherapy.

Summary

As the American population continues to age, we can anticipate increases in the numbers of older persons who develop lung cancer. Based on the available evidence, it is clear that age alone should not be a contraindication to treatment. Older persons should undergo the same comprehensive evaluation as their younger counterparts, with more focused attention on function, including assessments of performance status, cognition, and social environment, all of which may be issues in a geriatric population and may impact outcomes. Fit older persons can and should be offered the same state-of-the-art treatments for lung cancer as fit younger persons, with anticipated improvement in quality and quantity of life.

References

[1] Jemal A, Siegel R, Ward E, et al. Cancer statistics, 2007. CA Cancer J Clin 2007;57(1):43–66.
[2] Bach PB, Kattan MW, Thornquist MD, et al. Variations in lung cancer risk among smokers. J Natl Cancer Inst 2003;95(6):470–8.
[3] Woloshin S, Schwartz LM, Welch HG. Risk charts: putting cancer in context. J Natl Cancer Inst 2002; 94(11):799–804.
[4] Peto R, Darby S, Deo H, et al. Smoking, smoking cessation, and lung cancer in the UK since 1950: combination of national statistics with two case-control studies. BMJ 2000;321(7257):323–9.
[5] Alberg AJ, Samet JM. Epidemiology of lung cancer. Chest 2003;123(1 Suppl):21S–49S.
[6] Tanoue L, Matthay RA. Lung cancer: epidemiology and carcinogenesis. In: Shields T, Locicero JI,

Ponn R, et al, editors. General thoracic surgery. 6th edition. Philadelphia: Lippincott Williams & Wilkins; 2005. p. 1425–41.

[7] Webster's dictionary. New York: Lexicon Publications, Inc.; 1988.

[8] Zagonel V, Tirelli U, Serraino D, et al. The aged patient with lung cancer: management recommendations. Drugs Aging 1994;4(1):34–46.

[9] Chan ED, Welsh CH. Geriatric respiratory medicine. Chest 1998;114(6):1704–33.

[10] Johnson DH. Small cell lung cancer in the elderly patient. Semin Oncol 1997;24(4):484–91.

[11] Jennens RR, de Boer R, Irving L, et al. Differences of opinion: a survey of knowledge and bias among clinicians regarding the role of chemotherapy in metastatic non-small cell lung cancer. Chest 2004; 126(6):1985–93.

[12] Guadagnoli E, Weitberg A, Mor V, et al. The influence of patient age on the diagnosis and treatment of lung and colorectal cancer. Arch Intern Med 1990;150(7):1485–90.

[13] National Center for Health Statistics. Health, United States, 2006, with Chartbook on Trends in the Health of Americans. Hyattsville (MD): US Government Printing Office; 2006. p. 60–7, 113.

[14] ECOG performance status. Available at: http://www.ecog.org/general/perf_stat.html. Accessed July 10, 2007.

[15] Oken MM, Creech RH, Tormey DC, et al. Toxicity and response criteria of the Eastern Cooperative Oncology Group. Am J Clin Oncol 1982;5(6): 649–55.

[16] Hurria A, Kris MG. Management of lung cancer in older adults. CA Cancer J Clin 2003;53(6):325–41.

[17] Landi F, Zuccala G, Gambassi G, et al. Body mass index and mortality among older people living in the community. J Am Geriatr Soc 1999;47(9): 1072–6.

[18] Eagles JM, Beattie JA, Restall DB, et al. Relation between cognitive impairment and early death in the elderly. BMJ 1990;300(6719):239–40.

[19] Wolfson C, Wolfson DB, Asgharian M, et al. A reevaluation of the duration of survival after the onset of dementia. N Engl J Med 2001;344(15): 1111–6.

[20] Fukuse T, Satoda N, Hijiya K, et al. Importance of a comprehensive geriatric assessment in prediction of complications following thoracic surgery in elderly patients. Chest 2005;127(3): 886–91.

[21] Kris MG, Giaccone G, Davies A, et al. Systemic therapy of bronchioloalveolar carcinoma: results of the first IASLC/ASCO consensus conference on bronchioloalveolar carcinoma. J Thorac Oncol 2006;1(9 Suppl):S32–6.

[22] Sandler A, Gray R, Perry MC, et al. Paclitaxel-carboplatin alone or with bevacizumab for non-small-cell lung cancer. N Engl J Med 2006;355(24): 2542–50.

[23] Lynch TJ, Adjei AA, Bunn PA Jr, et al. Summary statement: novel agents in the treatment of lung cancer: advances in epidermal growth factor receptor-targeted agents. Clin Cancer Res 2006;12(14 Pt 2): 4365s–71s.

[24] Olaussen KA, Dunant A, Fouret P, et al. DNA repair by ERCC1 in non-small-cell lung cancer and cisplatin-based adjuvant chemotherapy. N Engl J Med 2006;355(10):983–91.

[25] Mountain CF. Revisions in the International System for Staging Lung Cancer. Chest 1997;111(6): 1710–7.

[26] Lababede O, Meziane MA, Rice TW. TNM staging of lung cancer: a quick reference chart. Chest 1999; 115(1):233–5.

[27] Martini N, Bains MS, Burt ME, et al. Incidence of local recurrence and second primary tumors in resected stage I lung cancer. J Thorac Cardiovasc Surg 1995;109(1):120–9.

[28] Henschke CI, Yankelevitz DF, Libby DM, et al. Survival of patients with stage I lung cancer detected on CT screening. N Engl J Med 2006; 355(17):1763–71.

[29] Kato H, Ichinose Y, Ohta M, et al. A randomized trial of adjuvant chemotherapy with uracil-tegafur for adenocarcinoma of the lung. N Engl J Med 2004;350(17):1713–21.

[30] Winton T, Livingston R, Johnson D, et al. Vinorelbine plus cisplatin vs. observation in resected non-small-cell lung cancer. N Engl J Med 2005; 352(25):2589–97.

[31] Douillard JY, Rosell R, De Lena M, et al. Adjuvant vinorelbine plus cisplatin versus observation in patients with completely resected stage IB-IIIA non-small-cell lung cancer (Adjuvant Navelbine International Trialist Association [ANITA]): a randomised controlled trial. Lancet Oncol 2006; 7(9):719–27.

[32] Bach PB, Jett JR, Pastorino U, et al. Computed tomography screening and lung cancer outcomes. JAMA 2007;297(9):953–61.

[33] Bach PB. CT screening for lung cancer. N Engl J Med 2007;356(7):744.

[34] Sato M, Saito Y, Endo C, et al. The natural history of radiographically occult bronchogenic squamous cell carcinoma: a retrospective study of overdiagnosis bias. Chest 2004;126(1):108–13.

[35] Motohiro A, Ueda H, Komatsu H, et al. Prognosis of non-surgically treated, clinical stage I lung cancer patients in Japan. Lung Cancer 2002;36(1): 65–9.

[36] Sobue T, Suzuki T, Matsuda M, et al. Survival for clinical stage I lung cancer not surgically treated: comparison between screen-detected and symptom-detected cases. The Japanese Lung Cancer Screening Research Group. Cancer 1992;69(3): 685–92.

[37] Beckles MA, Spiro SG, Colice GL, et al. The physiologic evaluation of patients with lung cancer

being considered for resectional surgery. Chest 2003;123(1 Suppl):105S–14S.

[38] Wyser C, Stulz P, Soler M, et al. Prospective evaluation of an algorithm for the functional assessment of lung resection candidates. Am J Respir Crit Care Med 1999;159(5 Pt 1):1450–6.

[39] Mery CM, Pappas AN, Bueno R, et al. Similar long-term survival of elderly patients with non-small cell lung cancer treated with lobectomy or wedge resection within the surveillance, epidemiology, and end results database. Chest 2005;128(1): 237–45.

[40] Peake MD, Thompson S, Lowe D, et al. Ageism in the management of lung cancer. Age Ageing 2003; 32(2):171–7.

[41] O'Rourke MA, Feussner JR, Feigl P, et al. Age trends of lung cancer stage at diagnosis. Implications for lung cancer screening in the elderly. JAMA 1987;258(7):921–6.

[42] Trimble EL, Carter CL, Cain D, et al. Representation of older patients in cancer treatment trials. Cancer 1994;74(7 Suppl):2208–14.

[43] Turner NJ, Haward RA, Mulley GP, et al. Cancer in old age: is it inadequately investigated and treated? BMJ 1999;319(7205):309–12.

[44] Cerfolio RJ, Bryant AS. Survival and outcomes of pulmonary resection for non-small cell lung cancer in the elderly: a nested case-control study. Ann Thorac Surg 2006;82(2):424–9 [discussion: 9–30].

[45] Teeter SM, Holmes FF, McFarlane MJ. Lung carcinoma in the elderly population: influence of histology on the inverse relationship of stage to age. Cancer 1987;60(6):1331–6.

[46] Bernet F, Brodbeck R, Guenin MO, et al. Age does not influence early and late tumor-related outcome for bronchogenic carcinoma. Ann Thorac Surg 2000;69(3):913–8.

[47] Mahoney FI, Barthel DW. Functional evaluation: the Barthel Index. Md State Med J 1965;14:61–5.

[48] Sainsbury A, Seebass G, Bansal A, et al. Reliability of the Barthel Index when used with older people. Age Ageing 2005;34(3):228–32.

[49] Folstein MF, Folstein SE, McHugh PR. Mini-mental state: a practical method for grading the cognitive state of patients for the clinician. J Psychiatr Res 1975;12(3):189–98.

[50] Crum RM, Anthony JC, Bassett SS, et al. Population-based norms for the mini-mental state examination by age and educational level. JAMA 1993; 269(18):2386–91.

[51] Holsinger T, Deveau J, Boustani M, et al. Does this patient have dementia? JAMA 2007;297(21): 2391–404.

[52] Zagonel V. Importance of a comprehensive geriatric assessment in older cancer patients. Eur J Cancer 2001;37(Suppl 7):S229–33.

[53] Repetto L, Fratino L, Audisio RA, et al. Comprehensive geriatric assessment adds information to

Eastern Cooperative Oncology Group performance status in elderly cancer patients: an Italian Group for Geriatric Oncology Study. J Clin Oncol 2002;20(2):494–502.

[54] van Rens MT, de la Riviere AB, Elbers HR, et al. Prognostic assessment of 2,361 patients who underwent pulmonary resection for non-small cell lung cancer, stage I, II, and IIIA. Chest 2000;117(2): 374–9.

[55] Jazieh AR, Hussain M, Howington JA, et al. Prognostic factors in patients with surgically resected stages I and II non-small cell lung cancer. Ann Thorac Surg 2000;70(4):1168–71.

[56] Ginsberg RJ, Hill LD, Eagan RT, et al. Modern thirty-day operative mortality for surgical resections in lung cancer. J Thorac Cardiovasc Surg 1983;86(5):654–8.

[57] Damhuis RA, Schutte PR. Resection rates and postoperative mortality in 7,899 patients with lung cancer. Eur Respir J 1996;9(1):7–10.

[58] Fan J, Wang XJ, Jiang GN, et al. Survival and outcomes of surgical treatment of the elderly NSCLC in China: a retrospective matched cohort study. Eur J Surg Oncol 2007;33(5):639–43.

[59] Sullivan V, Tran T, Holmstrom A, et al. Advanced age does not exclude lobectomy for non-small cell lung carcinoma. Chest 2005;128(4):2671–6.

[60] Yamamoto K, Alarcon J, Medina V, et al. Surgical results of stage I non-small cell lung cancer: comparison between elderly and younger patients. Eur J Cardiothorac Surg 2003;23:21–5.

[61] Sawada S, Komori E, Nogami N, et al. Advanced age is not correlated with either short-term or long-term postoperative results in lung cancer patients in good clinical condition. Chest 2005; 128(3):1557–63.

[62] Haffty BG, Goldberg NB, Gerstley J, et al. Results of radical radiation therapy in clinical stage I, technically operable non-small cell lung cancer. Int J Radiat Oncol Biol Phys 1988;15(1): 69–73.

[63] Sibley GS. Radiotherapy for patients with medically inoperable stage I non-small cell lung carcinoma: smaller volumes and higher doses: a review. Cancer 1998;82(3):433–8.

[64] Perez CA, Pajak TF, Rubin P, et al. Long-term observations of the patterns of failure in patients with unresectable non-oat cell carcinoma of the lung treated with definitive radiotherapy: report by the Radiation Therapy Oncology Group. Cancer 1987;59(11):1874–81.

[65] Decker RH, Tanoue LT, Colasanto JM, et al. Evaluation and definitive management of medically inoperable early-stage non-small-cell lung cancer. Part 1: assessment and conventional radiotherapy. Oncology (Williston Park) 2006; 20(7):727–36.

[66] Decker RH, Tanoue LT, Colasanto JM, et al. Evaluation and definitive management of medically

inoperable early stage non-small-cell lung cancer. Part 2: newer treatment modalities. Oncology (Williston Park) 2006;20(8):899–905 [discussion: 8, 13].

[67] Steinke K, Sewell PE, Dupuy D, et al. Pulmonary radiofrequency ablation: an international study survey. Anticancer Res 2004;24(1):339–43.

[68] VanSonnenberg E, Shankar S, Morrison PR, et al. Radiofrequency ablation of thoracic lesions, part 2. Initial clinical experience: technical and multidisciplinary considerations in 30 patients. AJR Am J Roentgenol 2005;184(2):381–90.

[69] Potters L, Steinberg M, Rose C, et al. American Society for Therapeutic Radiology and Oncology and American College of Radiology practice guideline for the performance of stereotactic body radiation therapy. Int J Radiat Oncol Biol Phys 2004;60(4): 1026–32.

[70] Hiraoka M, Nagata Y. Stereotactic body radiation therapy for early-stage non-small-cell lung cancer: the Japanese experience. Int J Clin Oncol 2004; 9(5):352–5.

[71] Onishi H, Araki T, Shirato H, et al. Stereotactic hypofractionated high-dose irradiation for stage I nonsmall cell lung carcinoma: clinical outcomes in 245 subjects in a Japanese multiinstitutional study. Cancer 2004;101(7):1623–31.

[72] Wulf J, Haedinger U, Oppitz U, et al. Stereotactic radiotherapy for primary lung cancer and pulmonary metastases: a noninvasive treatment approach in medically inoperable patients. Int J Radiat Oncol Biol Phys 2004;60(1):186–96.

[73] Strauss G, Herndon J, Maddaus M, et al. Adjuvant chemotherapy in stage IB non-small cell lung cancer (NSCLC): update of Cancer and Leukemia Group B (CALGB) protocol 9633. ASCO Meeting Abstracts 2006;24(18 Suppl):7007.

[74] Arriagada R, Bergman B, Dunant A, et al. Cisplatin-based adjuvant chemotherapy in patients with completely resected non-small-cell lung cancer. N Engl J Med 2004;350(4):351–60.

[75] Pepe C, Hasan B, Winton TL, et al. Adjuvant vinorelbine and cisplatin in elderly patients: National Cancer Institute of Canada and Intergroup Study JBR 10. J Clin Oncol 2007;25(12): 1553–61.

[76] Fruh M, Tribodet H, Pignon JP, et al. A pooled analysis of the effect of age on adjuvant cisplatin-based chemotherapy for completely resected non-small cell lung cancer (NSCLC). ASCO Annual Meeting Proceedings Part I. J Clin Oncol 2007;25: 18S.

[77] Dillman RO, Herndon J, Seagren SL, et al. Improved survival in stage III non-small-cell lung cancer: seven-year follow-up of cancer and leukemia group B (CALGB) 8433 trial. J Natl Cancer Inst 1996;88(17):1210–5.

[78] Sause W, Kolesar P, Taylor SI, et al. Final results of phase III trial in regionally advanced unresectable non-small cell lung cancer: Radiation Therapy Oncology Group, Eastern Cooperative Oncology Group, and Southwest Oncology Group. Chest 2000;117(2):358–64.

[79] Furuse K, Fukuoka M, Kawahara M, et al. Phase III study of concurrent versus sequential thoracic radiotherapy in combination with mitomycin, vindesine, and cisplatin in unresectable stage III non-small-cell lung cancer. J Clin Oncol 1999;17(9): 2692–9.

[80] Curran W, Scott C, Langer C. Long-term benefit is observed in a phase III comparison of sequential vs. concurrent chemoradiation for patients with unresected stage III non-small cell lung cancer: RTOG 9410. Proceedings of the American Society of Clinical Oncology 2003;22:621a.

[81] Langer C, Hsu C, Curran W. Elderly patients with locally advanced non-small cell lung cancer benefit from combined modality therapy: secondary analysis of Radiation Therapy Oncology Group (RTOG) 9410. Proceedings of the American Society of Clinical Oncology 2002;21:299a.

[82] Rocha Lima CM, Herndon JE 2nd, Kosty M, et al. Therapy choices among older patients with lung carcinoma: an evaluation of two trials of the Cancer and Leukemia Group B. Cancer 2002;94(1):181–7.

[83] Schild SE, Stella PJ, Geyer SM, et al. Phase III trial comparing chemotherapy plus once-daily or twice-daily radiotherapy in stage III non-small-cell lung cancer. Int J Radiat Oncol Biol Phys 2002;54(2): 370–8.

[84] Sgroi M, Neubauer M, Ansari R, et al. An analysis of elderly patients (pts) treated on a phase III trial of cisplatin (P) plus etoposide (E) with concurrent radiotherapy (CRT) followed by docetaxel (C) vs observation (O) in pts with stage III non small cell lung cancer (NSCLC). ASCO Meeting Abstracts 2007;25(18 Suppl):9037.

[85] Atagi S, Kawahara M, Tamura T, et al. Standard thoracic radiotherapy with or without concurrent daily low-dose carboplatin in elderly patients with locally advanced non-small cell lung cancer: a phase III trial of the Japan Clinical Oncology Group (JCOG9812). Jpn J Clin Oncol 2005;35(4):195–201.

[86] Schiller JH, Harrington D, Belani CP, et al. Comparison of four chemotherapy regimens for advanced non-small-cell lung cancer. N Engl J Med 2002;346(2):92–8.

[87] Lilenbaum RC, Herndon JE 2nd, List MA, et al. Single-agent versus combination chemotherapy in advanced non-small-cell lung cancer: the cancer and leukemia group B (study 9730). J Clin Oncol 2005;23(1):190–6.

[88] Sederholm C, Hillerdal G, Lamberg K, et al. Phase III trial of gemcitabine plus carboplatin versus single-agent gemcitabine in the treatment of locally advanced or metastatic non-small-cell lung cancer: the Swedish Lung Cancer Study Group. J Clin Oncol 2005;23(33):8380–8.

[89] Langer C, Vangel M, Schiller JH, et al. Age-specific subanalysis of ECOG 1594: fit elderly patients (70–80 YRS) with NSCLC do as well as young pts (<70). Proceedings of the American Society of Clinical Oncology 2003;22:2572.

[90] Ramalingam S, Dahlberg S, Langer C, et al. Outcomes for elderly advanced stage non-small cell lung cancer (NSCLC) patients (pts) treated with bevacizumab (V) in combination with carboplatin (C) and paclitaxel (P): analysis of Eastern Cooperative Oncology Group (ECOG) 4599 study. ASCO Meeting Abstracts 2007;25(Suppl 18):7535.

[91] Gridelli C. The ELVIS trial: a phase III study of single-agent vinorelbine as first-line treatment in elderly patients with advanced non-small cell lung cancer: Elderly Lung Cancer Vinorelbine Italian Study. Oncologist 2001;6(Suppl 1):4–7.

[92] The Elderly Lung Cancer Vinorelbine Italian Study Group. Effects of vinorelbine on quality of life and survival of elderly patients with advanced non-small-cell lung cancer. J Natl Cancer Inst 1999; 91(1):66–72.

[93] Gridelli C, Perrone F, Gallo C, et al. Chemotherapy for elderly patients with advanced non-small-cell lung cancer: the Multicenter Italian Lung Cancer in the Elderly Study (MILES) phase III randomized trial. J Natl Cancer Inst 2003;95(5): 362–72.

[94] Kudoh S, Takeda K, Nakagawa K, et al. Phase III study of docetaxel compared with vinorelbine in elderly patients with advanced non-small-cell lung cancer: results of the West Japan Thoracic Oncology Group Trial (WJTOG 9904). J Clin Oncol 2006;24(22):3657–63.

[95] Simon GR, Wagner H. Small cell lung cancer. Chest 2003;123(1 Suppl):259S–71S.

[96] Pignon JP, Arriagada R, Ihde DC, et al. A meta-analysis of thoracic radiotherapy for small-cell lung cancer. N Engl J Med 1992;327(23):1618–24.

[97] Turrisi AT 3rd, Kim K, Blum R, et al. Twice-daily compared with once-daily thoracic radiotherapy in limited small-cell lung cancer treated concurrently with cisplatin and etoposide. N Engl J Med 1999; 340(4):265–71.

[98] Yuen AR, Zou G, Turrisi AT, et al. Similar outcome of elderly patients in intergroup trial 0096: cisplatin, etoposide, and thoracic radiotherapy administered once or twice daily in limited stage small cell lung carcinoma. Cancer 2000;89(9): 1953–60.

[99] Schild SE, Bonner JA, Shanahan TG, et al. Long-term results of a phase III trial comparing once-daily radiotherapy with twice-daily radiotherapy in limited-stage small-cell lung cancer. Int J Radiat Oncol Biol Phys 2004;59(4):943–51.

[100] Schild SE, Stella PJ, Brooks BJ, et al. Results of combined-modality therapy for limited-stage small cell lung carcinoma in the elderly. Cancer 2005; 103(11):2349–54.

[101] Okamoto H, Watanabe K, Kunikane H, et al. Randomised phase III trial of carboplatin plus etoposide vs split doses of cisplatin plus etoposide in elderly or poor-risk patients with extensive disease small-cell lung cancer: JCOG 9702. Br J Cancer 2007;97(2):162–9.

[102] Ardizzoni A, Favaretto A, Boni L, et al. Platinum-etoposide chemotherapy in elderly patients with small-cell lung cancer: results of a randomized multicenter phase II study assessing attenuated-dose or full-dose with lenograstim prophylaxis. A Forza Operativa Nazionale Italiana Carcinoma Polmonare and Gruppo Studio Tumori Polmonari Veneto (FONICAP-GSTPV) study. J Clin Oncol 2005; 23(3):569–75.

[103] Auperin A, Arriagada R, Pignon JP, et al. Prophylactic cranial irradiation for patients with small-cell lung cancer in complete remission: Prophylactic Cranial Irradiation Overview Collaborative Group. N Engl J Med 1999;341(7):476–84.

[104] Slotman B, Faivre-Finn C, Kramer G, et al. Prophylactic cranial irradiation in extensive small-cell lung cancer. N Engl J Med 2007;357(7):664–72.

ELSEVIER
SAUNDERS

Clin Chest Med 28 (2007) 751–771

CLINICS
IN CHEST
MEDICINE

Pneumonia in the Older Patient

Michael S. Niederman, MD, FACP, FCCP[a,b,*], Veronica Brito, MD[c]

[a]Department of Medicine, Winthrop-University Hospital, 222 Station Plaza North,
Suite 509, Mineola, NY 11550, USA
[b]Department of Medicine, State University of New York at Stony Brook, NY, USA
[c]Pulmonary and Critical Care Medicine, Winthrop-University Hospital, 222 Station Plaza North,
Suite 509, Mineola, NY 11550, USA

Pneumonia is the leading cause of death from infectious diseases among older individuals and is among the ten leading causes of death for this population as a whole. Pneumonia is the second most frequent illness requiring hospitalization in older adults, being surpassed only by congestive heart failure. Sixty percent of patients admitted to the hospital with pneumonia are aged 65 or older [1]. In older patients, there is a disparity in the cost of care for community-acquired pneumonia (CAP) compared with a younger population, with more older patients requiring admission, which is a more costly form of care, than outpatient therapy. Niederman and colleagues [2] used Medicare and insurance company databases to evaluate the cost of treating patients with CAP in 1994. Of the 5.6 million people diagnosed with CAP in the United States, approximately one third (1.7 million), were older than age 65. Although most patients with CAP are managed out of the hospital, most inpatients are older. Older patients are hospitalized more often because they have more comorbid illness compared with a younger population. As a consequence of increased rates of hospitalization and increased length of stay when they are admitted, older patients account for $4.8 billion of the total $8.4 billion spent for the care of pneumonia [2]. They represent only approximately one third of all

* Corresponding author. Department of Medicine, Winthrop-University Hospital, 222 Station Plaza North, Suite 509, Mineola, NY 11550.
E-mail address: mniederman@winthrop.org (M.S. Niederman).

patients with CAP yet were responsible for more than half of the dollars spent on this illness. In fact, the average hospital stay for an older person with CAP is 7.8 days, which costs $7166, compared with a younger person with CAP staying 5.8 days, which costs $6042.

Older patients have an increased incidence of pneumonia and increased mortality compared with younger populations. In a large community-based study, Marston and colleagues [3] evaluated all residents of two Ohio counties who were hospitalized with CAP in a single year (total of 2776 patients). They found that the incidence and mortality of CAP increased with advancing age. The overall incidence of illness was 266.8 cases per 100,000, but patients aged 18 to 44 had an incidence of 92 cases per 100,000 population, compared with a rate of 1014 cases per 100,000 in patients over age 65. The mortality of CAP was 8.8% overall but was only 4.5% in individuals aged 18 to 44 compared with 12.5% in persons over age 65. The high frequency and enhanced mortality of pneumonia in older patients are well known, but controversy still continues about whether that is a consequence of aging itself or the result of the comorbid illnesses that become increasingly common in the aging population.

The mortality impact of pneumonia extends beyond the hospital stay in older individuals. Kaplan and colleagues [4] used a Medicare database to perform a matched case-control study to evaluate the long-term impact (1-year mortality rate) of CAP in older patients. A total of 158,960 patients with CAP were compared with 794,333 hospitalized controls (5 controls for each case) matched for age, sex, and race. Although the in-hospital mortality rate for CAP exceeded that of controls (11% versus 5.5%), the differences in 1-year mortality rates were even more dramatic (40.9% versus 29.1%). The high mortality rate could not be explained by the types of underlying disease, and these findings persisted, even if only the hospital survivors were examined. Although the exact cause of death was not examined in the study, the population included mostly older patients. Eighty-five percent were older than age 65, the population included nursing home patients, and 70% had comorbid medical illness. The findings expanded on an older Scandinavian study that reported a lower 10-year survival rate in patients with CAP over the age of 60 than in an age-matched population without CAP [5]. In that study, the relative risk for death in patients with CAP was 1.5 compared with patients without CAP, and the 10-year survival rate was 39% compared with 61% in the non-CAP population, with many of the deaths related to cardiovascular disease and subsequent pneumonia.

Although none of these studies directly examined the cause for the high long-term mortality rate in older patients with CAP, other studies have shown that mortality after hospital discharge is more likely to occur in patients who suffer a persistent (>3 months) functional decline as a result of pneumonia, already have poor functional status on admission, and have pre-existing coronary artery disease [6–8].

This article examines the bacteriology, clinical features, therapy for, and prevention of pneumonia in older patients. The discussion focuses on patients who develop pneumonia out of the hospital, including individuals with CAP and those with health care–associated pneumonia (HCAP). HCAP incorporates patients who live in nursing homes when they develop pneumonia, and in many instances requires management similar to nosocomial pneumonia. We have chosen not to discuss nosocomial pneumonia (other than HCAP) in older patients because it does not have distinctive features or a different management approach than when this illness arises in younger patients.

Pathophysiology

Pneumonia develops when an infecting pathogen overwhelms a patient's host defense system, whether because of a virulent pathogen, a large

inoculum of bacteria, impairment in the patient's ability to fight infection, or a combination of these factors. The increased risk of pneumonia in older patients is more often a consequence of the comorbid illnesses that are common with advanced age rather than aging itself. Many comorbid conditions can interfere with host defenses, as can the medications to treat these conditions. The presence of malnutrition, which can be a consequence of various illnesses (malignancy, emphysema, congestive heart failure, liver disease), also can interfere with immune function (Box 1). Certain illnesses, such as neurologic and gastrointestinal processes, can lead to an increased risk of aspirating large inocula of bacteria, whereas

---

Box 1. Risk factors for pneumonia in older persons

Comorbidities and patient habits
  Malignancy
  Chronic obstructive pulmonary
    disease (COPD)
  Heart failure
  Liver disease
  Malnutrition
  Cigarette smoking
Aging
  Poor cough
  Chest wall rigidity
  Impaired mucociliary clearance
  Poor cough reflex
  Immune impairment
  Loss of immune regulation
  Need for medications that interfere
    with immune function
Poor oral hygiene
  Xerostomia
  Age-related increases in
    oropharyngeal gram-negative
    colonization
  Drying of oral secretions because
    of medications, dehydration
  Poor dentition/dental plaque
Poor functional status
  Reduced mobility
  Impaired activities of daily living
Aspiration
  Impaired swallowing
  Stroke
  Dementia

residence in a nursing home can lead to exposure to virulent and drug-resistant organisms.

Aging itself can lead to certain deficiencies in host defense and can predispose to physiologic changes in the lung that interfere with bacterial clearance. With aging, there are associated reductions in the ability to expectorate and clear bacteria and reduced physiologic reserve, which makes it harder for patients to tolerate and overcome severe infection. The aging chest wall becomes more rigid, with an increase in the elastic work of breathing and a reduction in respiratory muscle endurance [9]. Advanced age and impaired FEV_1 have been shown to be significant risk factors for severe pneumonia [10]. Increased work of breathing means that physiologic reserves are reduced when a patient is faced with insults such as surgery or superimposed infection. Mucociliary transport also declines with age, which can lead to reduced clearance of organisms from the respiratory tract. Impaired mucociliary transport is compounded by a reduction in the cough reflex, which was found to be markedly depressed in older patients with pneumonia [11]. The greater the derangement of the cough reflex, the higher the risk for pneumonia [12]. It may not be age, per se, that causes the decrease in cough reflex but rather the comorbidities that are more prevalent in the older population.

In older adults, xerostomia can be present because of medications and as a consequence of oral or dental disease. Oral intake of fluids and oral hygiene can be decreased, depending on the patient's ability for self-care and the degree of support in the patient's place of residence. El-Solh and colleagues [13] found that gram-negative enteric bacteria and *Staphylococcus aureus* accounted for most dental plaque colonization by respiratory pathogens. The prevalence of colonization of dental plaque with aerobic respiratory pathogens was high in institutionalized patients who were critically ill. In general, oropharyngeal bacterial colonization is more common in older than younger populations. Organisms such as *S aureus, Klebsiella pneumoniae,* and *Escherichia coli* transiently colonize the oropharynx of older patients and serve as a harbinger of subsequent pneumonia [14]. Mechanisms that predispose to colonization in the older adults are complex, but Valenti and colleagues [15] found increased rates of gram-negative colonization in patients who were immobile and incontinent, had chronic cardiopulmonary comorbidities, and were clinically deteriorating. Many comorbid illnesses and malnutrition can predispose to oropharyngeal colonization by enteric gram-negative organisms, an event associated with a higher rate of pneumonia. Colonization can be associated with pneumonia because patients commonly aspirate their oropharyngeal flora, and these organisms can lead to lower respiratory tract infection.

Aspiration (small or large volume) is more common in older adults because of impaired swallowing reflexes, especially in persons with neurologic illness. Stroke and degenerative neurologic diseases, such as Alzheimer's disease, can lead to dysphagia. The entity known as silent cerebral infarction affects the basal ganglia and leads to subclinical aspiration, which can cause pneumonia. It also has been reported that patients with oropharyngeal dysphagia treated with ACE inhibitors have a decreased incidence of pneumonia, possibly related to the induction of cough by these medications [16,17]. Malnutrition is also a risk factor for host defense impairment, and Riquelme and colleagues [18,19] found that low serum albumin levels and other anthropometric variables of malnutrition correlated with the development of CAP in older patients, and other studies have found that malnutrition is commonly present in patients with dysphagia [20].

The frequency of comorbid illnesses in older pneumonia patients is high. Fry and colleagues [21] found that in hospitalized older patients with a discharge diagnosis of pneumonia, at least one underlying medical condition was reported in most medical records. Chronic cardiac disease was present in 56.9%, COPD in 47.25%, and diabetes mellitus in 19.5%. All of these comorbid conditions had increased in the time period from 2000 to 2002, compared with the interval between 1988 and 1990. In addition to comorbidity itself leading to host defense impairment, it also can lead to impaired mobility, and Riquelme and colleagues [18] found that diminished physical activity and bedridden status were predictors of increased risk of death in patients over age 65 with pneumonia. Better functional status—as measured by activities of daily living—was identified as a good prognostic factor in a case-control study of pneumonia in nursing home patients [22]. Another study examined 104 patients with pneumonia; when compared with controls, the patients with pneumonia had a correlation between the level of dependence, defined by impairment in activities of daily living, and increased mortality. Large volume aspiration and sedative medication administration were also found to be risk factors for pneumonia [23].

Various other impairments are present in the host immune system of certain older patients, which recently were summarized [24]. In addition to impaired mucociliary clearance and a higher risk of aspiration, older adults can have reduced oropharyngeal clearance, reduced numbers of T cells, reduced helper T-cell activity and response to antigens, reduced numbers of B cells and B-cell response to antigens, reduced antibody response, reduced phagocytosis, and reduced Toll-like receptors on phagocytic cells [24]. Certain older individuals may have a loss of immune regulation.

Clinical presentation and course

More than 100 years ago, Osler described pneumonia in older adults as being a frequent, painless, and often lethal event. Described as "the friend of the aged" and the "captain of the men of death," pneumonia was brought to attention not only in terms of morbidity and mortality but also in terms of its unusual and nonclassic clinical presentations. Osler observed that "in old age pneumonia may be latent, coming on without a chill; the cough and expectoration are slight, the physical signs ill-defined and changeable, and the constitutional symptoms out of all proportion" [25]. Osler also noted the high frequency of extrapulmonary manifestations, such as confusion, often in the absence of any respiratory findings.

Instead of classic pneumonic symptoms, an older patient can present with failure to thrive, confusion, falling, or worsening of a chronic illness (eg, congestive heart failure) (Table 1). These types of clinical presentations can lead to a delay in treatment, which in turn can adversely affect outcome, and presentation in this fashion has been reported to be a factor predicting mortality [19]. The presence of coexisting chronic diseases, such as COPD, diabetes mellitus, and congestive heart failure, not only can mask the presence of infection but also may become the disease processes that are decompensated as the first sign of the presence of pneumonia. Metlay and colleagues [26] evaluated 1812 patients with CAP and found that older patients reported fewer symptoms and that many symptoms (eg, cough, sputum, dyspnea, fatigue, anorexia, myalgias, and abdominal pain) were present for a longer time in older compared to younger patients. In patients over age 75, cough, dyspnea, and sputum production were present for 1 day longer before presentation than in patients aged 18 to 44. Although fever and pleuritic chest

Table 1
Clinical features of pneumonia in elderly persons

Feature	Comment
Fever	Less commonly seen than in younger patients
Tachypnea	Common and reliable feature of CAP
Mental status	Delirium, confusion more likely than in younger patients
Presentation	Cough, sputum production, and dyspnea may not be present
	Confusion, worsening of underlying illness are common
	May present with falling, incontinence, anorexia, reduction in daily activities
	Pleuritic chest pain is less common than in younger patients
	Nonclassic symptoms may lead to delay in diagnosis and delay in administration of antibiotics
Course	Delayed clinical and/or radiologic resolution is common, especially with comorbid illness and more severe illness

pain were more common in younger patients, tachypnea was more common with advancing age. For example, in persons aged 18 to 44, fever was present in 85% and tachypnea in 36%, compared with 53% and 65%, respectively, in persons older than 75 years. In another study of CAP in older patients, Marrie and Blanchard [27] found that fever was present in only 71% of 93 patients, productive cough in 61%, anorexia in 58%, chills in 58%, shortness of breath in 46%, confusion in 37% and pleuritic chest pain in 32%. Patients also had symptoms for a mean of 6.1 days before admission, again emphasizing the high frequency of delay in recognizing CAP in this population.

Riquelme and colleagues [19] studied the most common clinical symptoms in a cohort of 101 older patients with CAP and reported dyspnea in 71%, cough in 67%, and fever in 64%. Nineteen percent of patients did not present with cough, pleuritic chest pain, or purulent sputum, whereas delirium and acute confusion were present in 44.5% of this cohort. Fever is not as frequent in older patients who present with pneumonia, partly because of a baseline decrease in temperature in older adults, referred to as "the older, the colder." There is also a blunted febrile response in older patients caused by an impaired thermoregulatory capacity to produce and respond to endogenous pyrogens. For every decade increase in age, the average temperature during the first 3 days of illness in patients who had pneumonia was reported to be lower by 0.15°C. This difference may translate into a 1°C difference between the body temperature of a 20-year-old and an 80-year-old patient with pneumonia [28]. Muder and colleagues [29] reported that only approximately two thirds of patients from a nursing home with pneumonia had cough or fever. In another study that compared 1169 patients younger than 80—with 305 patients at least 80 years old (excluding those in nursing homes)—underlying illness was more common in very elderly persons, including COPD, chronic heart disease, and dementia, and clinical features were less distinct. The very old patients had more confusion, less pleuritic chest pain, fewer myalgias and headaches, more hypoxemia, more crackles on physical examination, and less multilobar illness [30]. At comparable degrees of severity of illness, as measured by prognostic scoring, the older patients had a higher mortality rate and more complications.

Waterer and colleagues [31] found that in patients with CAP with increased age seen in a hospital emergency department, the absence of fever and the presence of an altered mental status led to patients receiving antibiotics more than 4 hours after arrival, and this delay affected mortality. Although timely administration of antibiotics has become a standard of care for CAP endorsed as a "core measure " by Medicare and the Joint Commission on the Accreditation of Healthcare Organizations, achievement of this goal may be problematic in older patients because of the unusual clinical presentations of infection, which add to diagnostic uncertainty in this population. Some investigators have argued that comorbid illnesses in older patients contribute to this diagnostic uncertainty and that the enhanced mortality seen with delayed therapy is a consequence of the comorbid illnesses that lead to the delay, rather than a result of the delay itself [31,32].

Causative organisms and bacteriology

In the United States, the most frequent cause of CAP in all age groups is *Streptococcus pneumoniae*, which accounts for more than half of all identified cases. Identification of a specific etiologic diagnosis is difficult in the older population, because many individuals are not able to provide a good specimen of sputum for analysis. For individuals who reside in long-term care facilities and for patients with other types of exposure to the health care environment, the problem is even more complex because of the common presence of respiratory tract colonization with bacterial pathogens (including enteric gram-negative organisms), which can lead to confusion regarding the etiologic cause of pneumonia. Although *S pneumoniae* is the most common etiologic agent of CAP, there is an increased incidence of drug-resistant *S pneumoniae* (DRSP) in patients over age 65, in patients with a history of prior antibiotic therapy, and in patients with a history of alcoholism or immune suppression (including corticosteroid therapy), and in patients with multiple medical comorbidities (especially chronic cardiopulmonary disease) [33–39]. Other common CAP pathogens are *Legionella* sp., and *Haemophilus influenzae* (particularly in cigarette smokers), *Staphylococcus aureus* (after influenza and in individuals who have diabetes or chronic renal failure), anaerobes (in persons with aspiration caused by impaired swallowing or neurologic illness), and viruses. Gram-negative enteric bacilli and *Pseudomonas aeruginosa* are generally not common causes of CAP but may be present at a higher incidence in individuals who reside in nursing homes and persons with other exposures to the health care environment (eg, recent hospitalization or care in a hemodialysis center) [36].

The frequency of enteric gram-negative organisms in older patients with CAP is widely debated, but these organisms seem to be more related to the presence of comorbid illness than to age itself. In one study, the risk for infection with gram-negative bacteria was 4.4 times more for patients who were at least 60 years old and with any medical comorbidity [37]. When *P aeruginosa* was the pathogen, it occurred almost exclusively in this population. In another study of 559 patients with CAP, 60 patients had infection caused by gram-negative organisms (39 were caused by *P aeruginosa*). The risk factors for gram-negative infection were probable aspiration, prior hospitalization, and prior antibiotic therapy and pulmonary comorbidity, whereas the risks for pseudomonal infection were pulmonary comorbidity and prior hospitalization [38]. Atypical pathogens also have been found in older patients, and one study found that the frequency of infection with *Clamydophila pneumoniae*, *Mycoplasma pneumoniae*, and *Legionella pneumophila* was higher in patients aged 65 to 79 than in patients aged 18 to 34 [3]. Pathogens such as *C pneumoniae* can even occur in nursing home patients and in an epidemic fashion, spreading from one patient to another [40,41]. In some epidemics in nursing homes, colonization of the drinking water has led to Legionella infection, whereas in other nursing homes, viruses such as rhinovirus have affected up to 40% of patients hospitalized with pneumonia [42,43].

Riquelme and colleagues [18] evaluated 101 older patients (>65 years) with CAP with extensive diagnostic testing, including two sets of blood cultures, respiratory tract cultures (sputum in 47, bronchoscopy in 15, and needle aspirate or pleural fluid sampling in 5), and acute and convalescent serum to evaluate for influenza and other viruses, *M pneumoniae, C pneumoniae, Coxiella burnetti, and L pneumophila*. Using this diagnostic armamentarium, 53 patients had an etiologic diagnosis established, but only 18 of 47 sputum samples were considered valid for evaluation, and most diagnoses were made by blood cultures or serologic testing. In clinical practice, serologic testing results are not available for weeks, so in this population, few pathogen diagnoses can be made at the time of admission. Of the 42% of all patients who had an etiologic diagnosis established, *S pneumoniae* was the most common organism (36% of all diagnoses, 26% of which were penicillin resistant), followed by *C pneumoniae* (17%), *C burnetti* (11%), *L pneumophila* (6%) and *M pneumoniae* (4%). *P aeruginosa, Proteus mirabilis, Streptococcus viridans*, and *Moraxella catarrahlis* were recovered in 2% each of all patients with an etiologic diagnosis.

Similar data were reported by Metlay and colleagues [26] in a group of 583 hospitalized patients older than 65. In this population, 427 patients had no etiologic diagnosis established, although 164 patients had no diagnostic testing done. Of the patients with an established diagnosis, *S pneumoniae* was most common, followed by *H influenzae*, gram-negative organisms, *S aureus*, and atypical pathogens. Some patients also had mixed infection, an increasingly recognized pattern, especially involving atypical pathogens such as *C pneumoniae* and bacterial pathogens such as pneumococcus [26,44]. In another study that compared patients with CAP aged 80 and older with patients who were younger, both groups had pneumococcus as the most common pathogen, but aspiration was more common in older patients, as was gram-negative infection, but atypical pathogens were less frequently seen [30]. The likely pathogens that cause CAP in older adults are listed in Box 2.

Box 2. Likely etiologic pathogens for pneumonia in older persons (in order of decreasing frequency)

Community-acquired pneumonia
Outpatient and non–intensive care unit (ICU) inpatient
  Pneumococcus (including DRSP)
  H influenzae, M catarrhalis
  Atypical pathogens
  M pneumoniae, C pneumoniae, Legionella spp.
  Influenza and other viruses
  Enteric gram-negatives organisms (only if bronchiectasis, COPD with recent antibiotics, and/or corticosteroids)
  S aureus (including methicillin-resistant *S aureus* [MRSA])
  Anaerobes (if aspiration risks present)
ICU treated
  Pneumococcus (including DRSP)
  Atypical pathogens
  M pneumoniae, C pneumoniae, Legionella spp.
  Enteric gram-negative organisms (including *P aeruginosa*)
  H influenzae
  S aureus, including MRSA (especially after influenza)
  Influenza and other viruses

HCAP
If risks for drug resistance are not present
  Pneumococcus (including DRSP)
  Atypical pathogens
  M pneumoniae, C pneumoniae, Legionella spp.
  H influenzae
  Influenza and other viruses
  Enteric gram-negative organisms
  Esherichia coli
  K pneumoniae
If risks are present (recent antibiotic therapy, poor functional status)
  ALL OF THE ABOVE, PLUS
  Drug-resistant gram-negative organisms
  Pseudomonas aeruginosa
  Acinetobacter spp.
  S aureus, including MRSA

With severe forms of CAP, the pathogens are similar, but certain organisms are more common, particularly pneumococcus and Legionella. Rello and colleagues [45] evaluated 95 patients with severe CAP and found that pneumococcus was the most common organism, followed by gram negative organisms (including *P aeruginosa*), and *H influenzae*, with some patients being infected with the other pathogens listed in Box 2. El-Solh and colleagues [46–48] have conducted a series of studies in older patients with severe pneumonia. In one study of 104 patients aged 75 or older with severe pneumonia from either the community ($n = 57$) or a nursing home ($n = 47$), the bacteriology differed in the two populations [46]. For persons with traditional CAP, pneumococcus was the most common organism (in 14% of all), followed by Legionella spp. (9%), *S aureus* (7%), and *H influenzae* (7%). Gram-negative organisms, as a group, occurred in 17% of all patients, with *E coli* being the most common organism. Among patients admitted from the nursing home, *S aureus* was the most common organism, followed by pneumococcus, but with 18% having enteric gram-negative organisms. Infection with *P aeruginosa* was associated with residence in a nursing home and bronchiectasis. Interestingly, as patient functional status declined, the frequency of *S aureus* and enteric gram-negative organisms increased, whereas the frequency of pneumococcus declined [46].

In another study of 95 older patients living in nursing homes who had aspiration pneumonia (defined by the presence of neurologic, swallowing, or intestinal diorders), the most commonly identified pathogens using protected bronchoalveolar lavage sampling were enteric gram-negative organisms in nearly 50% and *S. aureus* in approximately 10%, and anaerobes were present in only 11 of the 95 patients, but they were often part of a mixed infection and served as the sole pathogen in only 5 patients [47]. In another study of 88 patients with severe pneumonia from nursing homes, El Solh and colleagues [48] found multidrug-resistant pathogens in only 19% of the population, and they were generally present when patients had, in addition to severe illness, either prior antibiotic therapy in the preceding 6 months or poor functional status as defined by an activities of daily living score.

Because many older individuals come in contact with the health care environment, many have been labeled as having a new form of pneumonia termed HCAP. HCAP refers to any patient who develops pneumonia at any time during a hospital stay but has a history of residing in a nursing home, being hospitalized in the past 90 days, getting home infusion therapy or home wound care, undergoing chronic dialysis, or being exposed to a family member with a multi–drug-resistant (MDR) pathogen [49,50]. In 2005, this definition was incorporated into guidelines for nosocomial pneumonia, with the recommendation that all patients with HCAP be treated similarly to patients with nosocomial pneumonia, with therapy directed at MDR gram-negative organisms and MRSA [49]. This recommendation is probably correct for patients with HCAP who have multiple other risk factors, typically at least two of the following three: severe pneumonia, prior antibiotic therapy in the past 3 to 6 months, and poor functional status [48]. Patients with fewer than two of these risks, even if they have HCAP and are coming from a nursing home, may not need therapy targeted at such a broad spectrum of pathogens and might best be treated similar to other older individuals by targeting common CAP organisms, including atypical pathogens (see Box 2). In clinical practice, many patients who reside in nursing homes and are treated in nursing homes do not need such a broad-spectrum approach to bacteriology and therapy and have recovered with a much more focused therapeutic approach [51].

Recommended diagnostic testing

In the new Infectious Diseases Society of America/American Thoracic Society (IDS/ATS) guidelines for CAP, all patients suspected of having infection should have a chest radiograph to define the presence of pneumonia and the severity of illness [33]. This approach is particularly important in older patients because clinical findings of respiratory infection may be subtle and a radiograph is a more definitive way to define the extent of pneumonia. Blood cultures are only recommended for patients with more severe illness, particularly patients who have not received antibiotics before admission. This recommendation is based on a study of Medicare patients, which found that this population was less likely to have a false-positive finding than patients with mild illness, and a false-positive blood culture result could lead to unnecessary changes in management [52]. Other recommended diagnostic tests are a sputum Gram stain and culture before antibiotic therapy if a good quality specimen is available and can be transported to the laboratory rapidly. This testing can be used to confirm the presence of an unusual or drug–resistant pathogen, if suspected.

In individuals with severe CAP, urinary antigen testing for Legionella and pneumococcal urinary antigen are recommended, along with an endotracheal aspirate or sputum sample for culture. Routine serologic testing is not recommended and has been valuable only in population studies and in epidemiologic investigations.

Prognostic factors, risk stratification, and defining site of care

Severity assessment is key in determining not only patient prognosis but also patient disposition and site of care, resource use, and the approach to management. Severity of illness generally has been assessed by two prognostic scoring systems: the Pneumonia Severity Index (PSI) and a modification of a rule developed by the British Thoracic Society, termed the CURB-65 [53–55]. The PSI measures age, comorbidity, certain laboratory data, and physical findings using a complex point scale to divide patients into five risk groups (I–V), each with a progressively increasing risk of mortality. CURB-65 is an acronym that refers to an assessment of five factors: (1) confusion, (2) elevated blood urea nitrogen (BUN) (>19.6 mg/dL), (3) elevated respiratory rate (≥ 30/min), (4) low systolic (<90 mm Hg) or diastolic (≤ 60 mm Hg) blood pressure, and (5) age (≥ 65) [54]. Each of these approaches has limitations, particularly in older patients, and it may be best to view them as complementary, ideally identifying patients at extreme ends of the disease spectrum [55]. The PSI has been best validated as a way to identify patients at low risk for mortality, and although it is an accurate predictor of mortality, it may not be an ideal means for assessing severity of illness in older patients because it heavily weights age and comorbidity rather than directly measures CAP-specific disease severity [55]. On the other hand, the CURB-65 approach may be ideal for identifying patients at high risk for mortality with severe illness caused by CAP who might otherwise be overlooked without formal assessment of subtle aberrations in key vital signs [55]. One deficiency of the CURB-65 approach is that it does not generally account for comorbid illness, however, and may not be easily applied in older patients who may have substantial mortality risk if even a mild form of CAP destabilizes a chronic, but compensated, disease process.

One of the reasons for a limited applicability of prognostic scoring systems for CAP in older patients is their variable clinical presentations of infection. When the CURB-65 criteria were applied to older patients, Lim and Macfarlane [56] showed that this rule did not perform as well as it did in younger patients. In one study, the rule had a 66% sensitivity rate and a 73% specificity rate for predicting mortality in a population that included 48% who were at least 75 years old. In that study, the predictors of mortality in a multivariate analysis were age more than 65 years, confusion, fever less than 37°C, respiratory rate more than 24/min, serum sodium less than 135 μmol/L, BUN more than 19.6 mg/dL, and effusion on chest radiograph [54]. Although the CURB criteria were not optimal in an older population and did not work as well as they did in other populations, the approach had a higher sensitivity for predicting mortality than the PSI [54]. In a subsequent study, the same investigators confirmed many of these findings, adding a pulse of more than 95 beats/min and bilateral infiltrates as prognostic factors for mortality [56].

When the PSI was used in a population of patients aged 80 and older, investigators found that placing patients into classes IV and V and defining them as high risk for mortality had poor discriminating value [57]. The best predictors for mortality were being in PSI class V and having a poor performance status, anorexia, and an arterial carbon dioxide level of 50 mm Hg or more [57]. Other studies have examined different criteria to predict outcome in older patients with CAP. In a study of 200 patients with pneumococcal bacteremia aged 65 years and older, predictors of mortality were the presence of coronary artery disease and immunocompromising conditions [7]. Other studies have emphasized the prognostic value of functional status on admission in older patients and functional decline during admission to the hospital. In one study of 99 patients with CAP aged 65 years and older, functional decline was observed in 23% of the survivors [8]. The best predictor of functional decline was the PSI, and higher functional status was protective against mortality, with functional status for activities of daily living being the best mortality predictor [8]. Other studies have tried to develop models for predicting mortality; one study derived a prediction model in more than 500 nursing home patients with lower respiratory tract infection and dementia [58]. Factors that predicted death were feeding dependency, male gender, respiratory rate more than 20 breaths/min, pulse more than 75 beats/min, decreased alertness, respiratory difficulty, poor fluid intake in the preceding week, and the presence of pressure sores. In another study, serum measurement of tumor necrosis factor was a useful predictor of functional impairment after hospitalization for CAP, and admission PSI class correlated with serum levels of tumor necrosis factor, functional status (measured by the Charlson comorbidity index), and functional decline after admission. The investigators also found that older patients with impaired cognitive function and underlying comorbid illness who had a delayed functional recovery at 3 months after discharge were at a high risk for death [6].

In one recent study that compared the PSI to the CURB-65 in 3181 patients seen in emergency departments in the United States, both were good for predicting mortality and identifying patients at low risk for mortality [59]. The PSI seemed to be more discriminating in identifying patients at low risk for mortality, whereas the CURB-65 may have been more valuable at the severe disease end of the spectrum. CURB-65 defined high-risk patients as having a score of 2, 3, 4, or 5, each with a progressively increasing risk of death, whereas the PSI was less discriminating and defined only two groups as being severely ill (PSI groups IV and V). In a similar study conducted in Europe, Capelastegui and colleagues [60] used the PSI and CURB-65 approach to evaluate a large number of inpatients and outpatients with CAP. They observed that the CURB-65 (and its simpler CRB-65 version, which excludes measurement of BUN and can be used in outpatients) could accurately predict 30-day mortality, need for mechanical ventilation, and, to some extent, the need for hospitalization. The CURB-65 criteria also correlated with the time to clinical stability; a higher score was predictive of a longer duration of intravenous therapy and a longer length of hospital stay. The PSI also worked well to predict mortality in that study.

Although the PSI and CURB-65 are good for predicting mortality, neither can be used to define the site of care without considering other clinical and social variables. This is a particular consideration in older patients, because even patients with severe illness may be electively treated at home out of a desire to avoid overly aggressive care because of the presence of serious comorbidity or dementia [61–63]. This approach has been used in the Netherlands, where patients who live in nursing homes and have severe dementia receive less aggressive care when they develop pneumonia than similar patients who reside in nursing homes in the United States [61,62]. Social factors may mitigate against hospital admission in certain older individuals, although they may favor inpatient care in others. In one study at a public hospital in the United States with many indigent patients, the PSI could not define need for admission if patients were homeless or acutely intoxicated or if they did not have a stable home environment that allowed them to be discharged on oral antibiotic therapy [64].

How to define the need for hospitalization

Hospitalization can be detrimental for older persons and can delay return to full activities when compared with outpatient-based care. Hospitalization is accompanied by increased bed rest and the attendant complications, including venous thromboembolic disease or catheter-related sepsis and exposure to drug-resistant pathogens. Hospitalization does not always need to be a prolonged stay but simply long enough to allow close observation and determine when it is safe for therapy to be continued in the outpatient setting. Home treatment for CAP is being increasingly recognized as an acceptable approach for certain patients depending on their stated therapeutic goals and desire for life support and advanced care [63]. Having a caregiver to provide support at home, including the availability of home nursing and home intravenous therapy, and the availability of an intermediate care site such as a subacute facility can enable a patient to be managed safely outside the hospital.

The decision to admit a patient to the hospital depends on the patient's stated goals and the balance between the benefits of home care compared with hospital care. Patients should be considered for admission on a medical basis if there are signs of severe illness, decompensated comorbidity, or a high risk of death as defined by prognostic scoring systems. It is important to recognize that need for hospitalization is not always synonymous with a high risk of dying and vice versa. Patients may require therapy that is best given in the hospital, even if the risk of mortality is not high. Hospitalization may be necessary if a patient needs hydration, frequent respiratory therapy, cardiac monitoring, or titration of oxygen therapy. When prognostic scoring systems are used to help with the admission decision, they must be viewed as supportive of clinical judgment and not a replacement for what is otherwise an "art of medicine" decision. When the PSI approach has been used to inform the admission decision, patients in classes IV and V are considered for hospitalization, recognizing that older patients, on the basis of age and comorbidities, fall into these categories regardless of the severity of their pneumonia. Similarly, the CURB-65 approach is not an infallible tool to guide the admission decision. In one study, the factors considered by the CURB criteria were found to be important predictors of mortality—but not the only important factors—in patients older than age 75 [56]. In that population, the tool had a positive predictive value of 56% for death, which seems to mean that many patients who have abnormal CURB criteria do poorly. The rule only had a 66% negative predictive value, however, which means that some patients died even without meeting all of these criteria. These findings indicate that older patients with CAP should have multiple factors included in the evaluation of need for hospitalization and mortality risk.

Need for intensive care unit admission

None of the proposed criteria for severe pneumonia is completely accurate for determining the need for ICU admission. In one study of 696 patients with CAP admitted to the hospital, 116 needed ICU admission. The PSI was not an accurate tool to guide this decision, because 37% of the patients admitted to ICU fell into low-risk classes I to III [65]. The best predictor of need for admission was the presence of one of two major criteria (need for mechanical ventilation or septic shock) or the presence of two of three minor criteria (systolic pressure <90 mm Hg, multilobar infiltrates, and a PaO_2/FiO_2 ratio <250). Use of this approach had a sensitivity of nearly 70%, a specificity of 98%, a positive predictive value of 87%, and a negative predictive value of 94%. The findings in this study are similar to the data from another study of older patients with CAP, which concluded that the best predictor of severe illness and death was the presence of two of four SOAR criteria: systolic blood pressure less than 90 mm Hg, PaO_2/FiO_2 of 250 or less, age 65 years or older, and respiratory rate 30/min or more. When two criteria were present, the sensitivity for predicting mortality was 81%, specificity was 60%, positive predictive value was 27%, and negative predictive value was 94% [66].

In the new IDSA/ATS guidelines, ICU admission is recommend if a patient has at least one major criteria of severity or three minor criteria [33]. The major criteria are the same as previously mentioned (need for mechanical ventilation or septic shock), and the minor criteria are respiratory rate 30/min or more, PaO_2/FiO_2 of 250 or less, multilobar infiltrates, confusion/disorientation, BUN of 20 mg/dL or more, white blood cell count less than 4000/mm^3, temperature less than 36°C, and hypotension requiring aggressive fluid resuscitation. Recently, a novel rule for identifying severe CAP was identified that requires the presence of one of two major criteria (arterial pH <7.30 or systolic blood pressure <90 mm Hg) or the presence of two of six minor criteria, including confusion, BUN more than 30 mg/dL, respiratory rate more than 30/min, multilobar infiltrates, PaO_2/FiO_2 ratio less than 250, and age at least 80 years [67]. When used, this rule was 92% sensitive for identifying patients needing ICU care. Unlike other rules, it gave different importance to the minor criteria, with systolic hypotension and elevated respiratory rate being the most important factors; however, age of at least 80 was as important as the presence of multilobar infiltrates.

Therapy

General approach

The initial therapy of pneumonia is necessarily empiric, based on targeting the most likely etiologic pathogens, because diagnostic testing is not usually rapid enough or definitive enough to allow for specific, organism-directed therapy. Older patients should be categorized as having either CAP or HCAP, and each of these populations has subgroups with different suspected pathogens and different recommended initial therapy (Box 3). Patients with CAP are those who reside at home and do not have any of the HCAP risk factors. Patients with CAP fall into three groups: outpatients, patients admitted to the hospital ward, and patients admitted to the ICU. Patients with HCAP can be divided into four groups based on first determining if a patient is severely ill or not and then determining how many risk factors are present for MDR pathogens (assessing for a history or prior antibiotics in the past 6 months and the presence of a poor functional status) (Fig. 1).

Empiric therapy of community-acquired pneumonia

All patients with CAP should be treated for pneumococcus and atypical pathogens, and older patients should be treated routinely for drug-resistant pneumococcus, because patients who are older than 65 years are at increased risk

---

Box 3. Suggested initial empiric therapy for pneumonia in older persons

CAP
Outpatient
  Fluoroquinolone orally (gemifloxacin, levofloxacin[a], moxifloxacin)
  Beta-lactam (high-dose amoxicillin[b], amoxicillin-clavulanate, cefuroxime, I cefpodoxime)
    with macrolide (azithromycin, clarithromycin) or doxycycline
Non-ICU inpatient
  Fluroquinolone intravenously (levofloxacin[a], moxifloxacin)
  Beta-lactam (ceftriaxone, cefotaxime, ampicillin/sulbactam, ertapenem) with a macrolide
    (azithromycin intravenously) or doxycycline
ICU-admitted
  No pseudomonal risks
Beta-lactam (cefotaxime, ceftriaxone, ampicillin/sulbactam) plus a macrolide (azithromycin)
  or quinolone (levofloxacin[a], moxifloxacin)
  Pseudomonal risks
Anti-pseudomonal beta-lactam (cefepime, imipenem, meropenem, piperacillin/tazobactam
  PLUS anti-pseudomonal quinolone (ciprofloxacin, levofloxacin[a])
OR
  Anti-pseudomonal beta-lactam (cefepime, imipenem, meropenem, piperacillin/
  tazobactam) PLUS aminoglycoside (amikacin, gentamicin, tobramycin) PLUS a macrolide
  (azithromycin) or a quinolone (levofloxacin[a], moxifloxacin)

HCAP
Nonsevere
  0–1 risks for MDR pathogens
Fluoroquinolone or beta-lactam/macrolide orally
  2 risk factors for MDR pathogens
Intravenous therapy with cefepime, ertapenem, levofloxacin[a] PLUS consider MRSA and/or
  additional gram-negative coverage
Severe
  0–1 risks for MDR pathogens
Treat the same as severe CAP in ICU with no pseudomonal risks
  2 risks for MDR pathogens
Dual pseudomonal therapy plus MRSA coverage using anti-pseudomonal beta-lactam
  (cefepime, imipenem, meropenem, piperacillin/tazobactam or if penicillin allergic
  aztreonam) PLUS an aminoglycoside (amikacin, gentamicin, tobramycin) or a quinolone
  (ciprofloxacin or levofloxacin[a], especially if concerned about atypical pathogens) PLUS
  linezolid or vancomycin

---

  [a]Levofloxacin is available in two doses, 500 mg and 750 mg daily. For patients with normal renal
function, the 750-mg dose is currently recommended.
  [b]High-dose amoxicillin is 1 g three times daily.

---

for this organism, as are persons with multiple medical comorbidities, including cardiopulmonary disease [33]. Enteric gram-negative organisms are not a major consideration in this group unless the patient has severe CAP, because most patients with risks for these organisms would be classified as having HCAP. Cigarette smokers need therapy for *H influenzae* and *M catarrhalis*.

Patients with severe CAP in the setting of recent influenza should be treated for *S aureus*, including the possibility of MRSA.

Patients with CAP who are treated out of the hospital should receive therapy with either an oral fluoroquinolone or the combination of a selected beta-lactam with a macrolide or doxycycline [33]. The oral quinolones that are currently available are

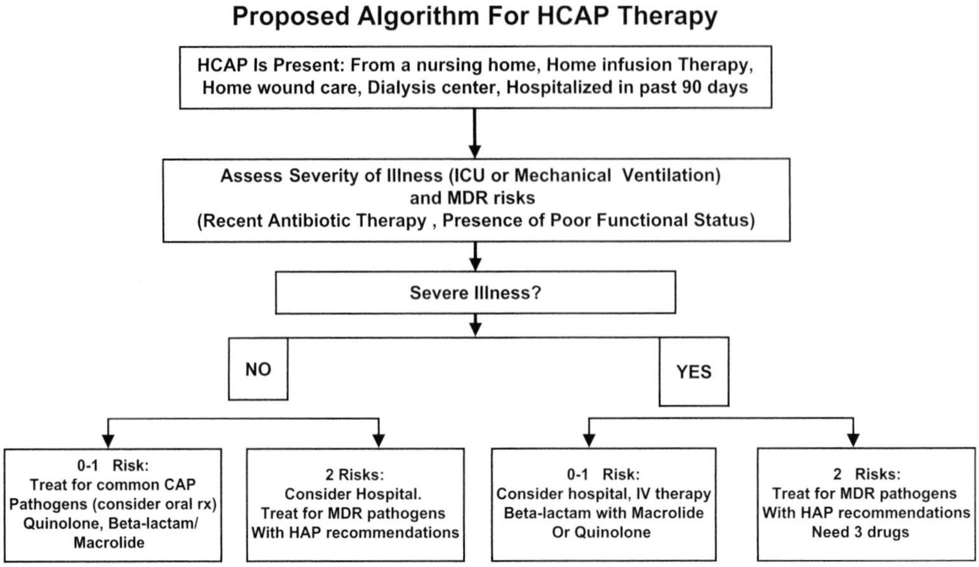

Proposed Algorithm For HCAP Therapy

HCAP Is Present: From a nursing home, Home infusion Therapy, Home wound care, Dialysis center, Hospitalized in past 90 days

Assess Severity of Illness (ICU or Mechanical Ventilation)
and MDR risks
(Recent Antibiotic Therapy , Presence of Poor Functional Status)

Severe Illness?

NO

YES

0-1 Risk:
Treat for common CAP
Pathogens (consider oral rx)
Quinolone, Beta-lactam/
Macrolide

2 Risks:
Consider Hospital.
Treat for MDR pathogens
With HAP recommendations

0-1 Risk:
Consider hospital, IV therapy
Beta-lactam with Macrolide
Or Quinolone

2 Risks:
Treat for MDR pathogens
With HAP recommendations
Need 3 drugs

Fig. 1. All patients with HCAP should be identified and then divided on the basis of severity of illness to guide initial therapy. Patients in each group are further divided based on whether they have risk factors for drug-resistant pathogens (MDR pathogens), which include recent antibiotic therapy in the past 3 to 6 months, and poor functional status, as defined by activities of daily living.

gemifloxacin, levofloxacin (the 750-mg dose is recommended for persons with normal renal function) and moxifloxacin. The selected oral beta-lactams are high-dose amoxicillin (1 g three times daily), amoxicillin-clavulanate, cefuroxime (500 mg twice daily), and cefpodoxime. The oral macrolides should be either azithromycin or clarithromycin, which are better tolerated than erythromycin. For patients admitted to the hospital but not the ICU, the choice is between a quinolone as monotherapy or a selected beta-lactam with a macrolide or doxycycline. The available intravenous quinolones are levofloxacin (750 mg for persons with normal renal function) or moxifloxacin. The recommended intravenous beta-lactams are cefotaxime, ceftriaxone (but not cefuroxime), ampicillin/sulbactam or ertapenem (especially for individuals who might be at risk for non-pseudomonal gram-negative organisms). The recommended intravenous macrolide is azithromycin, 500 mg daily.

Patients with severe CAP get treated differently, depending on whether risk factors for *P aeruginosa* are present. Although not all patients with severe CAP require therapy for *P aeruginosa* and enteric gram-negative organisms, it is necessary to cover these pathogens in patients with bronchiectasis and in patients with severe COPD and a history of recent antibiotic or corticosteroid therapy [33].

All patients in the ICU are treated for the possibility of DRSP and atypicals, including Legionella. No patient should receive monotherapy, including with a quinolone, because the safety, efficacy, and proper dosing of these agents in ICU patients with CAP have not been established [33]. If a patient has no pseudomonal risk factors, therapy should be with a beta-lactam (cefotaxime, ceftriaxone, or ampicillin-sulbactam) with either azithromycin or a fluoroquinolone (levofloxacin or moxifloxacin), or the combination of aztreonam and a quinolone if the patient is penicillin allergic. For patients with pseudomonal risks in the ICU, recommended therapy is with an anti-pneumococcal, anti-pseudomonal beta-lactam (cefepime, imipenem, meropenem, or piperacillin-tazobactam) combined with an aminoglycoside and either azithromycin or a quinolone. If the patient is penicillin allergic, aztreonam can be used in place of a beta-lactam in this regimen. An alternative approach would be to use one of these beta-lactams and combine it with either ciprofloxacin or levofloxacin (750-mg dose).

Need for atypical pathogen coverage in all patients with community-acquired pneumonia

For all patients with CAP, the recommended therapy regimens include coverage of atypical pathogens for all patients. This recommendation is based on retrospective analyses of several large databases, primarily in older Medicare patients, which showed that when hospitalized patients with CAP receive either a beta-lactam with a macrolide or a quinolone alone, mortality is lower than if a beta-lactam alone is used [68,69]. Even in patients with pneumococcal bacteremia, the use of dual therapy (generally directed at atypical pathogens and pneumococcus) has been associated with lower mortality than if monotherapy is used, including in patients with mild and severe CAP [70–72]. Five retrospective studies have shown reduced mortality in patients with pneumococcal bacteremia who receive combination therapy when compared with patients who received monotherapy [70]. In one of these studies, although multiple drugs were given to sicker patients as reflected by APACHE score and the PSI, the odds ratio for death was threefold higher than for patients who received single effective therapy [71]. Persons who got dually effective therapy generally received a beta-lactam plus either a macrolide or quinolone. The mechanism for benefit of combination therapy is not clear, with possibilities being atypical pathogen coverage in the setting of coinfection, synergistic effects of the two drugs, or an anti-inflammatory effect of macrolide therapy.

The impact of drug-resistant S pneumoniae on the choice of empiric therapy for community-acquired pneumonia

Although earlier studies have not shown an impact of in vitro penicillin resistance on the outcome of pneumococcal CAP, this may be changing, and in older patients, careful selection of beta-lactams is necessary, emphasizing adequate dosing. In guidelines, cefotaxime and ceftriaxone are preferred as empiric therapy because they are less likely than other agents to be "discordant" if DRSP organisms are present, and in some studies, discordant therapy has led to worse outcome [73]. In one study, when cefuroxime was used for pneumococcal bacteremia, if the organism had in vitro resistance the clinical outcome was worse; therefore it is not a recommended empiric beta-lactam for hospitalized patients [74]. The impact of DRSP may not be measured only by mortality, but in some studies, there has been an enhanced likelihood of suppurative complications, and a more prolonged hospital length of stay [75,76]. One of the reasons for uncertainty about the impact of DRSP has been that early studies examined

relatively few patients, many of whom did not have high levels of in vitro resistance. The issue may have been clarified by a large study that evaluated more than 5000 patients with pneumococcal bacteremia and CAP, however, which found an increased mortality for patients with a penicillin minimum inhibitory concentration of at least 4 mg/L or more or with a cefotaxime minimum inhibitory concentration of 2.0 mg/L or more [77]. This increased mortality was only present, however, if patients who died in the first 4 days of therapy were excluded from analysis. Fortunately, few patients have organisms with this magnitude of in vitro resistance, which may explain the conflicting findings in various studies. More recently, another study using cohort and matched control methods found that severity of illness—and not resistance or accuracy of therapy—was the most important predictor of mortality [78].

Recent antibiotic use

In choosing among the therapeutic options for patients with CAP or HCAP, it is important to know what antibiotics a patient has received in the past 3 months and then choose an agent from a different class. One of the clinical factors that drives pneumococcal resistance is antibiotic use, and therapy within the past 3 months is a risk factor for pneumococcal resistance to the agent that was recently received [79]. In a study of 3339 cases of invasive pneumococcal infection, of which 563 had a history of antibiotic therapy in the preceding 3 months and the identity of the therapy was known, investigators found that recent therapy with penicillin, macrolides, trimethoprim-sulfa, and quinolones (but not cephalosporins) was associated with a higher frequency of resistance to that same agent. Among all the classes of antibiotics, the one with the greatest effect on subsequent resistance was therapy with the quinolone levofloxacin [79]. This latter finding is consistent with case reports of quinolone failures in CAP that document recent quinolone therapy as a major risk factor [80]. All of these data lend further support to the recommendation that when choosing among all acceptable therapeutic alternatives, clinicians should choose an agent that differs from what a patient has received recently.

The role of quinolones in older patients with community-acquired pneumonia

Moxifloxacin has been used to treat CAP, and in an inpatient trial in older hospitalized patients, this agent had similar cardiac safety to levofloxacin, with a statistically significantly more rapid rate of clinical improvement at days 3 to 5[81,82]. The high bioavailability of quinolones may allow oral therapy to replace intravenous therapy, which keeps some patients out of the hospital with CAP. Using oral levofloxacin in a cluster-randomized protocol design, Loeb and colleagues [51] documented the safety of this approach in nursing home patients who had CAP but were able to eat and drink and had a pulse of 100 beats/min or less, a respiratory rate less than 30 breaths/min, a systolic pressure of 90 mm Hg or more, and an oxygen saturation of 92% or more. These patients may be classified as having nonsevere HCAP with zero to one risk factor for MDR pathogens, and quinolone monotherapy would be appropriate (see Fig. 1). One concern with quinolones has been their safety in older patients with CAP. Gatifloxacin recently was documented to cause hypo- and hyperglycemia, which limits its ability to be used safely in patients who have diabetes; this drug is no longer used [83]. Quinolones have caused QT prolongation and cardiac arrhythmias, which has limited the use of agents such as sparfloxacin. A randomized, double-blinded comparative study of levofloxacin and moxifloxacin, using clinical evaluation and Holter monitoring, found no difference in the frequency of clinically significant cardiac events between the two agents [81].

Empiric therapy of health care–associated pneumonia

In the 2005 ATS/IDSA nosocomial pneumonia guidelines, HCAP was considered an infection that should be treated similar to nosocomial pneumonia and not using a CAP antibiotic approach because patients are at risk for infection with MDR gram-negative organisms and MRSA [49]. When the guidelines suggested that HCAP be treated like nosocomial pneumonia with a focus on MDR pathogens, the implied assumption was that the patients being evaluated were patients in the hospital who would be treated with intravenous antibiotics. HCAP also includes patients who are not ill enough to require hospital admission, are not at risk for MDR pathogens (but are at risk for CAP pathogens, particularly atypical pathogens in the nursin home setting), are treated orally, and prefer to be treated at home or in a nursing home, regardless of the severity of illness present. Because of the heterogeneity of the HCAP population, initial empiric therapy should allow for the possibility that some subpopulations should be managed like HAP, some like CAP, and some with a hybrid approach (see Fig. 1). HCAP also includes many populations, some of which have been studied extensively, such as those with nursing home–acquired pneumonia, whereas other populations, such as those undergoing hemodialysis and those recently hospitalized, are less well described.

For several reasons, HCAP should not always be treated the same as HAP. Although some patients need this approach, others would unnecessarily receive too broad a spectrum of antibiotics if this approach were used routinely. In reality, for nursing home patients treated either in the hospital or in the nursing home, many studies have demonstrated the efficacy of monotherapy regimens that would not be recommended for patients with HAP at risk for MDR pathogens. Effective monotherapies in this population have included ciprofloxacin, levofloxacin, cefepime, and ertapenem [51,84,85]. HAP therapy also would not adequately treat some patients with HCAP who might be infected with community pathogens, such as *Legionella* spp. or *C pneumoniae*, which have been found in some epidemics of nursing home–acquired pneumonia.

Although some patients with HCAP are likely to be infected with MDR pathogens and would require therapy identical to HAP, these patients generally have at least two of three key risk factors, including severe pneumonia, prior antibiotic therapy in the past 3 to 6 months, and poor functional status [48]. Based on these considerations and as shown in Fig. 1, patients with HCAP should be divided into individuals with and without severe illness, with each population then being evaluated for the presence of risk factors for MDR pathogens.

If a patient has nonsevere illness and zero to one of the other risk factors (prior antibiotics, poor functional status), then MDR pathogens are unlikely, and these patients should receive oral therapy similar to outpatient CAP in older patients, but being sure to target DRSP and atypical pathogens. This therapy would require use of an oral fluoroquinolone or a beta-lactam/macrolide combination. If the patient has nonsevere illness but the other two risk factors are present, then therapy should be directed at the usual CAP pathogens and MDR gram-negative organisms and possibly MRSA. These patients may need to be treated in the hospital and covered with a monotherapy regimen using agents such as ertapenem, cefepime, or levofloxacin (the latter especially if atypicals are being considered) given intravenously, with consideration of additional coverage for MRSA with an agent such as vancomycin or linezolid. If *P aeruginosa* is likely (particularly because of structural lung disease or severe steroid-treated COPD), then it may be necessary to give dual pseudomonal coverage with a third agent added to cover MRSA. Dual pseudomonal therapy can be given using either an aminoglycoside (amikacin, gentamicin, or tobramycin) or an anti-pseudomonal quinolone (ciprofloxacin or levofloxacin, 750 mg) with an anti-pseudomonal beta-lactam (cefepime, imipenem, meropenem, piperacillin-tazobactam).

Unfortunately, no data verify these recommendations directly, but they are based on therapy studies in populations of patients with HCAP without severe illness. For example, in one cluster-randomized trial of 680 patients over the age of 65 with radiographic pneumonia and nonsevere illness at 20 nursing homes, patients were randomized to receive either usual care or a clinical pathway using oral therapy with levofloxacin, 500 mg, daily in the nursing home as long as the patient was able to eat and drink, had an oxygen saturation of at least 92%, and had stable vital signs [51]. Using this pathway, only 10% were hospitalized, compared with 22% with usual care (P=.001), and there was a substantial cost savings of at least $1000 per patient with the pathway, whereas mortality and functional status were similar in both groups. There are also studies of nonsevere HCAP in patients who are admitted to the hospital. In one prospective, double-blind, randomized study of 51 hospitalized patients with HCAP, none of whom had pseudomonal risks, 23 received intravenous monotherapy with ertapenem, whereas 28 received intravenous therapy with cefepime. Although nearly 80% had gram-negative organisms, the favorable responses with both therapies were high: 90% with cefepime and 75% with ertapenem [85].

In patients with HCAP with severe pneumonia, individuals with zero to one risk factor for MDR pathogens should be treated the same as patients with severe CAP using ceftotaxime, ceftriaxone, or ampicillin/sulbactam with either a quinolone (levofloxacin or moxifloxacin) or a macrolide (azithromycin). If a patient with severe HCAP has two risk factors for MDR pathogens, however, then therapy with three agents is needed, including dual pseudomonal therapy plus coverage of MRSA, as discussed previously. If a patient

is also thought to be at risk for atypical pathogen infection, then the dual pseudomonal therapy should include a quinolone rather than an aminoglycoside.

Resolution and response to therapy

The clinical response to therapy determines the total duration of therapy and the duration of intravenous therapy in hospitalized patients. The clinical response, in turn, depends on host factors (including the intensity of the immune response), the virulence of the pathogen, and the appropriateness of empiric therapy. Hospitalized patients with CAP typically respond to appropriate therapy with clinical stabilization and improvement over the first several days, with up to half of patients reaching clinical stability by day 3 of therapy [39,86–89]. Clinical stability is defined as improvement in the symptoms of cough, sputum production, dyspnea, and fever (becoming afebrile for at least two occasions 8 hours apart), having good oral intake, and having an improving white blood cell count. Once a patient becomes clinically stable, it is possible to switch to oral therapy and discharge the patient, after which continued clinical improvement can occur. In the new CAP guidelines, the recommended total duration of therapy is a minimum of 5 days, with patients being afebrile for at least 48 to 72 hours before stopping therapy [33].

Because of altered immune responses, older patients may improve slower than younger ones. In one study of CAP, the predictors of early clinical stability were adherence to guidelines with appropriate antibiotic choice, whereas delayed improvement occurred in the presence of concomitant congestive heart failure and COPD [87]. In another study of 1383 hospitalized patients with CAP, the independent factors associated with early clinical failure were older age (>65 years), multilobar pneumonia, PSI score more than 90, Legionella pneumonia, gram-negative pneumonia, and discordant antimicrobial therapy. Compared with treatment responders, patients with early failures had significantly higher rates of complications (58% versus 24%) and overall mortality (27% versus 4%) (P<.001 for both) [88].

Radiographic resolution lags behind clinical resolution, and most patients require 4 to 6 weeks for radiographic resolution, so it is usually not helpful to follow a chest film early in the course of illness unless a patient is not clinically improving.

Delays in radiographic resolution are common in older patients who have severe illness, alcoholism, COPD, bacteremia, or multiple medical comorbidities [39]. El-Solh and colleagues [89] examined the radiographic resolution of CAP in 74 patients older than 70 years by performing chest radiographs every 3 weeks until resolution or up to 12 weeks. They found that only 35% had normal radiographic findings at 3 weeks, 60.2% at 6 weeks, and 76% had normal radiographic findings at 12 weeks. Slower resolution occurred in patients with a high degree of comorbidity and in patients with multilobar involvement and bacteremia. In a multivariate analysis, multilobar pneumonia and comorbidity were associated with delayed resolution, but each comorbid process further slowed resolution, which implied that host factors—not disease severity—were the best predictors of radiographic response [89]. Of note, the authors examined the rate of resolution as a function of bacteriology. At 12 weeks, complete clearing occurred in 100% with pneumococcus ($n = 14$), 91.6% with H influenzae ($n = 12$), 54.75% with enteric gram-negative organisms ($n = 25$), and 100% with C pneumoniae ($n = 6$).

If a patient is not responding as expected, in addition to host immune considerations a broad differential diagnosis is needed, especially if there is no response to therapy. A delayed response to therapy can be the result of inadequate therapy (pathogen not covered by the agent chosen), an unusual and unsuspected pathogen (tuberculosis, fungus), a pneumonic complication (empyema, endocarditis, meningitis, pulmonary embolus), or the presence of a noninfectious illness that presents like a pneumonia (bronchiolitis obliterans and organizing pneumonia, pulmonary vasculitis) [39]. The evaluation of nonresponse depends on the timing of deterioration and the patient's overall health status. Patients over the age of 55 who have smoked and who have a focal pneumonia commonly take a long time to improve, and diagnostic evaluation often does not reveal a specific reason for delayed resolution [86]. In the evaluation of a patient who is slow to respond, diagnostic testing can include CT scan of the chest, bronchoscopy, serologic testing, and rarely, open lung biopsy.

Prevention

For all older patients it is important to address the presence of risk factors and comorbidities that add to the likelihood of respiratory infection,

including smoking cessation, attention to aspiration risks, and improvement of malnutrition. In one study of 46,237 persons over the age of 65 [90], not only was smoking a risk factor for pneumonia but also the authors estimated that when smokers developed pneumonia, approximately 31% of cases were the direct result of current smoking, which emphasizes the potential benefit of smoking cessation. In the same study, more than 10% of the population had stroke or dementia, diseases often associated with aspiration risk. For these patients and for those with dysphagia or esophageal or other swallowing problems, careful assessment of aspiration potential and intervention with feeding regimens and other efforts to avoid aspiration may be helpful. Finally, malnutrition has been identified as a risk for pneumonia in older patients, and attention to treatment of nutritional deficits may be valuable. The mainstay of CAP prevention is pneumococcal and influenza vaccination.

Influenza vaccination

Influenza can lead to secondary bacterial pneumonia, particularly with S aureus, and vaccination has been consistently identified as an effective means for reducing hospitalization and mortality from respiratory infection [91,92]. Influenza vaccine is revised annually to account for changes in the antigenic nature of the virus (antigenic drift) that varies each season, and patients need yearly vaccination (beginning in September and going until at least December). The vaccine should be given to all patients older than 65 years, patients with chronic medical illness (including nursing home residents), and persons who provide health care to patients at risk for complications of influenza. The vaccine includes three strains: two influenza A strains (H3N2 and H1N1) and one influenza B strain. If an epidemic is present, unvaccinated patients should be vaccinated immediately and given chemoprophylaxis with amantidine or rimantidine against influenza A. They also can receive oseltamivir or zanamivir, which are active against influenza A and B. These latter agents are generally preferred in older patients because of a lower risk of toxicity.

Pneumococcal vaccination

The current 23-valent vaccine has been demonstrated to be effective for preventing bacteremic pneumonia in healthy adults and military recruits, but controversy has persisted about its benefit in older patients and persons with serious comorbid illness. The vaccine's efficacy has ranged from 65% to 84% in patients who have diabetes mellitus, coronary artery disease, congestive heart failure, chronic pulmonary disease, and anatomic asplenia [39]. In immunocompetent patients over the age of 65, effectiveness has been documented to be 75%. In immunocompromised patients, however, effectiveness has not been proven, including patients who have sickle cell disease, chronic renal failure, immunoglobulin deficiency, Hodgkin's disease, lymphoma, leukemia, and multiple myeloma. A single re-vaccination is indicated in persons aged 65 years or older who initially received the vaccine more than 5 years earlier and were younger than age 65 on first vaccination [33]. If the initial vaccination was given at age 65 or older, repeat is not indicated unless a patient has anatomic or functional asplenia or has one of the immunocompromising conditions listed previously. In these patients, re-vaccination is indicated; the second dose is given at least 5 years after the original dose.

Some new data suggest clear benefit to pneumococcal vaccine in older patients. Recently, a new conjugate pneumococcal vaccine was introduced for children, and with increasing use the rate of invasive disease has dropped not only in the vaccinated children but also in adults, with an 18% decline in invasive pneumococcal disease in persons over age 65. These findings imply a type of "herd immunity" that protects older adults when the vaccine is used in children with whom they come in contact [93]. In another study, a database was evaluated to define the impact of prior pneumococcal vaccination on patients hospitalized with CAP. Only 12% of 62,918 hospitalized CAP patients had prior vaccination, but this group was less likely to die from any cause, had a lower risk of respiratory failure and other complications, and had a reduced length of stay compared with patients who were not vaccinated [94]. The benefit of the vaccine for reducing mortality was equal for patients in all age groups, and persons older than 65 who were vaccinated had an odds ratio of death of 0.29 compared with unvaccinated individuals.

Pneumococcal vaccine is generally not used widely enough, and recently the administration of the vaccine before hospital discharge for all patients hospitalized with CAP has become a standard of care for all Medicare patients. This effort could even be extended to all older patients in the hospital for any reason, and hospital-based immunization could be highly effective. One study found that among 1633 patients with pneumonia treated in the hospital, 62% were hospitalized in the preceding 4 years [95]. Eighty percent of these patients had a high-risk condition that would have qualified them to receive pneumococcal vaccine. Pneumococcal vaccine can be given simultaneously with other vaccines, such as influenza vaccine, but each should be given at a separate site. One concern with immunization in the hospital is the possibility that patients will receive repeated vaccination in less than the recommended 5-year interval because of the absence of a reliable history of vaccination, especially in persons who have been repeatedly admitted to different hospitals or treated in nursing homes. One policy to ensure widespread use would be to vaccinate all patients if there is any uncertainty about the history of prior vaccination. If this approach is used and the vaccine given too often, however, there has been concern about injection site and other reactions. In a study of 179 patients who received at least three vaccinations who were compared with 181 patients who received either one or two doses, there was no higher incidence of adverse reactions [96]. Although 54.6% of patients who were revaccinated received their repeat in less than 6 years, only one patient had an adverse reaction, which was described as tachycardia and arm redness. It seems to be safe to give repeat vaccination, and although this is not to be done indiscriminately, if it is done, the benefits are likely to outweigh any associated risks.

Summary

Pneumonia presents unique challenges to older patients. CAP occurs more commonly in older than younger patients and leads to a higher mortality. The disease carries a significant economic and clinical burden and will be more commonly encountered in the future as the American population ages. The natural history and clinical course of pneumonia may be different from that seen in younger patients, and the approach to management is different. Diagnosis may be obscured by nonclassic presentations, and clinicians must be especially suspicious of pneumonia whenever there is deterioration in the clinical status of an older patient. The site of care is important for appropriate management, but this determination is based not only on clinical factors but also on social factors. Some seriously ill patients choose home care or limited therapy in a nursing home because of a desire to avoid aggressive inpatient care. Timely and appropriate empiric therapy enhances the likelihood of a good clinical outcome, although clinical resolution may be more delayed in older patients than in younger patients.

When approaching the therapy of pneumonia in older patients, persons with CAP must be distinguished from persons with HCAP, and each group requires a specific approach to therapy (see Fig. 1). Depending on the population being considered, in addition to pneumococcus, other pathogens must be treated, including drug-resistant pneumococcus, MRSA, atypical pathogens, and drug-resistant enteric gram-negative organisms. Prevention always should be implemented, with a particular focus on smoking cessation, aspiration prevention, and pneumococcal and influenza vaccination.

References

[1] US Department of Health and Human Services. HHS News August 31, 1995:1–3.

[2] Niederman MS, McCombs JS, Unger AN, et al. The cost of treating community-acquired pneumonia. Clin Ther 1998;20:820–37.

[3] Marston BJ, Plouffe JF, File TM Jr, et al. Incidence of community-acquired pneumonia requiring hospitalization: results of a population-based active surveillance study in Ohio. The community-based pneumonia incidence study group. Arch Intern Med 1997;157(15):1709–18.

[4] Kaplan V, Clermont G, Griffin MF, et al. Pneumonia: still the old man's friend? Arch Intern Med 2003; 163:317–23.

[5] Koivula I, Sten M, Makela PH. Prognosis after community-acquired pneumonia in the elderly: a population-based 12 year follow-up study. Am J Med 1999; 159:1550–5.

[6] El Solh A, Pineda L, Bouquin P, et al. Determinants of short and long term functional recovery after hospitalization for community-acquired pneumonia in the elderly: role of inflammatory markers. BMC Geriatr 2006;6:12.

[7] Chi RC, Jackson LA, Neuzil KM. Characteristics and outcomes of older adults with community-acquired pneumococcal bacteremia. J Am Geriatr Soc 2006;54:115–20.

[8] Torres OH, Muñoz J, Ruiz D, et al. Outcome predictors of pneumonia in elderly patients: importance of functional assessment. J Am Geriatr Soc 2004;52: 1603–9.

[9] Feldman C. Pneumonia in the elderly. Clin Chest Med 1999;20:563–73.

[10] Lange P, Vestbo J, Nyboe J. Risk factors for death and hospitalization from pneumonia: a prospective study of a general population. Eur Respir J 1995;8: 1694–8.

[11] Sekizawa K, Ujiie Y, Itabashi S, et al. Lack of cough reflex in aspiration pneumonia. Lancet 1990;335: 1228–9.

[12] Nakajoh K, Nakagawa T, Sekizawa K, et al. Relation between incidence of pneumonia and protective reflexes in post-stroke patients with oral or tube feeding. J Intern Med 2000;247:39–42.

[13] El-Solh AA, Pietrantoni C, Bhat A, et al. Colonization of dental plaques: a reservoir of respiratory pathogens for hospital-acquired pneumonia in institutionalized elders. Chest 2004;126(5):1575–82.

[14] Niederman MS. Pathogenesis of airway colonization: lessons learned from studies of bacterial adherence. Eur Respir J 1994;8:1737–40.

[15] Valenti WM, Trudell RG, Bentlye DW. Factors predisposing to oropharyngeal colonization with gram negative bacilli in the aged. N Engl J Med 1978;298:1108–11.

[16] Arai T, Yasuda Y, Toshima S, et al. ACE inhibitors and pneumonia in elderly people. Lancet 1998;352: 1937–8.

[17] Arai T, Yasuda Y, Takaya T, et al. Angiotensin-converting enzyme inhibitors, angiotensin-II receptor antagonists, and pneumonia in elderly hypertensive patients with stroke. Chest 2001;119:660–1.

[18] Riquelme R, Torres A, El-Ebiary M, et al. Community acquired pneumonia in the elderly: a multivariate analysis of risk and prognostic factors. Am J Respir Crit Care Med 1996;154:1450–5.

[19] Riquelme R, Torres A, el Ebiary M, et al. Community acquired pneumonia in the elderly: clinical and nutritional aspects. Am J Respir Crit Care Med 1997;156:1908–14.

[20] Marik PE, Kaplan D. Aspiration pneumonia and dysphagia in the elderly. Chest 2003;124:328–36.

[21] Fry AM, Shay DK, Holman RC, et al. Trends in hospitalizations for pneumonia among persons aged 65 years or older in the United States, 1988–2002. JAMA 2005;294(21):2712–9.

[22] Mehr DR, Foxman B, Colombo P. Risk factors for mortality from lower respiratory infections in nursing home patients. J Fam Pract 1992;34(5):585–91.

[23] Vergis EN, Brennen C, Wagener M, et al. Pneumonia in long-term care: a prospective case-control study of risk factors and impact on survival. Arch Intern Med 2001;161(19):2378–81.

[24] Donowitz GR, Cox HL. Bacterial community-acquired pneumonia in older patients. Clin Geriatr Med 2007;23:515–34.

[25] Berk SL. Bacterial pneumonia in the elderly: the observations of Sir William Osler in retrospect. J Am Geriatr Soc 1984;32:683–5.

[26] Metlay JP, Schulz R, Li YH, et al. Influence of age on symptoms at presentation in patients with community-acquired pneumonia. Arch Intern Med 1997;157(13):1453–9.

[27] Marrie TJ, Blanchard W. A comparison of nursing home-acquired pneumonia patients with patients with community-acquired pneumonia and nursing

home patients without pneumonia. J Am Geriatr Soc 1997;45:50–5.

[28] Roghmann MC, Warner J, Mackowiak PA. The relationship between age and fever magnitude. Am J Med Sci 2001;322:68–70.

[29] Muder RR, Aghababian RV, Loeb MB, et al. Nursing home-acquired pneumonia: an emergency department treatment algorithm. Curr Med Res Opin 2004;8:1309–20.

[30] Fernández-Sabé N, Carratalà J, Rosón B, et al. Community-acquired pneumonia in very elderly patients: causative organisms, clinical characteristics, and outcomes. Medicine 2003;82:159–69.

[31] Waterer GW, Kessler LA, Wunderink RG. Delayed administration of antibiotics and atypical presentation in community-acquired pneumonia. Chest 2006;130(1):11–5.

[32] Meteresky ML, Sweeney TA, Getzow MB, et al. Antibiotic timing and diagnostic uncertainty in Medicare patients with pneumonia: is it reasonable to expect all patients to receive antibiotics within 4 hours? Chest 2006;130:16–21.

[33] Mandell L, Wunderink F, Anzueto A, et al. Infectious Diseases Society of America/American Thoracic Society Guidelines on the management for community-acquired pneumonia in adults. Clin Infect Dis 2007;44(Suppl 2):S27–72.

[34] Vanderkooi OG, Low DE, Green K, et al. Predicting antimicrobial resistance in invasive pneumococcal infections. Clin Infect Dis 1997;24:1052–9.

[35] Ho PL, Tse WS, Tsang KW, et al. Risk factors for acquisition of levofoxacin-resistant Streptococcus pneumoniae: a case-control study. Clin Infect Dis 2001;32:701–7.

[36] Ruhe JJ, Hasbun R. Streptococcus pneumoniae bacteremia: duration of previous antibiotic use and association with penicillin resistance. Clin Infect Dis 2003;36:1132–8.

[37] Ruiz M, Ewig S, Marcos MA, et al. Etiology of community-acquired pneumonia: impact of age, comorbidity, and severity. Am J Respir Crit Care Med 1999;160:397–405.

[38] Arancibia F, Bauer TT, Ewig S, et al. Community-acquired pneumonia due to gram-negative bacteria and Pseudomonas aeruginosa. Arch Intern Med 2002;162:1849–58.

[39] Niederman MS, Mandell LA, Anzueto A, et al. Guidelines for the management of adults with community-acquired pneumonia: diagnosis. Assessment of severity, antimicrobial therapy, and prevention. Am J Respir Crit Care Med 2001; 167:1730–54.

[40] Troy CJ, Peeling AG, Ellis JC, et al. Chlamydia pneumoniae as a new source of infectious outbreaks in nursing homes. JAMA 1997;277:1214–8.

[41] Nakashima K, Tanaka T, Kramer MH, et al. Outbreak of Chlamydia pneumoniae in a Japanese nursing home, 1999–2000. Infect Control Hosp Epidemiol 2006;27:1171–7.

[42] Seenivasan MH, Yu VL, Muder RR. Legionnaires' disease in long-term care facilities: overview and proposed solutions. J Am Geriatr Soc 2005;53:875–80.

[43] Wald TG, Shult P, Krause P, et al. A rhinovirus outbreak among residents of a long-term care facility. Ann Intern Med 1995;123:588–93.

[44] Lieberman D, Lieberman D, Schlaeffer F, et al. Community-acquired pneumonia in old age: a prospective study of 91 patients admitted from home. Age Ageing 1997;26:69–75.

[45] Rello J, Rodriguez R, Jubert P, et al. Severe community-acquired pneumonia in the elderly: epidemiology and prognosis. Clin Infect Dis 1996;23:723–8.

[46] El-Solh AA, Sikka P, Ramadan F, et al. Etiology of severe pneumonia in the very elderly. Am J Respir Crit Care Med 2001;163:645–51.

[47] El-Solh AA, Pietrantoni C, Bhat A, et al. Microbiology of severe aspiration pneumonia in institutionalized elderly. Am J Respir Crit Care Med 2003;167: 1650–4.

[48] El Solh AA, Pietrantoni C, Bhat A, et al. Indicators of potentially drug-resistant bacteria in severe nursing home-acquired pneumonia. Clin Infect Dis 2004; 39:474–80.

[49] Niederman MS, Craven DE, Bonten MJ, et al. Guidelines for the management of adults with hospital-acquired, ventilator-associated, and healthcare-associated pneumonia. Am J Respir Crit Care Med 2005;171:388–416.

[50] Kollef MH, Shorr A, Tabak YP, et al. Epidemiology and outcomes of health-care-associated pneumonia: results from a large US database of culture positive patients. Chest 2005;128:3854–62.

[51] Loeb M, Carusone SC, Goeree R, et al. Effect of a clinical pathway to reduce hospitalizations in nursing home residents with pneumonia: a randomized controlled trial. JAMA 2006;295:2503–10.

[52] Metersky ML, Sweeney TA, Getzow MB, et al. Predicting bacteremia in patients with community acquired pneumonia. Am J Respir Crit Care Med 2004;169:342–7.

[53] Neill AM, Martin IR, Weir R, et al. Community acquired pneumonia; aetiology and usefulness of severity criteria on admission. Thorax 1996;51:1010–6.

[54] Lim WS, Macfarlane JT, Boswell TC, et al. Severity prediction rules in community acquired pneumonia: a validation study. Thorax 2000;55:219–23.

[55] Niederman MS, Feldman C, Richards GA. Combining information from prognostic scoring tools for CAP: an American view on how to get the best of all worlds. Eur Respir J 2006;27:9–11.

[56] Lim WS, Macfarlane JT. Defining prognostic factors in the elderly with community acquired pneumonia: a case controlled study of patients aged > 75 years. Eur Respir J 2001;17:200–5.

[57] Naito T, Suda T, Yasuda K, et al. A validation and potential modification of the pneumonia severity index in elderly patients with community-acquired pneumonia. J Am Geriatr Soc 2006;54:1212–9.

[58] van der Steen JT, Mehr DR, Kruse RL, et al. Dementia, lower respiratory tract infection, and mortality. J Am Med Dir Assoc 2007;8:396–403.

[59] Aujesky D, Auble TE, Yealy DM, et al. Prospective comparison of three validated prediction rules for prognosis in community-acquired pneumonia. Am J Med 2005;118:384–92.

[60] Capelastegui A, Espana PP, Quintana JM, et al. Validation of a predictive rule for the management of community-acquired pneumonia. Eur Respir J 2006;27:151–7.

[61] van der Steen JT, Ribbe MW, Mehr DR, et al. Do findings of high mortality from pneumonia in the elderly make it the old man's friend? Arch Intern Med 2004;164:224–5.

[62] van der Steen JT, Kruse RL, Ooms ME, et al. Treatment of nursing home residents with dementia and lower respiratory tract infection in the United States and The Netherlands: an ocean apart. J Am Geriatr Soc 2004;52:692–9.

[63] Ramsdell J, Narsavage FL, Fink JB. Management for community-acquired pneumonia in the home: an American College of Chest Physicians clinical position statement. Chest 2005;127:1752–63.

[64] Goss CH, Rubenfeld GD, Park DR, et al. Cost and incidence of social comorbidities in low-risk patients with community-acquired pneumonia admitted to a public hospital. Chest 2003;124:2148–55.

[65] Ewig S, de Roux A, Bauer T, et al. Validation of predictive rule and indices of severity for community acquired pneumonia. Thorax 2004;59:421–7.

[66] Myint P, Kamath AV, Vowler SL, et al. Severity assessment criteria recommended by the British Thoracic Society for community-acquired pneumonia and older patients: should SOAR criteria be used in older people? A compilation study of two prospective cohorts. Age Ageing 2006;35:286–91.

[67] España PP, Capelastegui A, Gorordo I, et al. Development and validation of a clinical prediction rule for severe community-acquired pneumonia. Am J Respir Crit Care Med 2006; 174:1249–56.

[68] Houck PM, MacLehose RF, Niederman MS, et al. Empiric antibiotic therapy and mortality among Medicare pneumonia inpatients in 10 western states: 1993, 1995, and 1997. Chest 2001;119:1420–6.

[69] Gleason PP, Meehan TP, Fine JM, et al. Associations between initial antimicrobial therapy and medical outcomes for hospitalized elderly patients with pneumonia. Arch Intern Med 1999;159: 2562–72.

[70] Weiss K, TIllotson GS. The controversy of combination vs. monotherapy in the treatment of hospitalized community-acquired pneumonia. Chest 2005; 128:940–6.

[71] Waterer GW, Somes GW, Wunderink RG. Monotherapy may be suboptimal for severe bacteremic pneumococcal pneumonia. Arch Intern Med 2001; 161:1837–42.

[72] Baddour LM, Yu VL, Klugman KP, et al. Combination antibiotic therapy lower mortality among severely ill patients with pneumococcal bacteremia. Am J Respir Crit Care Med 2004;170:440–4.

[73] Lujan ML, Gallego M, Fontanals D, et al. Prospective observational study of bacteremic pneumococcal pneumonia: effect of discordant therapy on mortality. Crit Care Med 2004;32:625–31.

[74] Yu VL, Chiou CC, Feldman C, et al. An international prospective study of pneumococcal bacteremia: correlation with in vitro resistance, antibiotics administered and clinical outcome. Clin Infect Dis 2003;37: 230–7.

[75] Plouffe JF, Breiman RF, Facklam RR. Bacteremia with Streptococcus pneumoniae: implications for therapy and prevention. Franklin County pneumonia study group. JAMA 1996;275:194–8.

[76] Metlay JP, Hofmann J, Cetron MS, et al. Impact of penicillin susceptibility on medical outcomes for adult patients with bacteremic pneumococcal pneumonia. Clin Infect Dis 2000;30:520–8.

[77] Feikin DR, Schuchat A, Kolczak M, et al. Mortality from invasive pneumococcal pneumonia in the era of antibiotic resistance, 1995–1997. Am J Public Health 2000;90:223–9.

[78] Moroney JF, Fiore AE, Harrison LH, et al. Clinical outcomes of bacteremic pneumococcal pneumonia in the era of antibiotic resistance. Clin Infect Dis 2001;33:797–805.

[79] Vanderkooi OF, Low DE, Green K, et al. Predicting antimicrobial resistance in invasive pneumococcal infections. Clin Infect Dis 2005;40:1288–97.

[80] Fuller JD, Low DE. A review of Streptococcus pneumoniae infection treatment failures associated with fluoroquinolone resistance. Clin Infect Dis 2005;41: 118–21.

[81] Morganroth J, Dimarco JP, Anzueto A, et al. A randomized trial comparing the cardiac rhythm safety of moxifloxacin vs levofloxacin in elderly patients hospitalized with community-acquired pneumonia. Chest 2005;128:3398–406.

[82] Anzueto A, Niederman MS, Pearle J, et al. Community-acquired pneumonia recovery in the elderly (CAPRIE): efficacy and safety of moxifloxacin therapy versus that of levofloxacin therapy. Clin Infect Dis 2006;42:73–81.

[83] Park-Wyllie LY, Jurlink DN, Kopp A, et al. Outpatient gatifloxacin therapy and dysglycemia in older adults. N Engl J Med 2006;354:1352–61.

[84] Hirata-Dulas CA, Stein DJ, Guay DR, et al. A randomized study of ciprofloxacin versus ceftriaxone in the treatment of nursing home-acquired lower respiratory tract infections. J Am Geriatr Soc 1991;39: 979–85.

[85] Yakovlev SV, Stratchounski LS, Woods GL, et al. Ertapenem versus cefepime for initial empirical treatment of pneumonia acquired in skilled-care facilities or in hospitals outside the intensive care unit. Eur J Clin Microbiol Infect Dis 2006;25:633–41.

[86] Feinsilver SH, Fein AM, Niederman MS, et al. Utility of fiberoptic bronchoscopy in nonresolving pneumonia. Chest 1990;98:1322–6.

[87] Menendez R, Torres A, Rodriguez de Castro F, et al. Reaching stability in community-acquired pneumonia: the effects of the severity of disease, treatment and the characteristics of patients. Clin Infect Dis 2004;39:1783–90.

[88] Rosón B, Carratalà J, Fernández-Sabé N, et al. Causes and factors associated with early failure in hospitalized patients with community-acquired pneumonia. Arch Intern Med 2004;164:502–8.

[89] El Solh AA, Aquilaina AT, Gulen H, et al. Radiographic resolution of community-acquired bacterial pneumonia in the elderly. J Am Geriatr Soc 2004;52:224–9.

[90] Jackson ML, Neuzil KM, Thompson WW, et al. The burden of community-acquired pneumonia in seniors: results of a population-based study. Clin Infect Dis 2004;39:1642–50.

[91] Gross PA, Hermogenes AW, Sacks HS, et al. The efficacy of influenza vaccine in elderly persons: a meta analysis and review of the literature. Ann Intern Med 1995;123:518–27.

[92] Jefferson R, Rivetti D, Rivetti A, et al. Efficacy and effectiveness of influenza vaccines in elderly people: a systematic review. Lancet 2005;366:1165–74.

[93] Whitney CG, Farley MM, Hadler J, et al. Decline in invasive pneumococcal disease after the introduction of protein-polysaccharide conjugate vaccine. N Engl J Med 2003;348:1737–46.

[94] Fisman DN, Abrutyn E, Spaude KA, et al. Prior pneumococcal vaccination is associated with reduced death, complications, and length of stay among hospitalized adults with community-acquired pneumonia. Clin Infect Dis 2006;42:1093–101.

[95] Fedson DS, Harward MP, Reid RA, et al. Hospital-based pneumococcal immunization: epidemiologic rationale from the Shenandoah study. JAMA 1990;264:1117–22.

[96] Walker FJ, Singleton RJ, Bulkow LR, et al. Reactions after 3 or more doses of pneumococcal polysaccharide vaccine in adults in Alaska. Clin Infect Dis 2005;40:1730–5.

ELSEVIER
SAUNDERS

Clin Chest Med 28 (2007) 773–781

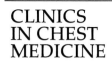

Tuberculosis and Nontuberculous Mycobacterial Infections in Older Adults

Neil W. Schluger, MD[a,b,*]

[a]Division of Pulmonary, Allergy, and Critical Care Medicine, Columbia University Medical Center, PH-8 East, Room 101,
622 West 168th Street, New York, NY 10032, USA
[b]Epidemiology and Environmental Health Sciences, Columbia University, Mailman School of Public Health,
722 West 168th Street, New York, NY 10032, USA

Tuberculosis

Epidemiology

Tuberculosis is one of the world's great public health crises. It is estimated by the World Health Organization that roughly one third of the world's population, or some 2 billion people, are infected with *Mycobacterium tuberculosis*, the causative agent. More than 8 million people every year develop active tuberculosis disease, and 2 million die as a result [1].

The vast majority of cases of tuberculosis occur in the 22 so called high burden countries of the world. China and India contribute together nearly 3 million cases per year, and the remaining high burden countries are primarily poor nations with limited resources to devote to tuberculosis or health care in general. The annual incidence of active tuberculosis in these high burden countries ranges from 100 per 100,000 to as high as 1000 per 100,000 [2]. In contrast, rates of tuberculosis in most established market economy countries are in the range of 15 to 35 per 100,000, and in the United States in 2006, there were only 13,700 cases of active tuberculosis, for an incidence rate of 4.6 per 100,000. This rate is among the lowest of any country, and it represents a historical low for the United States.

In terms of sheer numbers, older patients (defined here completely arbitrarily as persons

aged 65 years and older) account for a significant number of tuberculosis cases in the world each year. According to the most recent statistical report from the World Health Organization, 9.8% of sputum smear-positive cases of tuberculosis occur in this age group [2]. Older patients account for more than 234,000 cases of smear-positive tuberculosis in the world. Although this is lower than for younger age groups (the mode of the age group distribution for prevalent cases is 25–34 years), the incident rate (cases of active, smear-positive tuberculosis per 100,000 population) in the older than 65 year age group is similar to most other age groups around the world.

In the United States, there is a more even distribution of tuberculosis among older age groups. In 2005, the most recent year for which data are available from the Centers for Disease Control and Prevention (CDC), 20% of all tuberculosis cases occurred in persons older than 65 years [3]. Furthermore, incidence rates (cases per 100,000 persons) among persons in the older than 65 years age group in the United States are the highest for any age group in this country. The incidence rate for tuberculosis among men older than 65 years is just more than 10 per 100,000 and the rate for women is just more than 5 per 100,000. For males, this is considerably higher than the incidence rate in any other age group, and for females it is a slightly higher rate than observed in the 25- to 44-year age group, which is the next highest. By way of comparison, the overall rate of tuberculosis in the United States is roughly 4.6 per 100,000.

Among members of all racial and ethnic minority groups, the trend toward a higher rate of tuberculosis is seen in older age groups, but the

* Corresponding author. Division of Pulmonary, Allergy, and Critical Care Medicine, Columbia University Medical Center, PH-8 East, Room 101, 622 West 168th Street, New York, NY 10032.
E-mail address: ns311@columbia.edu

effect of age on tuberculosis incidence seems most pronounced in Asians, who in general have the highest rates of tuberculosis of all racial or ethnic groups in the United States. There is nearly a fourfold increase in case rates in the over 65-years age group (more than 80 cases per 100,000 persons) as compared with the 15- to 25-year-old cohort, for example. Even the 25- to 44-year age group among Asians have only half the rate of tuberculosis compared with the over 65-years group. The reasons for the much more pronounced effect of age on tuberculosis rates among Asians are not clear. Overall the higher rate of tuberculosis in this group is probably because many Asians have come to the United States from countries in which tuberculosis is common, and so the rates of latent infection are high, but this does not explain the striking increase in rates among the older Asian population in the United States.

Clinical presentation and diagnosis of tuberculosis in older adults

In general there has been an assumption that the vast majority of tuberculosis in older populations results from reactivation of latent infection. The determination as to whether a case is the result of reactivation of latent infection or of recently acquired infection, however, is often inaccurate when made on clinical or radiographic grounds, as a recent molecular epidemiologic analysis of this issue has demonstrated [4]. Certainly, however, it is true that immune function, and in particular cellular immune function, declines with age, and there is every reason to think that older persons are in fact more susceptible to developing tuberculosis by whatever mechanism than are younger persons [5,6].

The effect of age on the clinical presentation of tuberculosis has been examined in several studies, although most of these studies are several years old [7–12]. Several points seem clear from these studies. Extrapulmonary tuberculosis, including miliary tuberculosis, seems to be more common in older patients. Features commonly identified in patients who have tuberculosis, such as fever, cough, hemoptysis, and weight loss, seem to occur less frequently in older patients, and nonspecific complaints, such as fatigue, loss of appetite, or even worsening cognitive function, may be presenting complaints, as is the case with many infectious syndromes among older individuals.

Pulmonary disease is still the most common manifestation of tuberculosis in older patients,

but here too the clinical and radiographic presentation may be somewhat different from that typically seen in younger persons. Older patients who have pulmonary tuberculosis may have few symptoms, so clinicians need to have a high index of suspicion to make a diagnosis. In particular, for patients who have been in congregate settings such as nursing homes, clinicians should take care to obtain a history of sick contacts or other residents who have had similar respiratory illnesses.

Overall one of the most thorough reviews of the clinical presentation of tuberculosis in older patients was a meta-analysis done by Perez-Guzmán and colleagues [13], in which they examined characteristics associated with tuberculosis in persons older than age 60 years as compared with all other age groups. After conducting a thorough search and review of the literature, they found that certain characteristics, including the prevalence of cough, sputum, weight loss, and fatigue or malaise, were similar across all age groups. Fever, night sweats, and hemoptysis, however, were all less common in persons older than age 60 years. Not surprisingly, comorbid conditions, such as cardiovascular disease, diabetes mellitus, chronic obstructive pulmonary disease, and history of gastrectomy, were all more common in older patients.

After a history and physical examination are completed, the first diagnostic examination to be performed is usually a chest radiograph. The radiology of tuberculosis in older persons has been well described. Certainly upper lobe, cavitary disease is often seen in this age group, but somewhat more atypical manifestations can be seen also. Again, Perez-Guzmán and colleagues have examined the range of radiographic findings across age groups. They found that upper lobe predominant disease was no more common in older patients than in younger, but that cavities, at least as assessed by plain chest radiography, were less common.

Diagnostic evaluation

The approach to the diagnosis of tuberculosis has been extensively described and written about [14]. In the United States and other resource-rich countries, the diagnostic approach generally includes radiography and sputum examination by smear and culture, whereas in resource-poor countries, radiography and sputum culture are often too expensive to be performed on a routine basis [15].

Tuberculin skin testing (TST) with purified protein derivative has a more limited role to play in the diagnosis of active tuberculosis than it does in identifying patients who have latent tuberculosis infection, and this is particularly true in older individuals [16–19]. In patients who have tuberculosis in general, TST can be negative approximately 20% of the time in the setting of active disease, and the skin test is negative even more often in older patients [13]. A negative TST thus should not be taken as strong evidence against the diagnosis of active tuberculosis in an older patient if epidemiologic, clinical, and radiographic features support the diagnosis. The higher frequency of negative TST in older patients probably reflects a higher prevalence of anergy in this population because of impaired T-cell function.

More recently interferon gamma release assays (IGRAs) have been introduced as a diagnostic tool for the detection of tuberculosis [20]. These tests rely on the in vitro production of interferon gamma by peripheral blood mononuclear cells after stimulation with *M. tuberculosis*-specific antigens to identify persons who have been exposed to tuberculosis. Sensitivity of this test for active tuberculosis is also roughly 80%, although specificity for active disease (as opposed to latent infection) is considerably lower [21]. As recent guidelines from the CDC point out, however, IGRAs have not been evaluated thoroughly in patients at extremes of age, and at present there seems to be little role for these assays in the diagnosis of active tuberculosis in older individuals [22].

Most studies suggest that sputum acid-fast smears are equally likely to be positive in older and younger patients who have tuberculosis, and overall approximately 50% to 60% of patients who have pulmonary tuberculosis have a positive smear. It is possible, however, that older persons may be less able to produce an adequate sputum sample by spontaneous expectoration for examination. A substantial literature suggests that sputum induction is an extremely useful approach to obtaining sputum samples in patients who are unable to produce an expectorated sample, and this should be the next diagnostic maneuver in older patients who have suspected tuberculosis [23,24]. In general, bronchoscopy should be reserved for patients who are unable to produce a satisfactory sputum sample, even through induction, or for patients in whom substantial clinical uncertainty exists concerning the diagnosis [25]. This may likely be the case in older patients in whom a diagnosis of primary or metastatic carcinoma is high on the differential list. If this is the case, a more aggressive evaluation is certainly warranted.

Treatment

The basic approach to treatment of tuberculosis in older persons is the same as in younger patients [26]. Standard therapy of drug-susceptible disease consists of a 2-months' duration intensive phase of treatment with isoniazid (INH), rifampin, pyrazinamide, and ethambutol followed by a 4-month continuation phase of only isoniazid and rifampin. Vitamin B6 (pyridoxine) is usually given as a supplement to prevent the peripheral neuropathy that may occur from isoniazid-induced losses. This may be especially important in older persons, because there is evidence that dietary intake of vitamin B6 is lower in this patient group [27].

The major concerns related to treatment of tuberculosis in older age groups are those of adverse effects of drugs, because treatment efficacy should not be greatly different in tuberculosis patients as a function of age. Isoniazid is a well-known cause of drug-induced hepatitis. As many as 10% to 20% of patients who take INH develop a transient increase in liver function tests (predominantly transaminases), but fortunately in most cases this increase is transient and asymptomatic and does not require an alteration of therapy. Serious and even life-threatening liver injury, however, may occur as a result of INH treatment. The incidence of this is difficult to determine with precision, but may be as high as 0.1% to 2.0%. Patients at higher risk for INH-induced liver damage include those who have prior liver disease and persons older than 50 years of age [28,29]. In such patients, prudent practice is to obtain baseline and monthly liver function tests. Patients should also be educated about the signs and symptoms of liver damage and should be encouraged to report promptly to their physician any of these complaints.

Rifampin and pyrazinamide also may be associated with liver injury, and the same caveats apply.

Ethambutol is in general a safe and well-tolerated drug. The major adverse effect of this drug is ocular toxicity, with optic neuritis and impairment of visual acuity and color vision. This is generally uncommon at dose ranges in current clinical use (generally 15–25 mg/kg). In general, it is felt that much of the ocular toxicity caused by ethambutol is reversible. Some reports indicate, however, that ocular changes caused by ethambutol may be more frequent and less reversible in older patients [30]. Because most patients who have tuberculosis receive ethambutol for only 1 to 2 months, the risk for serious injury is probably still low, but visual acuity and color vision should be monitored monthly in patients on prolonged ethambutol-containing regimens. The problem of ethambutol ocular toxicity may be much greater in patients treated for nontuberculous mycobacterial infections, because treatment in these cases is prolonged [31].

Nontuberculous mycobacteria

A discussion of syndromes caused by infection with all the numerous species of nontuberculosis mycobacteria (NTM) is beyond the scope of this article. Instead the discussion largely focuses on disease caused by *M. avium* complex, because this is the most frequently encountered of the NTM in clinical practice.

Epidemiology

The epidemiology of infection and disease caused by NTM in general and *M. avium* complex organisms in particular is difficult to describe with the same precision as that of tuberculosis for several reasons. First and most significant is that NTM infections are not reportable in the United States, because they are generally not believed to be communicable diseases whose severity warrants a major public health response. Second, there has often been confusion (and undoubtedly a great deal of this confusion persists today) regarding issues of colonization, infection, and disease in patients from whom NTM have been isolated. There has been a lack of consensus regarding the definition of clinical syndromes caused by NTM, and there is great heterogeneity among reports and case series of these conditions. As a result, there is considerable uncertainty regarding the true epidemiology of disease caused by NTM. A recent statement by the American Thoracic Society notes that in industrialized countries the rate of disease caused by NTM is believed to be in the range of 1.0 to 1.8 per 100,000, but the statement also notes that in most mycobacteriology

laboratories, isolation of NTM is now more common than isolation of *M. tuberculosis* [32]. In the United States the rate of tuberculosis is 4.6 per 100,000, so there seems to be a discrepancy between the number of positive NTM cultures and the number of patients diagnosed with disease. A recent survey based on skin testing with NTM antigens suggests, however, that 1 in every 6 Americans is now exposed to NTM, as opposed to 1 in 9 approximately 30 years ago [33].

NTM seems to be widely distributed in the environment, and soil and water represent natural reservoirs for these organisms [34–37]. It is generally believed that there is little if any human-to-human transmission of NTM. In recent years, it seems that there may be an increase in the number of persons who have NTM infection, and there may be several reasons for this. First, better culture methods, primarily using broth-based systems, have been used in more and more laboratories, and there is evidence that these systems are more sensitive than solid media-based systems for recovering NTM [38]. To a certain extent, the increase in cases of disease caused by NTM thus may be partially an artifact of better detection. There are also reasons to think that exposure to NTM may in fact be higher, however, and that the increase in cases may be real. Cultural shifts from bathtubs to showers and more time spent in hot tubs and Jacuzzis may be associated with a true increase in infection, because these warm water sources are well known to be reservoirs of NTM, and persons using them are exposed to fine aerosols that may aid in transmission of mycobacteria.

Clinical syndromes

This and remaining sections focus exclusively on *M. avium* complex (MAC). There are several clinical syndromes associated with MAC infection [39,40]. These include hypersensitivity pneumonitis, the Lady Windermere syndrome, bronchiectasis, and pulmonary nodules with the well-described "tree-in-bud" appearance.

Hypersensitivity pneumonitis (HP) caused by MAC (occasionally called hot tub lung) is usually a disease of younger persons, and it is not discussed at length here. Cases have been described in persons exposed to MAC in the settings of showers, saunas, Jacuzzis, and hot tubs [41–45]. The presentation is similar to other HP syndromes, and patients usually improve when they are no longer in contact with the offending antigen, in this case MAC. Treatment therefore is generally avoidance of the source of the hypersensitivity, and occasionally prednisone is added. There is some controversy about the usefulness of antibiotic treatment for MAC in patients who have hot tub lung, but it seems that most patients improve without this.

More important in older patients are the syndromes of bronchiectasis and pulmonary nodules (often in the "tree-in-bud" pattern mentioned previously) which are well known to pulmonary physicians but which also pose great challenges in diagnosis and treatment. The term "Lady Windermere syndrome" was first used in 1992 by Reich and Johnson [46] to describe six older women who presented with right middle lobe or lingular infiltrates and evidence of infection with MAC. The name they assigned to the syndrome was drawn from a play by Oscar Wilde and was chosen to reflect the authors' contention that the patients in their series had voluntary suppression of cough, a behavior they ascribed to Wilde's character. Since that initial description, the entire spectrum of MAC pulmonary disease in apparently immunocompetent hosts has been increasingly recognized.

The symptoms of pulmonary disease caused by MAC in immunocompetent patients are nonspecific. Cough, dry or productive of sputum, is the predominant complaint, but patients also often note fatigue and malaise, weight loss, nonspecific chest pain, and fever.

Plain chest radiographs may mimic tuberculosis closely, and TB must be excluded as a diagnostic possibility. Computerized tomography (CT), particularly using the high-resolution technique (HRCT), has dramatically altered the understanding of pulmonary disease caused by MAC, and this is an extremely helpful tool in the evaluation of patients who have *M. avium* complex in respiratory secretions. HRCT studies demonstrate that disease is generally more diffuse than generally appreciated on the basis of plain chest radiographs [47–49]. In addition, HRCT studies often demonstrate what have come to be viewed as characteristic findings of MAC infection, namely, multiple small nodules and associated bronchiectasis [48,50,51]. The nodules are usually numerous and smaller than 1 cm in diameter. They occasionally can be larger, however, and in older patients who have a history of tobacco use there is often a question of whether one nodule among many could represent a malignancy.

Diagnosis of Mycobacterium avium complex

The diagnosis of pulmonary disease in patients who have MAC has been the source of some controversy that has mainly focused on the issue of differentiating infection (or colonization) from disease. The recently revised American Thoracic Society statement on NTM requires clinical and microbiologic criteria to be met [32]. The criteria are as follows:

1. Clinical
   a. Pulmonary symptoms, nodular or cavitary opacities on chest radiograph, or an HRCT scan that shows multifocal bronchiectasis with multiple nodules

   AND

   b. Appropriate exclusion of other diagnoses (particularly TB and malignancy)

2. Microbiologic
   a. Positive culture results from at least two separate expectorated sputum samples

   OR

   b. Positive culture result from at least one bronchial wash or lavage

   OR

   c. Transbronchial or other lung biopsy with granulomatous inflammation or AFB and positive culture from bronchoscopy or sputum

The most important aspect of the new ATS guidelines, however, is the following statement: "Making the diagnosis of NTM lung disease does not, per se, necessitate the institution of therapy, which is a decision based on potential risks and benefits of therapy for individual patients." In fact, it is the belief of the author that diagnosis has been somewhat overemphasized until recently, when the most difficult issues center on treatment.

Treatment of Mycobacterium avium complex pulmonary disease in older patients

The decision to initiate therapy for MAC disease, particularly in older patients, can be an extremely difficult one. The beneficial effects of therapy are uncertain, and there are considerable adverse effects associated with the drugs commonly used to treat these infections.

The most commonly used regimen in the treatment of pulmonary MAC disease in the immunocompetent host consists of a rifamycin (usually rifampin or rifabutin), a macrolide (clarithromycin or azithromycin), and ethambutol. There have been efforts to rely on regimens that substitute agents such as clofazimine for rifamycins in an effort to reduce toxicity of treatment, but the published experience with these approaches is limited [52]. Unlike treatment of tuberculosis, reliance on drug susceptibility testing is of much less certain value in developing a treatment regimen for MAC, with the possible exception of testing for macrolide susceptibility.

Several small studies have been published that describe outcomes, mostly microbiologic, in patients treated with macrolide-containing regimens, which are generally believed to be the most potent for treating these infections [53–58]. These studies taken together establish that drug susceptibility testing results have meaning for use of macrolides, but probably not for other agents. They also suggest that sputum culture conversion can be achieved in most patients whose isolates are in fact susceptible to macrolides, but little in the way of meaningful long-term clinical response and outcomes can be gleaned from these reports.

Recently a larger experience was reported on the outcomes of patients who had MAC treated with the three-drug regimen of a macrolide, rifamycin, and ethambutol. Lam and colleagues described results of patients who had pulmonary MAC who were treated as the control arm of a study designed to examine the role of adjunctive immunotherapy with interferon gamma [59]. In this study, 91 patients who had pulmonary MAC (diagnosed according to the ATS guidelines) were treated with a thrice weekly regimen of clarithromycin (or azithromycin), ethambutol, and rifampin (or rifabutin). Patients who had HIV infection were excluded from the study, as were patients who had cystic fibrosis, sarcoidosis, or malignancy. Patients underwent rigorous clinical, radiographic, and bacteriologic assessments, and sputum samples were collected frequently throughout the study.

The mean age of patients enrolled in the study was 60.9 years for those who had cavitary disease and 67.8 years for those who did not. Most patients had a history of prior bronchiectasis and COPD, and bronchiectasis and nodules were common findings on HRCT. Patients had evidence of moderate airflow limitation on pulmonary function testing, with a mean FEV_1/FVC of 61% in the cavitary group and 66% in the noncavitary group. Dyspnea was reported by most patients, and one quarter to one half reported consistent sputum production. Overall this patient group was representative of sicker patients who had MAC, and most clinicians would agree with treatment.

Results from this study were revealing. With culture conversion defined as going from a positive to a negative culture, only 13% of patients who had baseline positive cultures overall had a satisfactory response (4% in the cavitary group and 24% in the noncavitary group). Overall, the study reported that 60.4% of patients had improvement in HRCT findings of disease, and 52.5% had symptomatic improvement. These benefits were not immediate, however. Mean time for HRCT improvement was between 164 and 340 days, depending on the presence of cavities, and the mean time for symptom improvement was 252 days. Adverse events were common in the study. More than 90% of patients reported at least one side effect, with nearly one third of subjects reporting nausea.

What can this and other studies teach us about the treatment of MAC pulmonary disease in this older (and certainly representative) cohort of patients who had more severe disease? On the whole, bacteriologic response rates were low, and radiographic and clinical improvement was modest and often took a long time to achieve. Side effects were common. These data are helpful in framing expectations about treatment responses in patients who had pulmonary MAC, but they also raise further questions. The study was limited by the lack of an untreated control group. Is it possible that symptomatic therapy alone (chest physiotherapy, drainage maneuvers and assists, bronchodilators) would have achieved similar results, without the antibiotic therapy? Also, what about patients who have less advanced disease? Would results be better or worse? It is not uncommon for pulmonary physicians to encounter patients well into their seventies who have cough and sputum cultures positive for MAC but fairly localized bronchiectasis or a few nodules on HRCT, and normal or near normal pulmonary function. The author's approach to such patients is generally not to institute triple antibiotic therapy with the attendant side effects, but rather to follow them closely and to implement drug treatment only if there is a marked change in clinical or radiographic status. In general, rifampin-containing regimens are better tolerated in older patients than are rifabutin-containing regimens, and intermittent (thrice-weekly) therapy also seems better tolerated, and perhaps no less efficacious, than daily therapy [60].

Summary

Mycobacterial infections remain extraordinarily common around the world, and older persons are particularly vulnerable. Tuberculosis can be diagnosed and treated in a straightforward way in most instances, but infections with non-tuberculous mycobacteria pose greater challenges. Treatment of these latter infections is often associated with significant adverse effects and uncertain clinical outcomes. Physicians' judgment has an important role to play in selecting patients for treatment and in choosing an optimal drug regimen.

References

[1] Dye C, Watt CJ, Bleed DM, et al. Evolution of tuberculosis control and prospects for reducing tuberculosis incidence, prevalence, and deaths globally. JAMA 2005;293(22):2767–75.

[2] WHO. Global tuberculosis control—surveillance, planning, financing. Geneva (Switzerland): WHO; 2007.

[3] CDC. Reported tuberculosis in the United States, 2005. Atlanta (GA): Department of Health and Human Services; 2006.

[4] Geng E, Kreiswirth B, Burzynski J, et al. Clinical and radiographic correlates of primary and reactivation tuberculosis: a molecular epidemiology study. JAMA 2005;293(22):2740–5.

[5] Pawelec G. Immunity and ageing in man. Exp Gerontol 2006;41(12):1239–42.

[6] Vallejo AN. Age-dependent alterations of the T cell repertoire and functional diversity of T cells of the aged. Immunol Res 2006;36(1–3):221–8.

[7] Davies PD. Tuberculosis in the elderly. J Antimicrob Chemother 1994;34(Suppl A):93–100.

[8] Davies PD. Tuberculosis in the elderly. Epidemiology and optimal management. Drugs Aging 1996; 8(6):436–44.

[9] Nagami P, Yoshikawa TT. Aging and tuberculosis. Gerontology 1984;30(5):308–15.

[10] Stead WW. Special problems in tuberculosis. Tuberculosis in the elderly and in residents of nursing homes, correctional facilities, long-term care hospitals, mental hospitals, shelters for the homeless, and jails. Clin Chest Med 1989;10(3):397–405.

[11] Stead WW. Tuberculosis among elderly persons, as observed among nursing home residents. Int J Tuberc Lung Dis 1998;2(9 Suppl 1):S64–70.

[12] Yoshikawa TT. Tuberculosis in aging adults. J Am Geriatr Soc 1992;40(2):178–87.

[13] Perez-Guzman C, Vargas MH, Torres-Cruz A, et al. Does aging modify pulmonary tuberculosis?: A meta-analytical review. Chest 1999;116(4):961–7.

[14] Brodie D, Schluger NW. The diagnosis of tuberculosis. Clin Chest Med 2005;26(2):247–71, vi.

[15] Perkins MD, Kritski AL. Diagnostic testing in the control of tuberculosis. Bull World Health Organ 2002;80(6):512–3.

[16] Targeted testing and treatment of latent tuberculosis infection. Am J Respir Crit Care Med 2000;161(4 Pt 2): S221–47.

[17] Leduc Y, Drapeau S, Samson I, et al [Prevalence of positive tuberculin test in a population of patients requiring long-term care in a hospital setting]. Can Fam Physician 1997;43:2143–7 [in French].

[18] Woo J, Chan HS, Hazlett CB, et al. Tuberculosis among elderly Chinese in residential homes: tuberculin reactivity and estimated prevalence. Gerontology 1996;42(3):155–62.

[19] Nisar M, Williams CS, Ashby D, et al. Tuberculin testing in residential homes for the elderly. Thorax 1993;48(12):1257–60.

[20] Menzies D, Pai M, Comstock G. Meta-analysis: new tests for the diagnosis of latent tuberculosis infection: areas of uncertainty and recommendations for research. Ann Intern Med 2007;146(5): 340–54.

[21] Kang YA, Lee HW, Yoon HI, et al. Discrepancy between the tuberculin skin test and the whole-blood interferon gamma assay for the diagnosis of latent tuberculosis infection in an intermediate tuberculosis-burden country. JAMA 2005;293(22): 2756–61.

[22] Mazurek GH, Jereb J, Lobue P, et al. Guidelines for using the QuantiFERON-TB Gold test for detecting *Mycobacterium* tuberculosis infection, United States. MMWR Recomm Rep 2005;54(RR-15):49–55.

[23] Al Zahrani K, Al Jahdali H, Poirier L, et al. Yield of smear, culture and amplification tests from repeated sputum induction for the diagnosis of pulmonary tuberculosis. Int J Tuberc Lung Dis 2001; 5(9):855–60.

[24] Schoch OD, Rieder P, Tueller C, et al. Diagnostic yield of sputum, induced sputum, and bronchoscopy after radiologic tuberculosis screening. Am J Respir Crit Care Med 2007;175(1):80–6.

[25] Patel YR, Mehta JB, Harvill L, et al. Flexible bronchoscopy as a diagnostic tool in the evaluation of pulmonary tuberculosis in an elderly population. J Am Geriatr Soc 1993;41(6):629–32.

[26] Blumberg HM, Burman WJ, Chaisson RE, et al. American Thoracic Society/Centers for Disease Control and Prevention/Infectious Diseases Society of America: treatment of tuberculosis. Am J Respir Crit Care Med 2003;167(4):603–62.

[27] de Groot CP, van den Broek T, van Staveren W. Energy intake and micronutrient intake in elderly Europeans: seeking the minimum requirement in the SENECA study. Age Ageing 1999;28(5): 469–74.

[28] Maddrey WC. Drug-induced hepatotoxicity: 2005. J Clin Gastroenterol 2005;39(4 Suppl 2):S83–9.

[29] Gronhagen-Riska C, Hellstrom PE, Froseth B. Predisposing factors in hepatitis induced by

isoniazid-rifampin treatment of tuberculosis. Am Rev Respir Dis 1978;118(3):461–6.

[30] Tsai RK, Lee YH. Reversibility of ethambutol optic neuropathy. J Ocul Pharmacol Ther 1997;13(5): 473–7.

[31] Griffith DE, Brown-Elliott BA, Shepherd S, et al. Ethambutol ocular toxicity in treatment regimens for *Mycobacterium avium* complex lung disease. Am J Respir Crit Care Med 2005;172(2):250–3.

[32] Griffith DE, Aksamit T, Brown-Elliott BA, et al. An official ATS/IDSA statement: diagnosis, treatment, and prevention of nontuberculous mycobacterial diseases. Am J Respir Crit Care Med 2007;175(4): 367–416.

[33] Khan K, Wang J, Marras TK. Nontuberculous mycobacterial sensitization in the United States: national trends over three decades. Am J Respir Crit Care Med 2007;176:306–13.

[34] Fordham von Reyn C, Arbeit RD, Tosteson AN, et al. The international epidemiology of disseminated *Mycobacterium avium* complex infection in AIDS. International MAC Study Group. AIDS 1996;10(9):1025–32.

[35] von Reyn CF, Waddell RD, Eaton T, et al. Isolation of *Mycobacterium avium* complex from water in the United States, Finland, Zaire, and Kenya. J Clin Microbiol 1993;31(12):3227–30.

[36] Primm TP, Lucero CA, Falkinham JO 3rd. Health impacts of environmental mycobacteria. Clin Microbiol Rev 2004;17(1):98–106.

[37] Vaerewijck MJ, Huys G, Palomino JC, et al. Mycobacteria in drinking water distribution systems: ecology and significance for human health. FEMS Microbiol Rev 2005;29(5):911–34.

[38] Tortoli E, Cichero P, Piersimoni C, et al. Use of BACTEC MGIT 960 for recovery of mycobacteria from clinical specimens: multicenter study. J Clin Microbiol 1999;37(11):3578–82.

[39] Waller EA, Roy A, Brumble L, et al. The expanding spectrum of *Mycobacterium avium* complex-associated pulmonary disease. Chest 2006;130(4): 1234–41.

[40] Field SK, Fisher D, Cowie RL. *Mycobacterium avium* complex pulmonary disease in patients without HIV infection. Chest 2004;126(2):566–81.

[41] Aksamit TR. Hot tub lung: infection, inflammation, or both? Semin Respir Infect 2003;18(1):33–9.

[42] du Moulin GC, Stottmeier KD, Pelletier PA, et al. Concentration of *Mycobacterium avium* by hospital hot water systems. JAMA 1988;260(11): 1599–601.

[43] Embil J, Warren P, Yakrus M, et al. Pulmonary illness associated with exposure to *Mycobacterium-avium* complex in hot tub water. Hypersensitivity pneumonitis or infection? Chest 1997;111(3): 813–6.

[44] Hanak V, Kalra S, Aksamit TR, et al. Hot tub lung: presenting features and clinical course of 21 patients. Respir Med 2006;100(4):610–5.

[45] Parker BC, Ford MA, Gruft H, et al. Epidemiology of infection by nontuberculous mycobacteria. IV. Preferential aerosolization of *Mycobacterium intracellulare* from natural waters. Am Rev Respir Dis 1983;128(4):652–6.

[46] Reich JM, Johnson RE. *Mycobacterium avium* complex pulmonary disease presenting as an isolated lingular or middle lobe pattern. The Lady Windermere syndrome. Chest 1992;101(6):1605–9.

[47] Chung MJ, Lee KS, Koh WJ, et al. Thin-section CT findings of nontuberculous mycobacterial pulmonary diseases: comparison between *Mycobacterium avium*-intracellulare complex and *Mycobacterium abscessus* infection. J Korean Med Sci 2005;20(5): 777–83.

[48] Jeong YJ, Lee KS, Koh WJ, et al. Nontuberculous mycobacterial pulmonary infection in immunocompetent patients: comparison of thin-section CT and histopathologic findings. Radiology 2004;231(3): 880–6.

[49] Hollings NP, Wells AU, Wilson R, et al. Comparative appearances of non-tuberculous mycobacteria species: a CT study. Eur Radiol 2002;12(9):2211–7.

[50] Erasmus JJ, McAdams HP, Farrell MA, et al. Pulmonary nontuberculous mycobacterial infection: radiologic manifestations. Radiographics 1999; 19(6):1487–505.

[51] Patz EF Jr, Swensen SJ, Erasmus J. Pulmonary manifestations of nontuberculous *Mycobacterium*. Radiol Clin North Am 1995;33(4):719–29.

[52] Field SK, Cowie RL. Treatment of *Mycobacterium avium*-intracellulare complex lung disease with a macrolide, ethambutol, and clofazimine. Chest 2003;124(4):1482–6.

[53] Frothingham R. Clarithromycin treatment for *Mycobacterium avium*-intracellulare complex lung disease. Am J Respir Crit Care Med 1996;153(6 Pt 1): 1990–1.

[54] Griffith DE, Brown BA, Girard WM, et al. Azithromycin-containing regimens for treatment of *Mycobacterium avium* complex lung disease. Clin Infect Dis 2001;32(11):1547–53.

[55] Griffith DE, Brown BA, Murphy DT, et al. Initial (6-month) results of three-times-weekly azithromycin in treatment regimens for *Mycobacterium avium* complex lung disease in human immunodeficiency virus-negative patients. J Infect Dis 1998;178(1): 121–6.

[56] Kobashi Y, Matsushima T. The effect of combined therapy according to the guidelines for the treatment of *Mycobacterium avium* complex pulmonary disease. Intern Med 2003;42(8):670–5.

[57] Shimokata K. Treatment of pulmonary disease caused by *Mycobacterium avium* complex. Intern Med 2003;42(8):627–8.

[58] Kobashi Y, Yoshida K, Miyashita N, et al. Relationship between clinical efficacy of treatment of pulmonary *Mycobacterium avium* complex disease and drug-sensitivity testing of *Mycobacterium avium*

complex isolates. J Infect Chemother 2006;12(4): 195–202.

[59] Lam PK, Griffith DE, Aksamit TR, et al. Factors related to response to intermittent treatment of *Mycobacterium avium* complex lung disease. Am J Respir Crit Care Med 2006;173(11):1283–9.

[60] Griffith DE, Brown BA, Girard WM, et al. Adverse events associated with high-dose rifabutin in macrolide-containing regimens for the treatment of *Mycobacterium avium* complex lung disease. Clin Infect Dis 1995;21(3):594–8.

ELSEVIER
SAUNDERS

Clin Chest Med 28 (2007) 783–791

CLINICS
IN CHEST
MEDICINE

Mechanical Ventilation and Acute Respiratory Distress Syndrome in Older Patients

Jonathan M. Siner, MD[a],*, Margaret A. Pisani, MD, MPH[b]

[a]Section of Pulmonary and Critical Care Medicine, Department of Internal Medicine,
Yale University School of Medicine, P.O. Box 208057, TAC S441C, New Haven, CT 06520-8057, USA
[b]Section of Pulmonary and Critical Care Medicine, Department of Internal Medicine,
Yale University School of Medicine, P.O. Box 208057, TAC S425C, New Haven, CT 06520-8057, USA

As the population of the United States ages, an increasing number of elderly adults will be cared for in intensive care units (ICUs) [1]. An understanding of how aging affects the respiratory system is important for patient care and ongoing research. The incidence rates of acute respiratory failure and of acute respiratory distress syndrome (ARDS) increase dramatically with age, and therefore understanding the relationship between age and ARDS is important [2,3]. From a diagnostic and management standpoint, understanding the ways in which age affects disease and interventions allows better care to be delivered to older adults. In the absence of data, assumptions are often made about the impact of age on mechanical ventilation and diseases causing respiratory failure. These assumptions have often been shown to be incorrect [4]. This article focuses on the age-specific changes in respiratory function. We present a discussion of the management of acute lung injury (ALI) and ARDS with a focus on the role of mechanical ventilation. We conclude with what is known about age and its impact on mortality and functional outcomes after mechanical ventilation.

Age and respiratory function

The respiratory system undergoes many changes with aging that affect susceptibility to

disease and the response to it. Older patients have a multifactorial decrease in ventilatory reserve. Age has a significant impact on chest wall mechanics and the mechanisms of airway protection. Changes in the shape and function of the chest wall, including osteoporosis, kyphosis, and rib–vertebral articulations, lead to decreases in volume and compliance [5]. Total lung capacity remains unchanged as a result of the balancing forces of decreased outward chest wall force and decreased inward elastic recoil (elastance), but because elastance decreases more than chest wall recoil, there is an age-related increase in residual volume with a stable total lung capacity; therefore, there is a resultant steady decline in vital capacity with aging [5]. The decrease in elastance also leads to a decrease in maximal expiratory flow rates measured as a decline in forced expiratory volume in 1 second [6]. The combination of increased residual volume and decreased maximal flow rates means that augmentation of minute ventilation is increasingly achieved by a more rapid respiratory rate rather than increased tidal volume (Vt). It has been observed that although the response of the respiratory system to physical exertion seems to be preserved, the response to hypoxia and hypercapnia is less vigorous in older adults [7]. Aspiration is a frequent cause of pneumonia in older adults. Despite the many changes in the respiratory system, healthy older adults do not seem to have an increased risk of aspiration. They do have to swallow more slowly, and patients who have dementia or pneumonia have been documented to have significantly increased rates of silent aspiration [8,9]. Common diseases

---

* Corresponding author.
E-mail address: jonathan.siner@yale.edu (J.M. Siner).

in the elderly population may compound age-related dysphasia, and respiratory changes are likely the source for the increase risk of aspiration. For example, patients who have a history of stroke are at dramatically increased risk of aspiration pneumonia [10].

Acute respiratory failure in the elderly population

Acute respiratory failure is a common complication of critical illness in older adults due in large part to the increase in prevalence of chronic illnesses, major organ dysfunction, and an increased risk of acquired causes of respiratory failure [11,12]. The incidence rates of pulmonary embolism, chronic obstructive pulmonary disease, congestive heart failure, and community-acquired pneumonia rise with age [12,13]. Furthermore, as many as 47% of patients over the age of 65 who have acute respiratory failure have two diagnoses as the etiology of their respiratory decompensation, in large part due to the high incidence of congestive heart failure and chronic obstructive pulmonary disease in this population. The increased incidence of major organ dysfunction combined with decreased pulmonary reserve is likely responsible for the exponential increase in respiratory failure from the third through the ninth decade of life [2,14].

Etiology and incidence of acute lung injury and acute respiratory distress syndrome

ALI and ARDS are the continuum of a disease resulting in acute hypoxemic respiratory failure associated with bilateral pulmonary infiltrates that are not due to left-sided atrial hypertension [15]. Common causes of ALI include nonpulmonary sepsis, pneumonia, aspiration, trauma, pancreatitis, and transfusion of allogeneic blood products. The injury of ALI involves the alveolar epithelium and the lung capillary endothelium.

The criteria, as defined by the American-European Consensus Conference on ARDS, include a ratio of partial pressure of arterial to fractional inspired oxygen less than 200 (<300 for ALI) and left atrial pressure less than 18 mm Hg. In adult populations, 26% of acute respiratory failure is the result of ALI [3], and 16% to 18% of ventilated ICU patients have ALI [16]. Estimates of the incidence of ALI and ARDS have varied significantly, with earlier estimates from several European studies ranging from 1.5 to 3.5 $\times$ 10^5 per person-years to 16.0 $\times$ 10^5 person-years for ALI/ARDS [17–19]. Overall, the estimates have increased steadily, with a recent larger prospective study from the United States showing an incidence of 78.9 $\times$ 10^5 person-years for ALI and 58.7 $\times$ 10^5 person-years for ARDS [3,20]. It is clear from the two recent prospective trials that the incidence of ALI increases significantly with age from approximately 16 cases per 100,000 person-years in persons who are 15 to 19 years of age to 306 cases per 100,000 person-years in those 74 to 85 years of age [3]. The increased incidence of ALI/ARDS associated with older age is likely in part due to the fact that the incidence of sepsis, which is the primary risk factor in older adults for ALI, increases steadily with age [21]. The one group where ARDS plateaus with age is in trauma patients. A recent study showed that in the trauma population the incidence of ARDS increases with age but plateaus in the 60- to 69-year-old population and thereafter declines [22].

Treatment of acute lung injury and acute respiratory distress syndrome

Conventional mechanical ventilation

ALI and ARDS are inflammatory conditions of the lung that occur in response to injury. Clinically, they are associated with severe hypoxemia and a decrease in lung compliance and functional area usually requiring intubation and mechanical ventilation. Mechanical ventilation is life saving as a supportive measure because it allows the use of positive end expiratory pressure (PEEP) and allows delivery of a high fractional level of inspired oxygen. Extensive animal data have demonstrated that it also can contribute to lung injury in a process termed ventilator-induced lung injury (VILI). VILI involves parenchymal inflammation, atelectasis, and further elaboration of inflammatory cytokines [23,24]. After several smaller studies with conflicting results, the ARDS Network (ARDSnet) investigators published a large randomized trial comparing conventional Vt (12 mL/kg) with low-volume Vt (6 mL/kg). In this trial, the authors demonstrate a reduction in mortality from 40% to 31% with a relative risk reduction of 22% [25]. In addition to being adequately powered for the size of effect being investigated, the ARDSnet trial had two specific features that contributed to its success. First, it had a specific design that eliminated variations in PEEP as part of the protocol. Second, the investigators used ideal body weight to determine the appropriate Vt for each subject [25]. A second trial by the same ARDSnet investigators examined whether the addition of a high PEEP strategy to a low Vt strategy improved outcomes, but this study was terminated prematurely because of lack of efficacy. Mean airway pressures and plateau pressures were elevated in the intervention, and it is thought that this may have negated any beneficial effect from the PEEP [26]. Furthermore, there was an imbalance between the control and intervention group, with the intervention group being significantly older (54.0 ± 17 years versus 49 ± 17 years). An additional study by the ARDSnet group also examined the role of a liberal as compared with restrictive strategy for fluid management and found no difference but also no harm [27]. In all the preceding ARDSnet studies, the mean age was in the early sixth decade.

Both studies from the ARDSnet trial network investigating strategies for ventilator management were performed on populations that were young from a medical critical care standpoint. In all groups studied in the ARDSnet protocol, the mean age was close to 50 years [28]. Given that the incidence of ARDS increases with age, the significance of these large, randomized trials having enrolled a higher fraction of younger adults is unclear. Significant chronic lung disease was an exclusion criteria, and this would include a substantial portion of the older ICU population. Specific exclusion criteria were stringent and included forced expiratory volume in 1 second <20 ml/kg of ideal body weight, radiographic evidence of hyperinflation or interstitial lung disease, and arterial O_2 pressure less than 55 on room air (all those meeting standard criteria for O_2 therapy). One of the strengths of the original ARDSnet study protocol was the use of predicted body weight, which would potentially be advantageous in a population of older adults because use of unadjusted weight leads to increased Vt because lean body mass decreases with aging. The strategy in the ARDS studies was to use a combination of Vt and maximal plateau pressures as surrogates for alveolar volume. The presumption is that the physiologic response to a predetermined pressure is the same across the spectrum of normal population. Because older adults have increased lung compliance but decreased chest wall compliance, the impact of these ventilatory strategies in older patients is hard to determine. Analysis of data from these ARDSnet trials showed that patients over 70 years of age recovered from the acute phase of ARDS in equal proportions to those less than 70 years of age [29]. Despite apparent equivalent physiologic recovery rates, older patients had greater difficulty remaining extubated and being successfully discharged from the intensive care unit and had a lower survival rate as a result. Although these studies were not designed to determine the etiology of this decrease in survival to discharge, the decrease in respiratory reserve, including decreased muscle strength and ability to protect the airway, and increased incidence of delirium may have played a role [29].

Nonconventional mechanical ventilation

The ARDSnet protocol was a significant advancement in the management of patients who haves ARDS; however, whether it is the optimal strategy for all patients is unknown. Conventional mechanical ventilation has been paired with PEEP to augment end-expiratory airway pressures, preventing atelectasis and thereby improving oxygenation. Because animal data show that excess airway pressures and volumes can lead to VILI, alternate modes of ventilation, such as high-frequency oscillatory ventilation (HFOV) and airway pressure release ventilation (APRV), have been developed that use alternate methods of targeting "open lung" but limit VILI. HFOV has been used extensively in the neonatal population. The data from randomized controlled trials in the adult population are limited to two randomized controlled trials containing significant numbers of subjects. HFOV uses rapid pressure oscillations to mix the gas in the airway and allow for enhanced diffusion. In 2002, Derdak and colleagues [30] studied HFOV in ARDS and showed no difference compared with conventional ventilation. The mean age of the patients (48 years of age) was similar to that in the ARDSnet trials; however, the control group did not receive a low Vt strategy because it preceded the initial ARDSnet study. In addition, the study was underpowered for the size of the effect they were investigating [30]. The second randomized controlled trial of HFOV was smaller in size and had significant crossover between groups. No significant differences were observed between the HFOV group and the conventional group [31]. Due to patient discomfort, HFOV often requires increased levels of sedation, which could be more detrimental in an older population of patients who have increased sensitivity to sedative agents and a higher risk for delirium. HFOV is considered for use in those who have failed conventional ventilation, and given the limited data it is hard to make a recommendation for its use in an older population [32].

APRV has been used as an alternative to the ARDSnet protocol in patients who have ARDS. It functions by using continuous positive airway pressures and then using a release phase to augment ventilation. In addition, the patient is able to initiate spontaneous breaths [32]. Potential benefits of APRV are thought to accrue through several physiologic mechanisms. First, the continuous positive airway pressure portion with a prolonged hold is thought to maximize recruitment of injured lung. Second, spontaneous breathing can be effective at preventing collapse and consolidation at the dorsal and dependent regions of the lung. One of the earlier randomized controlled trials with APRV showed improved oxygenation and lung compliance with decreased sedation in a young population of trauma patients (mean age of 40 years) [33], and other studies have demonstrated improved hemodynamics as a result of spontaneous breathing and decreased vasopressor and sedative use [34]. Despite the promising animal and physiologic studies, subsequent studies have not clearly confirmed these benefits in larger populations [35]. Despite many potential benefits, APRV has yet to be shown to be superior to conventional mechanical ventilation in a randomized controlled trial. In summary, APRV has many potential benefits regarding lung and cardiopulmonary physiology and has the promise of decreased sedation. The studies performed thus far have been on a heterogeneous population and shed little light on actual benefits or risks for the older adult population. Based on our understanding of the prevalence of comorbid conditions and the relationship of delirium and dementia to poor outcomes, APRV might warrant additional investigation in older patients. The potential for spontaneous ventilation and therefore decreased sedation would be of great potential benefit in an older population.

Corticosteroids

Despite the severity of hypoxemia associated with ALI, during the acute phase the majority of patients do not succumb from refractory respiratory failure but rather from sepsis or nonpulmonary organ dysfunction [36,37]. This likely explains why interventions that improve oxygenation without addressing the underlying inflammatory disorder have not been successful [38]. The impact of low Vt ventilation on reducing in levels of circulating proinflammatory cytokines may be

the mechanism of improved outcomes seen with the ARDSnet protocol [25]. In part, the morbidity and mortality of ALI can be attributed to the complications that arise in patients who improve but do not resolve the insult enough to have mechanical ventilation discontinued or leave the ICU or hospital. Severe respiratory failure can be supported with mechanical ventilation, but unless it resolves, the prognosis for the patient is poor.

Many antiinflammatory strategies have been evaluated in ARDS, including the use of corticosteroids. One of the initial studies of corticosteroids examined patients who had nonresolving ARDS, which was defined as lack of improvement in the Lung Injury Score after 7 days. Although this study showed benefit, it was small and was criticized for a crossover study design [39]. A larger study performed by the ARDSnet investigators with a similar protocol found improvement in early cardiopulmonary performance. The significant incidence of neuromuscular weakness leading to reinitiation of mechanical ventilation, often in the setting of sepsis, negated the early observed improvement [40]. As with the previously cited studies, the mean age in these investigations of corticosteroids was in the early sixth decade, which is substantially below what is considered an older adult population. Older adults seem to tolerate the acute phase of ARDS well but have difficulty with recovery of multiorgan failure and other complications that arise from their acute illness that affect hospital discharge [29]. Given the difficulty of liberating older patients who have ARDS from the mechanical ventilator in a timely and permanent fashion, the significant increase in reintubation with corticosteroids is a major concern in this population. Given that the mean age of the patients enrolled in most of the ARDS studies has been fairly low, the benefit of corticosteroids for ARDS warrants specific investigation in older adults.

Weaning from mechanical ventilation

Surviving ALI and its associated complications leaves the patient a candidate for discontinuation from mechanical ventilation. The initial factor considered when determining whether a patient is a candidate for weaning and extubation is whether the initial process requiring mechanical ventilation has resolved. Once this determination has been made, then a host of factors are considered regarding respiratory function and the likelihood of maintaining a patent airway if the endotracheal tube is removed. There should be evidence that the primary cause of respiratory failure is improving or has resolved, be it ARDS, pneumonia, or sepsis. Airway factors, such as quantity and quality of secretions, ability to handle secretions, strength of cough, and the ability to protect the airway, are assessed. Additional factors, such as the patient's volume status and mental status, need to be assessed. Most ICUs use standardized protocols for assessing these factors and then proceed with spontaneous breathing trials (SBTs) once the acute process has resolved and mental status is appropriate. Most ICU protocols suggest a spontaneous breathing trial with monitoring of basic vital signs and respiratory status parameters, including arterial blood gas and weaning parameters and commonly the respiratory frequency to Vt ratio (f/Vt). Despite extensive research examining predictors to suggest readiness to remove mechanical ventilation, determining whether a SBT is successful remains as much an art as a science. A recent study has suggested that following the f/Vt rather than routinely available vital signs may inhibit successful weaning [41].

There are several physiologic changes associated with aging that may affect the decisions a physician makes regarding extubation. First, older adults at baseline tend to have a more rapid and shallow breathing pattern then younger adults [5,42]. Given that physicians generally regard the rapid shallow breathing pattern as evidence of compromised respiratory function, there is a concern that older adult patients were being judged as having failed an SBT when they had not. A complicating factor is that older adults have a diminished response to hypoxia and hypercapnia, and therefore a patient on an SBT might seem to be comfortable despite having developed significant hypercapnia or hypoxia [7]. These observations suggest that routine use of arterial blood gases might have greater utility in the older adult population to confirm failure in the setting of rapid shallow breathing and to insure effective respiration in a patient who seems to be comfortable on a SBT. Data regarding weaning in the older population after ARDS are sparse, but much can be gleaned from the general literature regarding recovering from respiratory failure. Two of the initial studies that promoted the use of routine daily SBTs examined populations where the mean age was at the low end of the seventh decade [43,44]. The trial performed by Esteban and colleagues [43] to examine SBT as compared with other ventilatory modes for weaning is notable because

a high percentage of the patients had ALI. In a medical ICU population, El Solh [45] observed that patients over the age of 70, as compared with a younger matched cohort, were much more likely to fail extubation because of the inability to handle secretions (20%) and that those who did had a high risk of developing nosocomial pneumonia. This study highlights the risk that nosocomial pneumonia is associated with the use of corticosteroids in ARDS and subsequent neuromuscular weakness. The most direct data regarding the older persons and extubation comes from the study by Ely and colleagues [29] investigating outcomes of the older patients in the large multicentered trial on ARDS. They reported that although older persons achieved physiologic recovery from ALI in equal proportions to younger patients, their ICU length of stay and duration of mechanical ventilation was increased because of a higher reintubation rate.

Outcomes: mortality, functional capacity, and quality of life after acute respiratory distress syndrome

Increasing age is a risk factor for mortality in patients who have ALI. Although older adult patients may resolve the lung injury as well as younger patients, their overall mortality is increased in multiple studies [29,46]. Comorbid conditions, age, and sepsis contribute to the mortality of ARDS [47]. Chelluri and colleagues looked at 2-month outcomes in 817 patients with a median age of 65 years who required at least 48 hours of mechanical ventilation and found that 2-month mortality was 43% [48]. Independent predictors of 2-month mortality were age, number of comorbidities, and prehospital functional status. For every additional comorbidity, the odds of dying at 2 months increased by 24% [48].

Although new therapies and improved supportive care may continue to reduce the mortality in ARDS, survivors will be discharged from the ICU and hospital, and the results of residual organ dysfunction may have a significant impact on health-related quality of life and functional status, especially in older patients. A large body of outcomes research over the past decade has clearly delineated the mental and physical sequelae of ARDS and associated critical illness. The mortality of ARDS is not predominantly associated with refractory respiratory failure but from sepsis and nonpulmonary organ failure and other complications of critical illness [36,37].

Major complications include neuromuscular complications, neurocognitive dysfunction, and psychiatric sequelae [49–52]. Other complications include respiratory limitations, heterotopic calcification, tracheostomy, and other airway complications. Pulmonary dysfunction has been the best studied complication of ARDS, with a wide range of studies documenting several abnormalities, including restrictive and obstructive lung dysfunction and most commonly a decreased diffusing capacity. One of the major difficulties of understanding the relative decrement in function across all the spectrum of disabilities is the fact that premorbid data are rarely available.

Muscle weakness and myopathy are some of the most significant disabilities affecting survivors. Given the impact of frailty on older patients' ability to remain independent, weakness and myopathy play an important role in long-term outcomes in this population. Critical illness, polyneuropathy, and myopathy are common, although the exact incidence is hard to define. The incidence in patients who have received corticosteroids or neuromuscular blockade is even higher. Herridge and colleagues [53] studied the 1-year outcomes of patients who had ARDS and noted that survivors on average had lost 18% of their baseline body weight, of which a substantial portion was loss of muscle mass. The survivors were also observed to have decrements in spirometry and diffusion capacity, although the most prominent abnormality was the decrease in functional capacity as demonstrated by their abnormal 6-minute walk tests. The abnormalities improved during the 12-month follow-up period, but longer duration studies have shown continued disability at 2 years [54]. It is unlikely that the decrease in functional capacity is related to abnormal pulmonary function but likely includes a significant component of muscle weakness and generalized deconditioning. Increased organ dysfunction was associated with worse outcomes, and the mortality during the 1-year follow-up period was significant at 11%.

Neuropsychologic disability is one of the major after-affects of receiving care in the ICU. One of the earliest prospective studies of this phenomenon documented specific cognitive deficits at discharge in all survivors of ARDS [55]. Additional assessment 1 year after discharge showed that 30% of survivors continued to have impaired intellectual functioning, and 78% of the survivors had impairment of memory and concentration [50]. Hopkins and colleagues [50] correlated these deficits with increased severity of hypoxemia as recorded during the ICU, suggesting that CNS hypoxia was a potential mechanism. As with some of the randomized controlled trials in ARDS, the mean age in this study was 45, and the subjects seemed to have severe disease as implied by the high prevalence of pneumothoraces. The normative data used for comparison was not from an ICU population or from medically ill patients; therefore, the specificity of these findings is unclear. Hopkins examined neurocognitive and psychologic outcomes at 2 years after an episode of ARDS in 66 survivors who had a mean age of 46 years (range 18–81 years). Seventy percent of patients had neurocognitive sequelae at hospital discharge. These patients demonstrated significant improvement at 1 year post-ICU discharge with a reduction in neurocognitive impairment to 43% at 1 year. Although the numbers in this study were small and the mean age was young, we know from other research that older patients may have preexisting cognitive impairment before ICU admission—up to 30% in one study of older patients—and that age and dementia are important risk factor for delirium [56,57]. Further research needs to be done examining the impact of delirium on neurocognitive outcomes after an ICU admission.

Psychiatric abnormalities are common in ARDS survivors and have a significant impact on quality of life (QOL). The incidence of depression is significant in survivors of ARDS, with initial studies suggesting that 16% of survivors had moderate to severe depression at 1 year and up to 23% at 2-year follow-up [58]. Post-traumatic stress disorder (PTSD) also has a significant impact on QOL and has a prolonged impact [59]. Another study reported that additional risk factors for PTSD after ARDS may include female sex and possibly increased use of lorazepam [60]. In this study, age greater than 50 seemed to be protective. The protective effect of age is likely real given that similar observations have been made in studies of PTSD in nonmedical populations. The incidence of PTSD in older patients after an episode of ARDS and critical illness needs to be investigated further.

Health care provider and surrogate decision makers

The vast majority of patients receiving care in an ICU have decisions regarding their medical treatment made by a proxy or surrogate decision maker in conjunction with the health professionals caring for them. Therefore, in the intensive care setting, understanding the attitudes and knowledge of proxy decision makers and physicians is essential to understanding how care decisions are made for older ICU patients. When using substituted judgment, one needs to carefully consider the patient's goals and wishes and what is medically appropriate. It is well documented that older adults receive reduced intensity of care in the ICU [55]. In the SUPPORT cohort, it was demonstrated that mechanical ventilation was withheld at a higher rate in patients who were 70 years of age or older [4]. When Scales and colleagues [61] examined the relationship between premorbid health-related QOL as estimated by surrogate decision makers and as described by the patients who had ARDS, there were significant differences. Specifically, patients routinely assessed their QOL as higher than that of their surrogate decision makers. As noted in many studies, it is often the comorbidities associated with age that confer the increased risk of poor outcomes.

Summary

ALI is a common disease among critically ill patients, and the incidence and mortality rise with age. Despite the prevalence of disease in the older adult population, most studies of this disease have focused on a younger population as a result of their design. Based on the available data, there is reason to believe that age and comorbid conditions affect all aspects of outcomes in critically ill patients who have ARDS. Furthermore, patients' own preferences may be different than the substituted judgments commonly used in the ICU. Taken together, these studies emphasize the importance of being cautious when making inferences regarding the relationship between age, utility of treatment, and outcomes in older patients. Given the preponderance of ALI in the general ICU population, all major studies should be designed to include older patients so that we may improve our understanding of the impact of age, comorbidities, and treatment on outcomes. Further research should continue to include patient-centered outcomes for older survivors of ALI and ARDs, including functional and cognitive status, PTSD, and QOL.

References

[1] Angus DC, Kelley MA, Schmitz RJ, et al. Caring for the critically ill patient. Current and projected workforce requirements for care of the critically ill and patients with pulmonary disease: can we meet the requirements of an aging population? JAMA 2000;284(21):2762–70.

[2] Behrendt CE. Acute respiratory failure in the United States: incidence and 31-day survival. Chest 2000; 118(4):1100–5.

[3] Rubenfeld GD, Caldwell E, Peabody E, et al. Incidence and outcomes of acute lung injury. N Engl J Med 2005;353(16):1685–93.

[4] Hamel MB, Teno JM, Goldman L, et al. Patient age and decisions to withhold life-sustaining treatments from seriously ill, hospitalized adults. Support investigators. Study to understand prognoses and preferences for outcomes and risks of treatment. Ann Intern Med 1999;130(2):116–25.

[5] Sprung J, Gajic O, Warner DO. Review article: age related alterations in respiratory function: anesthetic considerations [Article de synthese: les modifications de fonction respiratoire liees a l'age - considerations anesthesiques]. Can J Anaesth 2006;53(12):1244–57 [in French].

[6] Knudson RJ, Slatin RC, Lebowitz MD, et al. The maximal expiratory flow-volume curve: normal standards, variability, and effects of age. Am Rev Respir Dis 1976;113(5):587–600.

[7] Peterson DD, Pack AI, Silage DA, et al. Effects of aging on ventilatory and occlusion pressure responses to hypoxia and hypercapnia. Am Rev Respir Dis 1981;124(4):387–91.

[8] Sekizawa K, Ujiie Y, Itabashi S, et al. Lack of cough reflex in aspiration pneumonia. Lancet 1990; 335(8699):1228–9.

[9] Kikuchi R, Watabe N, Konno T, et al. High incidence of silent aspiration in elderly patients with community-acquired pneumonia. Am J Respir Crit Care Med 1994;150(1):251–3.

[10] Nakagawa T, Sekizawa K, Nakajoh K, et al. Silent cerebral infarction: a potential risk for pneumonia in the elderly. J Intern Med 2000;247(2):255–9.

[11] Ray P, Birolleau S, Lefort Y, et al. Acute respiratory failure in the elderly: etiology, emergency diagnosis and prognosis. Crit Care 2006;10(3):1–12.

[12] Marrie TJ. Community-acquired pneumonia in the elderly. Clin Infect Dis 2000;31(4):1066–78.

[13] Rich MW. Heart failure in the 21st century: a cardiogeriatric syndrome. J Gerontol A Biol Sci Med Sci 2001;56(2):M88–96.

[14] El Solh AA, Ramadan FH. Overview of respiratory failure in older adults. J Intensive Care Med 2006; 21(6):345–51.

[15] Bernard GR, Artigas A, Brigham KL, et al. The American-European Consensus Conference on ARDS. Definitions, mechanisms, relevant outcomes, and clinical trial coordination. Am J Respir Crit Care Med 1994;149(3 Pt 1):818–24.

[16] Roupie E, Lepage E, Wysocki M, et al. Prevalence, etiologies and outcome of the acute respiratory

distress syndrome among hypoxemic ventilated patients. SRLF collaborative group on mechanical
ventilation. Societe de Reanimation de Langue
Francaise. Intensive Care Med 1999;25(9):920–9.

[17] Hughes M, MacKirdy FN, Ross J, et al. Acute respiratory distress syndrome: an audit of incidence and
outcome in Scottish intensive care units. Anaesthesia
2003;58(9):838–45.

[18] Villar J, Slutsky AS. The incidence of the adult respiratory distress syndrome. Am Rev Respir Dis 1989;
140(3):814–6.

[19] Avecillas JF, Freire AX, Arroliga AC. Clinical epidemiology of acute lung injury and acute respiratory
distress syndrome: incidence, diagnosis, and outcomes [abstract vii]. Clin Chest Med 2006;27(4):
549–57.

[20] Manzano F, Yuste E, Colmenero M, et al. Incidence of acute respiratory distress syndrome and
its relation to age. J Crit Care 2005;20(3):
274–80.

[21] Angus DC, Linde-Zwirble WT, Lidicker J, et al.
Epidemiology of severe sepsis in the United States:
analysis of incidence, outcome, and associated costs
of care. Crit Care Med 2001;29(7):1303–10.

[22] Johnston CJ, Rubenfeld GD, Hudson LD. Effect
of age on the development of ARDS in trauma
patients. Chest 2003;124(2):653–9.

[23] Slutsky AS. Ventilator-induced lung injury: from
barotrauma to biotrauma. Respir Care 2005;50(5):
646–59.

[24] Ramnath VR, Hess DR, Thompson BT. Conventional mechanical ventilation in acute lung injury
and acute respiratory distress syndrome [abstract
viii]. Clin Chest Med 2006;27(4):601–13.

[25] Ventilation with lower tidal volumes as compared
with traditional tidal volumes for acute lung injury
and the acute respiratory distress syndrome. The
Acute Respiratory Distress Syndrome Network.
N Engl J Med 2000;342(18):1301–8.

[26] Brower RG, Lanken PN, MacIntyre N, et al. Higher
versus lower positive end-expiratory pressures in patients with the acute respiratory distress syndrome.
N Engl J Med 2004;351(4):327–36.

[27] Wiedemann HP, Wheeler AP, Bernard GR, et al.
Comparison of two fluid-management strategies in
acute lung injury. N Engl J Med 2006;354(24):
2564–75.

[28] Bernard GR, Vincent JL, Laterre PF, et al. Efficacy
and safety of recombinant human activated protein
C for severe sepsis. N Engl J Med 2001;344(10):
699–709.

[29] Ely EW, Wheeler AP, Thompson BT, et al. Recovery rate and prognosis in older persons who develop acute lung injury and the acute respiratory
distress syndrome. Ann Intern Med 2002;136(1):
25–36.

[30] Derdak S, Mehta S, Stewart TE, et al. High-frequency oscillatory ventilation for acute respiratory
distress syndrome in adults: a randomized,

controlled trial. Am J Respir Crit Care Med 2002;
166(6):801–8.

[31] Bollen CW, van Well GT, Sherry T, et al. High frequency oscillatory ventilation compared with conventional mechanical ventilation in adult
respiratory distress syndrome: a randomized controlled trial [ISRCTN24242669]. Crit Care 2005;
9(4):R430–9.

[32] Fan E, Stewart TE. New modalities of mechanical
ventilation: high-frequency oscillatory ventilation
and airway pressure release ventilation [abstract
viii-ix]. Clin Chest Med 2006;27(4):615–25.

[33] Putensen C, Zech S, Wrigge H, et al. Long-term
effects of spontaneous breathing during ventilatory
support in patients with acute lung injury. Am
J Respir Crit Care Med 2001;164(1):43–9.

[34] Kaplan LJ, Bailey H, Formosa V. Airway pressure
release ventilation increases cardiac performance in
patients with acute lung injury/adult respiratory distress syndrome. Crit Care 2001;5(4):221–6.

[35] Varpula T, Valta P, Niemi R, et al. Airway pressure
release ventilation as a primary ventilatory mode in
acute respiratory distress syndrome. Acta Anaesthe-
siol Scand 2004;48(6):722–31.

[36] Montgomery AB, Stager MA, Carrico CJ, et al.
Causes of mortality in patients with the adult respiratory distress syndrome. Am Rev Respir Dis 1985;
132(3):485–9.

[37] Stapleton RD, Wang BM, Hudson LD, et al. Causes
and timing of death in patients with ARDS. Chest
2005;128(2):525–32.

[38] Troncy E, Collet JP, Shapiro S, et al. Inhaled nitric
oxide in acute respiratory distress syndrome: a pilot
randomized controlled study. Am J Respir Crit Care
Med 1998;157(5 Pt 1):1483–8.

[39] Meduri GU, Headley AS, Golden E, et al. Effect
of prolonged methylprednisolone therapy in unre-
solving acute respiratory distress syndrome: a randomized controlled trial. JAMA 1998;280(2):
159–65.

[40] Steinberg KP, Hudson LD, Goodman RB, et al. Efficacy and safety of corticosteroids for persistent
acute respiratory distress syndrome. N Engl J Med
2006;354(16):1671–84.

[41] Tanios MA, Nevins ML, Hendra KP, et al. A randomized, controlled trial of the role of weaning predictors in clinical decision making. Crit Care Med
2006;34(10):2530–5.

[42] Zaugg M, Lucchinetti E. Respiratory function in the
elderly. Anesthesiol Clin North America 2000;18(1):
47–58, vi.

[43] Esteban A, Frutos F, Tobin MJ, et al. A comparison
of four methods of weaning patients from mechanical ventilation. Spanish lung failure collaborative
group. N Engl J Med 1995;332(6):345–50.

[44] Ely EW, Baker AM, Dunagan DP, et al. Effect on
the duration of mechanical ventilation of identifying
patients capable of breathing spontaneously. N Engl
J Med 1996;335(25):1864–9.

[45] El Solh AA, Bhat A, Gunen H, et al. Extubation failure in the elderly. Respir Med 2004;98(7): 661–8.

[46] Brun-Buisson C, Minelli C, Bertolini G, et al. Epidemiology and outcome of acute lung injury in European intensive care units: results from the ALIVE study. Intensive Care Med 2004;30(1): 51–61.

[47] Zilberberg MD, Epstein SK. Acute lung injury in the medical ICU: comorbid conditions, age, etiology, and hospital outcome. Am J Respir Crit Care Med 1998;157(4 Pt 1):1159–64.

[48] Quality of Life After Mechanical Ventilation in the Aged Study Investigators. 2-month mortality and functional status of critically ill adult patients receiving prolonged mechanical ventilation. Chest 2002; 121(2):549–58.

[49] Rubenfeld GD, Herridge MS. Epidemiology and outcomes of acute lung injury. Chest 2007;131(2): 554–62.

[50] Hopkins RO, Weaver LK, Pope D, et al. Neuropsychological sequelae and impaired health status in survivors of severe acute respiratory distress syndrome. Am J Respir Crit Care Med 1999;160(1): 50–6.

[51] Jackson JC, Hart RP, Gordon SM, et al. Post-traumatic stress disorder and post-traumatic stress symptoms following critical illness in medical intensive care unit patients: assessing the magnitude of the problem. Crit Care 2007;11(1):1–11.

[52] Jackson JC, Hart RP, Gordon SM, et al. Six-month neuropsychological outcome of medical intensive care unit patients. Crit Care Med 2003;31(4): 1226–34.

[53] Herridge MS, Cheung AM, Tansey CM, et al. One-year outcomes in survivors of the acute respiratory distress syndrome. N Engl J Med 2003;348(8): 683–93.

[54] Cheung AM, Tansey CM, Tomlinson G, et al. Two-year outcomes, health care use, and costs of survivors of acute respiratory distress syndrome. Am J Respir Crit Care Med 2006;174(5):538–44.

[55] Boumendil A, Aegerter P, Guidet B. Treatment intensity and outcome of patients aged 80 and older in intensive care units: a multicenter matched-cohort study. J Am Geriatr Soc 2005;53(1):88–93.

[56] Ely EW, Siegel MD, Inouye SK. Delirium in the intensive care unit: an under-recognized syndrome of organ dysfunction. Semin Respir Crit Care Med 2001;22(2):115–26.

[57] Pisani MA, Inouye SK, McNicoll L, et al. Screening for preexisting cognitive impairment in older intensive care unit patients: use of proxy assessment. J Am Geriatr Soc 2003;51(5):689–93.

[58] Hopkins RO, Weaver LK, Collingridge D, et al. Two-year cognitive, emotional, and quality-of-life outcomes in acute respiratory distress syndrome. Am J Respir Crit Care Med 2005;171(4):340–7.

[59] Kapfhammer HP, Rothenhausler HB, Krauseneck T, et al. Posttraumatic stress disorder and health-related quality of life in long-term survivors of acute respiratory distress syndrome. Am J Psychiatry 2004;161(1):45–52.

[60] Girard TD, Shintani AK, Jackson JC, et al. Risk factors for post-traumatic stress disorder symptoms following critical illness requiring mechanical ventilation: a prospective cohort study. Crit Care 2007;11(1):R28.

[61] Scales DC, Tansey CM, Matte A, et al. Difference in reported pre-morbid health-related quality of life between ARDS survivors and their substitute decision makers. Intensive Care Med 2006;32(11):1826–31.

ELSEVIER
SAUNDERS

Clin Chest Med 28 (2007) 793–800

CLINICS
IN CHEST
MEDICINE

Noninvasive Ventilation in the Older Patient Who Has Acute Respiratory Failure

Layola Lunghar, MD,
Carolyn M. D'Ambrosio, MD, MS[a,b,*]

[a]Pulmonary, Critical Care and Sleep Medicine Division, Tufts University School of Medicine,
750 Washington Street Box 369, Boston, MA 02111, USA
[b]The Center for Sleep Medicine, Tufts University School of Medicine, Tufts-New England Medical Center,
750 Washington Street #257, Boston, MA 02111, USA

Noninvasive positive pressure ventilation in the older population

Noninvasive mechanical ventilation (NIV) is the delivery of ventilatory support without the establishment of an invasive artificial airway. NIV was first used during the polio outbreak in the 1950s with the iron lung. Other forms of NIV have been tried since that time, such as pneumobelts and rocking beds [1]. NIV was not used much after the polio outbreak because of concerns about airway protection in patients with other causes of respiratory failure. When the nasal interface was introduced, however, it became much more popular [1]. NIV allows for the creation of a transpulmonary pressure gradient either by creating a subatmospheric, intrapulmonary pressure during inspiration in relation to an atmospheric oral pressure (also known as noninvasive negative pressure ventilation, such as the iron lung) or introducing positive pressure (noninvasive positive pressure ventilation [NPPV]) delivered by a nasal, oral, or oronasal device. NPPV is unique in its ability to create this transpulmonary pressure gradient either by using a volume-cycled or pressure-cycled ventilator. Because of its effectiveness and ease of use, NPPV has become the predominant form of NIV worldwide.

* Corresponding author. Pulmonary, Critical Care and Sleep Medicine Division, Tufts University School of Medicine, 750 Washington Street, Box 369, Boston, MA 02111.

E-mail address: cdambrosio@tufts-nemc.org (C.M. D'Ambrosio).

NPPV can be used either as a primary ventilation mode for respiratory failure in the acute or chronic setting or as a weaning device for patients who have difficulty being liberated from conventional mechanical ventilation. As life expectancy increases and the comorbidities associated with aging manifest, the need for acute mechanical ventilation and admissions to intensive care unit (ICU) will increase. Nearly two thirds of all ICU days are accounted for by patients over 65 years of age [2]. This article reviews the use of NPPV in acute respiratory failure and addresses specifically the use of NPPV in critically ill geriatric patients.

By virtue of its noninvasive interface, NIV leaves the upper airway intact and preserves airway defense mechanisms. The noninvasive interface also allows patients to speak, eat (in some settings), and clear secretions independently. NPPV has been associated with reduced infections, such as hospital-acquired pneumonia and sinusitis, when compared with traditional mechanical ventilation delivered via an endotracheal tube [3,4]. For similar reasons, NPPV was shown in some studies to be beneficial to immunocompromised patients with hypoxic respiratory failure by reducing the need for intubation and was associated with an overall reduced mortality [5].

Importantly, NPPV also reduces the amount of sedation needed when compared with invasive mechanical ventilation. Older patients have increased fatty tissue and decreased total body water, which affects drug metabolism. Higher doses of sedatives potentially lead to longer stays in the ICU, time on mechanical ventilation, and

0272-5231/07/$ - see front matter © 2007 Elsevier Inc. All rights reserved.
doi:10.1016/j.ccm.2007.08.001

chestmed.theclinics.com

incidence of delirium. The use of benzodiazepines and anticholinergic medications in older patients is associated with a higher risk of severe pulmonary aspiration [6]. Narcotics used in conjunction with benzodiazepines for sedation in mechanically ventilated patients are respiratory suppressants and may not be needed if a patient is treated with NPPV.

Noninvasive positive pressure ventilation: mechanism of action for acute respiratory failure

NPPV and invasive positive pressure ventilation both apply a supra-atmospheric pressure intermittently to the airways to inflate the lungs. This action increases transpulmonary pressure and augments tidal volume: unloading the muscles of inspiration reduces work of breathing [1]. During an acute exacerbation of chronic obstructive pulmonary disease (COPD), significant auto–positive end expiratory pressure (auto-PEEP) can develop. NPPV counteracts the effects of auto–positive end expiratory pressure, which reduces the work of breathing and lowers diaphragmatic pressure swings [7]. This action leads to rapid stabilization of the respiratory rate, reduction in sternocleidomastoid muscle activity, reduction in the symptom of dyspnea, and improved CO_2 levels. The application of positive pressure to the airways also increases functional residual capacity. This increase is related to opening collapsed alveoli and improving ventilation/perfusion ratios in specific types of acute respiratory failure (eg, acute cardiogenic pulmonary edema) [8]. Continuous positive airway pressure (CPAP) has been shown to reduce afterload in patients with acute cardiogenic pulmonary edema simply by increasing intrathoracic pressure [9]. This reduction can lead to improved left ventricular function in patients with dilated, hypocontractile left ventricles and improve overall status [10].

Noninvasive positive pressure ventilation use in critically ill older patients

Older adults have a higher risk of acute respiratory failure. In 2000, Behrendt [11] examined the incidence of acute respiratory failure in more than 300,000 patients. Her results showed an almost exponential increase in the incidence of acute respiratory failure each decade until age 85 years. Patients over the age of 65 had a particularly high incidence (493.5 cases per 100,000)

(Fig. 1). The causes of respiratory failure in older adults are similar to those in younger adults: COPD, congestive heart failure (CHF), pneumonia, and adult respiratory distress syndrome [12,13]. Older patients, however, are at increased risk for respiratory failure caused by nonpulmonary reasons, such as delirium, dementia, stroke, malnutrition, and other comorbidities [12].

NPPV has many benefits for patients who have acute respiratory failure. Studies have demonstrated reduced complications related to intubation, reduced hospital stays, decreased hospital readmission rates, and overall reductions in morbidity and mortality [3,4,14–16]. NPPV is successful when applied in carefully selected patients. The patient profile and cause of the respiratory failure are important predictors of success for NPPV (Boxes 1 and 2) [17,18]. As these overviews demonstrate, several features more prominent in older patients (eg, dementia, confusion, lack of dentition) may make NPPV more difficult to use. It is important to remember that significant improvement in the first 2 hours is important. If that improvement is not present, NPPV should be abandoned and endotracheal intubation should be strongly considered [1]. Although many studies include older patients, few address this issue specifically. This article focuses on data extrapolated from studies on NPPV in critically ill patients that included older patients and addresses specific concerns for these patients regarding NPPV use.

Respiratory mechanics and control of ventilation

Respiratory mechanics change with aging and lead to an overall decline in respiratory function [19]. Elastic tissue decreases and collagen increases in lung parenchyma with normal aging, which inevitably lead to early collapse of small distal airways and fewer gas exchange surfaces. Consequently, lung compliance increases, as does the size of the trachea and large bronchi [20]. In contrast, the chest wall stiffens with age. Calcification of cartilage, kyphosis, and osteoarthritis of the vertebrae all contribute to reduced compliance of the thoracic cage [20]. These changes often lead to the "barrel chest" with an increase in the anteroposterior diameter of the chest and subsequently flatten the diaphragm to some degree. A flatter diaphragm then requires more muscle power and energy to generate the same negative inspiratory pressure [21]. Normal aging leads to

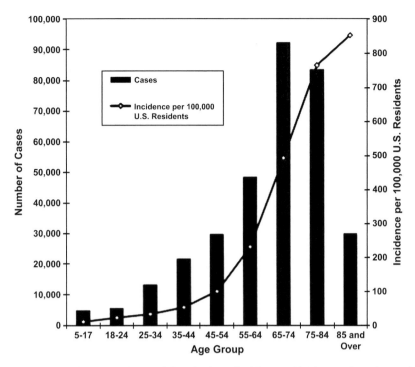

Fig. 1. Cases and incidence of acute respiratory failure in the United States, 1994, by age. Bars denote the numbers of acute respiratory failure cases; diamonds indicate incidence per 100,000 US residents. Age-specific incidence estimates are—from left to right—9.7, 21.6, 32.3, 52.3, 99.9, 231.3, 493.5, 765.5, and 852.9 cases per 100,000. (*From* Behrendt CE. Acute respiratory failure in the United States. Chest 2000;118:1100–05; with permission).

a 10% to 20% reduction in diaphragmatic strength and up to a 50% reduction in maximum pressures during full inhalation and expiration [21]. Although these changes in overall lung function do not seem to cause any significant problems in otherwise healthy older adults, they may become important when older patients develop acute respiratory failure.

The aging process also affects the control of breathing. Specifically, hypercarbic hypoxemia results in a reduced ventilatory response in older adults compared with younger adults [22]. This reduction seems to be mostly secondary to decreases in peripheral carbon dioxide sensitivity rather than oxygen sensitivity. During sleep, however, the response to hypoxia in REM sleep is much more impaired than in young adults [22]. These changes may be important in an older patient's ability to respond to increased respiratory load and gas exchange abnormalities during acute respiratory failure. NPPV may be an important part of the management of acute respiratory failure in older patients, especially if applied promptly.

Obstructive lung diseases

NPPV is most often used in patients with COPD exacerbations and has been well studied in older patients [1,12]. In particular, patients who have COPD have been shown to achieve maximal benefit from NPPV. Several studies have shown that patients who have acute COPD exacerbations and receive NPPV have lower rates of endotracheal intubation, shorter number of ventilator days, and shorter stays in the ICU [23–25]. Overall, reports are that NPPV leads to reduced mortality by 10% to 20% [15]. The prevalence of COPD increases with age, and acute exacerbations of chronic obstructive lung disease account for most patients with respiratory failure requiring mechanical ventilation [12]. Kramer and colleagues [26] found a dramatic decrease in the incidence of endotracheal intubation from 67% in control patients to 9% in the NPPV-treated COPD group. One of the reasons cited by the authors for the great success was early intervention. Four of the studies that have included patients aged 65 or older are shown in Table 1. Brochard

Box 1. Predictors of success during acute applications of noninvasive positive pressure ventilation

Younger age
Lower acuity of illness
Able to cooperate; better neurologic function
Able to coordinate breathing with ventilator
Less air leaking, intact dentition
Hypercarbia, but not too severe (Paco$_2$ > 45 mm Hg, < 92 mm Hg)
Acidemia, but not too severe (pH < 7.35, > 7.10)
Improvements in gas exchange and heart and respiratory rates within first 2 hours

From Mehta S, Hill NS. Noninvasive ventilation: state of the art. Am J Respir Crit Care Med 2001;163:540–77; with permission. Copyright © 2001, American Thoracic Society.

Box 2. Selection guidelines: noninvasive ventilation for patients with chronic obstructive pulmonary disease and acute respiratory failure

Step 1: Identify patients in need of ventilatory assistance
 A. Symptoms and signs of acute respiratory distress
  a. Moderate to severe dyspnea, increased over usual and
  b. Respiratory rate > 24, accessory muscle use, paradoxical breathing
 B. Gas exchange abnormalities
  a. Paco$_2$ > 45 mm Hg, pH < 7.35 or
  b. Pao$_2$/Fio$_2$ < 200
Step 2: Exclude persons at increased risk with noninvasive ventilation
 A. Respiratory arrest
 B. Medically unstable (hypotensive shock, uncontrolled cardiac ischemia or arrhythmias)
 C. Unable to protect airway (impaired cough or swallowing mechanism)
 D. Excessive secretions
 E. Agitated or uncooperative
 F. Facial trauma, burns, or surgery, or anatomic abnormalities interfering with mask fit

From Mehta S, Hill NS. Noninvasive ventilation: state of the art. Am J Respir Crit Care Med 2001;163:540–77; with permission. Copyright © 2001, American Thoracic Society.

and colleagues [15] were the first to show a reduction in the rate of intubation with the use of NPPV. Subsequent studies had larger subject enrollment and better controls for analysis and demonstrated similar findings [27,28]. Barbe and colleagues [24] showed no improvement with NPPV versus standard therapy, but the patients in this study had less severe blood gas abnormalities when compared with the larger studies with favorable outcomes. The authors of this study felt that their results demonstrated that NPPV was not helpful in acute exacerbations of COPD. Although larger studies have demonstrated more favorable outcomes when using NPPV for COPD exacerbations, one may conclude that perhaps NPPV may not be beneficial in mild COPD exacerbations.

Given the differing findings among studies, patient selection is important in determining if an older patient may benefit from NPPV. Severity or degree of respiratory compromise seems to make a difference in the success of NPPV in

Table 1
Summary of randomized studies using noninvasive positive pressure ventilation in acute respiratory failure caused by chronic obstructive pulmonary disease that included data on patients aged 65 or older

Author	Yr	Reference	# Control	# NPPV	Average age
Brochard	1995	[21]	42	43	71 ± 9 C, 69 ± 10 N
Plant	2000	[24]	118	118	69C, 69N
Barbe	1996	[22]	10	14	65 ± 3C, 70 ± 2N
Tobin	2000	[25]	29	32	58 ± 18C, 64 ± 17N

Abbreviations: C, controls; N, NPPV.

patients with COPD exacerbations. Squadrone and colleagues [29] studied the use of NPPV in patients who had COPD with advanced hypercapnic respiratory failure. Although they found a higher rate of NPPV failure than other studies, the NPPV group had fewer serious complications. Overall, NPPV is well tolerated and has a good success rate in older patients. The global mortality associated with NPPV is comparable to that of the general population, and NPPV is effective in disabled and demented patients [30,31]. These studies and others suggest that NPPV is an attractive alternative to endotracheal intubation in older patients with acute exacerbation of COPD and may be better for some hypercarbic patients.

Acute cardiogenic pulmonary edema/congestive heart failure

Older patients often have underlying cardiac disease and are at risk for acute cardiogenic pulmonary edema or CHF. In fact, CHF is currently the leading cause of hospitalizations in patients older than 65 years [32]. Several studies have been conducted to evaluate the role of CPAP and NPPV in these patients. Although CPAP is technically not a form of mechanical ventilation, it is similar in some ways and deserves mention as treatment for this form of acute respiratory failure. CPAP has been studied since 1938 in the treatment of acute pulmonary edema and found to be effective [33]. Several studies have shown that patients treated with CPAP had improved vital signs, gas exchange, and an overall dramatic reduction in intubation rates. The average intubation rates for these studies were 47% for controls compared with 19% for patients treated with CPAP (average pressures used 10–12.5 cm H$_2$O) [34–37]. Other studies have reported a trend toward decreased mortality when CPAP is compared with standard therapy [38]. CPAP increases intrathoracic pressure and decreases transmural pressure (the difference between left ventricular systolic pressure and intrathoracic pressure). This action leads to reduced afterload and improved left ventricular function in patients who have CHF [9,10]. Other studies have shown CPAP to improve cardiac output in patients who have CHF, which is in contrast to patients with normally functioning hearts. The failing heart is much more sensitive to reductions in afterload than to preload. CPAP reductions in transmural pressure can improve cardiac output in patients

who have CHF [39,40]. It is currently considered standard of care to use CPAP (10–12.5 cm H$_2$O) in many patients who have acute pulmonary edema. Caution should be exercised in patients with acute myocardial infarction, however [1].

NPPV also has been investigated as a treatment for acute pulmonary edema. The rationale for using NPPV instead of CPAP is that it may help reduce the work of breathing and improve dyspnea. In a study that compared 130 elderly patients, NPPV improved Pao$_2$/Fio$_2$, respiratory rate, and dyspnea more quickly than standard medical care [41]. There was no difference in the rate of intubation or outcomes, however. Other studies that compared NPPV and CPAP have shown benefits and potential harm when choosing NPPV over CPAP. One study by Mehta and colleagues [42] compared CPAP and NPPV in the treatment of acute pulmonary edema. In this study, the NPPV group had more rapid improvement in respiratory rate and hypercapnia and dyspnea scores compared with CPAP but also had a higher rate of myocardial infarction. Subsequent randomized studies of NPPV and CPAP did not have similar differences in the rate of myocardial infarction but did show benefits in mortality with CPAP and no clear benefit to NPPV [43,44]. Overall, CPAP at levels of 10 to 12.5 cm H$_2$O should be considered as first-line therapy in patients who have acute pulmonary edema and NPPV should be reserved for patients who fail CPAP or have significant hypercapnia or dyspnea. CPAP and NPPV should be used with great caution in patients who have active ischemia or acute myocardial infarction.

Pneumonia

Pneumonia is the sixth leading cause of death in the United States and the leading infectious cause of death [45]. Older adults have a particularly high risk of developing pneumonia for many reasons, one being the presence of COPD. Because pneumonia increases the work of breathing and by definition adversely affects ventilation/perfusion matching, ventilatory assistance is often needed. NPPV has been studied in older patients with respiratory failure from pneumonia with mixed results. In one randomized study of patients with community-acquired pneumonia (many of whom were older), NPPV was associated with a reduction in respiratory rate, ICU decreased length of stay, and need for intubation when compared with conventional therapy [46]. Importantly in this study, only the patients with pre-existing COPD showed benefit from NPPV. A subgroup analysis revealed no difference for the patients who did not have COPD. A subsequent study by Jolliet and colleagues [47] prospectively evaluated NPPV efficacy in patients who did not have COPD and had severe community-acquired pneumonia. Although improvements in oxygenation and respiratory rates were found initially, 66% of the patients required intubation eventually. One of the problems with NPPV use in patients with pneumonia is the inability to adequately clear secretions while NPPV is in use. NPPV should be reserved for treatment of acute respiratory failure caused by pneumonia only in patients who have COPD and when adequate staffing is available to assist with pulmonary secretion clearance.

Do not intubate patients

Experts have debated the role of NPPV in patients with do-not-intubate (DNI) orders since its popularity grew. Management of a critically ill patient with a DNI order is more likely to occur in older patients, often because of their multiple premorbid conditions. Although technically it is a form of life support, NPPV does not carry the same implications and complications as mechanical ventilation via an endotracheal tube. In one study of 30 older men who declined endotracheal intubation, NPPV was used for treatment of their severe respiratory failure from COPD [48]. NPPV was initially successful in 60% of these patients. Other uncontrolled studies have reported similar findings in hypercapnic and hypoxemic respiratory failure [25,49]. A more recent prospective study of 114 patients (age > 63 years) with DNI orders revealed that survival to hospital discharge was heavily influenced by underlying cause of respiratory failure, presence of a strong cough, and mental status [50]. In this study, Levy and colleagues [50] reported survival to hospital discharge of 72% for patients with acute pulmonary edema and 52% for patients who had COPD. Worse survival was seen in patients with pneumonia or cancer. This study not only supports the use of NPPV in some patients with DNI orders but also reinforces the overall recommendation that patient selection is important for success of NPPV. Among patients with DNI orders, the ability to be awake and have an effective

cough was an important predictor of success [50]. To date, no studies have focused on patient comfort or family satisfaction with NPPV in patients with DNI orders. NPPV may reduce dyspnea and allow for verbal communication with patients, which may be important for end-of-life care and patient autonomy. Others argue that NPPV in the DNI population simply prolongs the dying process and unnecessarily increases use of hospital resources, however [51]. Overall, the data available support the use of NPPV in select patient populations with DNI orders.

Mask interface

One of the most common problems with NPPV clinically is getting the mask interface to fit well and be comfortable for the patient. Nasal masks are the most commonly used because they are considered to be the most comfortable and come in multiple sizes. One of the major problems with nasal masks is mouth leak, which may be most prevalent in patients with acute respiratory failure because they are likely to be mouth breathing. Many institutions use oronasal masks (interfaces that cover both the nose and mouth) for acute respiratory failure. Although the oronasal mask prevents air leaking through the mouth, it also interferes with speaking, eating, and expectorating secretions [1]. They also may work better in older patients, especially if a patient is edentulous. In a comparison of nasal masks, nasal pillows, and oronasal masks in patients with either COPD or restrictive thoracic disease, the nasal mask was considered more comfortable [52]. It was the least effective for correcting hypercapnia, however, likely because of mouth leak. Oral interfaces have been used in patients on NPPV but are better suited for chronic respiratory failure. Oral interfaces take some time to adjust and may need to be custom fit.

References

[1] Mehta S, Hill NS. Noninvasive ventilation: state of the art. Am J Respir Crit Care Med 2001;163: 540–77.
[2] Angus DC, Kelley MA, et al. Current and projected workforce requirements for care of the critically ill and patients with pulmonary disease: can we meet the requirements of an aging population? JAMA 2000;284(21):2762–70.
[3] Nourdine K, Combes P, Carton MJ, et al. Does noninvasive ventilation reduce the ICU nosocomial

infection risk? A prospective clinical survey. Intensive Care Med 1999;25 567–57.

[4] Girou E, Brun-Buisson C, Taille S, et al. Secular trends in nosocomial infections and mortality associated with noninvasive ventilation in patients with exacerbation of COPD and pulmonary edema. JAMA 2003;290(22):2985–91.

[5] Hilbert G, Gruson D, Vargas F, et al. Noninvasive ventilation in immunosuppressed patients with pulmonary infiltrates, fever, and acute respiratory failure. N Engl J Med 2001;344(7):481–7.

[6] Feinberg M, Knebl J, Tully J, et al. Aspiration and the elderly. Dysphagia 1990;5:61–71.

[7] Appendini L, Palessio A, Zanaboni S, et al. Physiologic effects of positive end-expiratory pressure and mask pressure support during exacerbations of chronic obstructive pulmonary disease. Am J Respir Crit Care Med 1994;149:1069–76.

[8] Hill NS. Noninvasive mechanical ventilation. In: Tobin M, editor. Principles and practices of mechanical ventilation. 2nd edition. Columbus (OH): McGraw-Hill; 2006.

[9] Bradley TD. Hemodynamic and sympathoinhibitory effects of nasal CPAP in congestive heart failure. Sleep 1996;19(10 Suppl):S232–5.

[10] Naughton MT, Rahman MA, Hara K, et al. Effect of continuous positive airway pressure on intrathoracic and left ventricular transmural pressures in patients with congestive heart failure. Circulation 1995; 91(6):1725–31.

[11] Behrendt CE. Acute respiratory failure in the United States. Chest 2000;118:1100–5.

[12] El Solh AA, Ramadan FH. Overview of respiratory failure in older adults. J Intensive Care Med 2006;21: 345–51.

[13] Janssens JP, Cicotti E, Fitting JW, et al. Non-invasive home ventilation in patients over 75 years of age: tolerance, compliance, and impact on quality of life. Respir Med 1998;92(12):1311–20.

[14] Jones SE, Packham S, Hebden M, et al. Domiciliary nocturnal intermittent positive pressure ventilation in patients with respiratory failure due to severe COPD: long term follow up and effect on survival. Thorax 1998;53(6):495–8.

[15] Brochard L, Mancebo J, Wysocki M, et al. Noninvasive ventilation for acute exacerbations of chronic obstructive pulmonary disease. N Engl J Med 1995;333:817–22.

[16] Balami JS, Packham SM, Gosney MA. Non-invasive ventilation for respiratory failure due to acute exacerbations of chronic obstructive pulmonary disease in older patients. Age Ageing 2006;35(1):75–9.

[17] Anton A, Guell R, Gomez J, et al. Predicting the result of noninvasive ventilation in severe acute exacerbations of patients with chronic airflow limitation. Chest 2000;117(3):828–33.

[18] Keenan SP, Sinuff T, Cook DJ, et al. Which patients with acute exacerbation of chronic obstructive pulmonary disease benefit from noninvasive positive-pressure ventilation? A systematic review of the literature. Ann Intern Med 2003;138(11):861–70.

[19] Enright P, Kronmal R, Higgins M, et al. Spirometry reference values for women and men 65-85 years of age. Am Rev Respir Dis 1993;147:125–33.

[20] Zaugg M, Lucchinetti E. Respiratory function in the elderly. Anesthesiol Clin North America 2000;18: 47–58.

[21] Polkey MI, Harris ML, Hughes PD, et al. The contractile properties of the elderly human diaphragm. Am J Respir Crit Care Med 1997;155: 1560–4.

[22] Poulin MJ, Cunningham DA, Paterson D, et al. Ventilatory sensitivity to CO_2 in hyperoxia and hypoxia in older aged humans. J Appl Physiol 1993;75: 2209–16.

[23] Brochard L, Isabey D, Piquet J, et al. Reversal of acute exacerbations of chronic obstructive lung disease by inspiratory assistance with a face mask. N Engl J Med 1990;95:865–70.

[24] Barbe F, Togores B, Rubi M, et al. Noninvasive ventilatory support does not facilitate recovery from acute respiratory failure in chronic obstructive pulmonary disease. Eur Respir J 1996;9:1240–5.

[25] Bott J, Carroll MP, Conway JH, et al. Randomized controlled trial of nasal ventilation in acute ventilatory failure due to chronic obstructive airways disease. Lancet 1993;341:1555–7.

[26] Kramer N, Meyer T, Meharg J, et al. Randomized, prospective trial of noninvasive positive pressure ventilation in acute respiratory failure. Am J Respir Crit Care Med 1995;151:1799–806.

[27] Plant PK, Owen JL, Elliott MW. Early use of noninvasive ventilation for acute exacerbations of chronic obstructive pulmonary disease on general respiratory wards: a multicenter randomized controlled trial. Lancet 2000;355:1931–5.

[28] Tobin T, Hovis J, Constantino J, et al. A randomized, prospective evaluation of positive pressure ventilation for acute respiratory failure. Am J Respir Crit Care Med 2000;161:807–13.

[29] Squadrone E, Frigerio P, Fogliati C, et al. Noninvasive vs invasive ventilation in COPD patients with severe acute respiratory failure deemed to require ventilatory assistance. Intensive Care Med 2004;30: 1303–10.

[30] Lightowler JV, Wedzicha JA, Elliot MW, et al. Non-invasive positive pressure ventilation to treat respiratory failure resulting from exacerbations of chronic obstructive pulmonary disease: Cochrane systemic review and meta-analysis. BMJ 326(7382):185.

[31] Rozzini R, Sabatini T, et al. Non-invasive ventilation for respiratory failure in elderly patients. Age Ageing 35(5):546–7.

[32] Yan AT, Bradley TD, Liu PP. The role of continuous positive airway pressure in the treatment of congestive heart failure. Chest 2001;120:1675–85.

[33] Barach AL, Martin J, Eckman M. Positive pressure respiration and its application to the treatment of

acute pulmonary edema. Ann Intern Med 1938;12: 754–95.

[34] Rasanen J, Heikkila J, Downs J, et al. Continuous positive airway pressure by face mask in acute cardiogenic pulmonary edema. Am J Cardiol 1985;55: 296–300.

[35] Vaisanen IT, Rasanen J. Continuous positive airway pressure and supplemental oxygen in the treatment of cardiogenic pulmonary edema. Chest 1987;92: 481–5.

[36] Bersten AD, Holt AW, Vedig AE, et al. Treatment of severe cardiogenic pulmonary edema with continuous positive airway pressure delivered by face mask. N Engl J Med 1991;325:1825–30.

[37] Lin M, Yang Y, Chiany H, et al. Reappraisal of continuous positive airway pressure therapy in acute cardiogenic pulmonary edema: short-term results and long-term follow-up. Chest 1995;107:1379–86.

[38] Pang D, Keenan SP, Cook DJ, et al. The effect of positive pressure airway support on mortality and the need for intubation in cardiogenic pulmonary edema: a systemic review. Chest 1998;114: 1185–92.

[39] De Hoyos A, Liu PP, Benard DC, et al. Haemodynamic effects of continuous positive airway pressure in humans with normal and impaired left ventricular function. Clin Sci 1995;88:173–8.

[40] Pinsky MR, Summer WR, Wise RA, et al. Augmentation of cardiac function by elevation of intrathoracic pressure. J Appl Physiol 1983;54:950–5.

[41] Nava S, Carbone G, DiBattista N, et al. Noninvasive ventilation in cardiogenic pulmonary edema: a multicenter randomized trial. Am J Respir Crit Care Med 2003;168:1432–7.

[42] Mehta S, Jay G, Woolard RH, et al. Randomized, prospective trial of bilevel versus continuous positive airway pressure in acute pulmonary edema. Crit Care Med 1997;25:620–8.

[43] Crane SD, Elliott MW, Gilligan P, et al. Randomized controlled comparison of continuous positive airways pressure, bilevel non-invasive ventilation, and standard treatment in emergency department patients with acute cardiogenic pulmonary oedema. Emerg Med J 2004;21:155–61.

[44] Bellone A, Monari A, Cortellaro F, et al. Myocardial infarction rate in acute pulmonary edema: noninvasive pressure support ventilation versus continuous positive airway pressure. Crit Care Med 2004;32:1860–5.

[45] Minino AM, Smith BL. Deaths: preliminary data for 2000. Natl Vital Stat Rep 2001;49(12):1–40.

[46] Confalonieri M, Potena A, Carbone G, et al. Acute respiratory failure in patients with severe community-acquired pneumonia: a prospective randomized evaluation of noninvasive ventilation. Am J Respir Crit Care Med 1999;160:1585–91.

[47] Jolliet P, Abajo B, Pasquina P, et al. Non-invasive pressure support ventilation in severe community-acquired pneumonia. Intensive Care Med 2001; 27(5):812–21.

[48] Benhamou D, Girault C, Faure C, et al. Nasal mask ventilation in acute respiratory failure: experience in elderly patients. Chest 1992;102(3):912–7.

[49] Meduri GU, Fox RC, Abou-Shala N, et al. Noninvasive mechanical ventilation via face mask in patients with acute respiratory failure who refused endotracheal intubation. Crit Care Med 1994;22: 1584–90.

[50] Levy M, Tanios MA, Nelson D, et al. Outcomes of patients with do-not-intubate orders treated with noninvasive ventilation. Crit Care Med 2004;32: 2002–7.

[51] Clarke DE, Vaughan L, Raffin TA. Noninvasive positive pressure ventilation for patients with terminal respiratory failure: the ethical and economic costs of delaying the inevitable are too great. Am J Crit Care 1994;3:4–5.

[52] Navalesi P, Fanfulla F, Frigeiro P, et al. Physiologic evaluation of noninvasive mechanical ventilation delivered with three types of masks in patients with chronic hypercapnic respiratory failure. Chest 2000;28:1785–90.

ELSEVIER
SAUNDERS

Clin Chest Med 28 (2007) 801–811

CLINICS
IN CHEST
MEDICINE

End-of-Life Considerations in Older Patients Who Have Lung Disease

Renee D. Stapleton, MD, MSc[a,b,*], J. Randall Curtis, MD, MPH[a,b]

[a]Division of Pulmonary and Critical Care Medicine, Department of Medicine, School of Medicine,
University of Washington, Seattle, WA, USA
[b]Harborview Medical Center, Box 359762,
325 Ninth Avenue, Seattle, WA 98104-2499, USA

The United States population and populations throughout the world are aging at increasing rates, and the proportion of people over age 65 is growing faster than any other age group [1]. It has been estimated that by 2030, more than 20% of Americans will be age 65 or older [2]. This increase in longevity, however, means that the geriatric population comprises a larger proportion of people nearing the end of life and translates into more deaths resulting from chronic, rather than acute, illnesses [3]. The median age at death in the United States is currently 77 years, with most deaths occurring after age 65 [2]. Some literature has suggested that the last year of life is often associated with multiple unpleasant symptoms and marked reductions in quality of life [4]. Improvements in palliative care for older patients are an important public health issue [5].

With the aging population, lung disease has become a major cause of morbidity and mortality worldwide. Chronic obstructive pulmonary disease (COPD) is the fourth leading cause of death in the United States—exceeded only by heart disease, cancer, and stroke [6,7]. While mortality from cardiovascular disease, stroke, and cancer has decreased over the last two decades, COPD mortality in the United States has doubled and is increasing worldwide [8–10]. Although

mortality and morbidity from COPD vary considerably around the world, it is the leading cause of death in developed and developing countries [7,10]. Lung cancer, another category of lung disease that substantially contributes to mortality, is the leading cause of cancer deaths in the United States, and its death rate is rapidly increasing in developing countries [11,12].

Along with mortality, health care use among patients with lung disease is also increasing exponentially. Patients who have COPD in developed countries are often hospitalized three or four times per year, and many of these hospitalizations are in an intensive care unit (ICU) [13–15]. In 2005, the National Heart, Lung, and Blood Institute reported that the annual direct health care costs for COPD were almost $22 billion, and the indirect costs (lost productivity and work days) were approximately $17 billion [16].

Palliative care includes management of symptoms, preservation of quality of life, communication with patients and their loved ones, and support of the physical, emotional, and spiritual well-being for patients and families [17]. As the population ages, the prevalence of lung disease and other chronic diseases increases, the burden of symptoms enlarges, and—because there are more deaths from lung disease—there is a strong and increasing need for palliative care and end-of-life services for these patients [18,19]. Some research, mostly in patients who have cancer, has shown that delivery of palliative care is associated with reductions in pain and other symptoms, improvements in quality of life, and enhanced family and patient satisfaction [20–24]. A recent study

---

* Corresponding author. Division of Pulmonary and Critical Care Medicine, Harborview Medical Center, Box 359762, 325 Ninth Avenue, Seattle, WA 98104-2499.

E-mail address: rstaplet@u.washington.edu (R.D. Stapleton).

also showed that receipt of hospital-based palliative care services is associated with significantly lower likelihood of admission to an ICU and lower inpatient costs [25]. Available data suggest that high-quality palliative care leads to improved patient- and family-centered outcomes and decreased costs. This article highlights the major factors involved in providing palliative and end-of-life care to older patients with lung diseases.

Quality of life and burden of symptoms in older patients with lung diseases

Much literature over the past few decades has focused on symptom management and palliative care in patients who have cancer [26]. In contrast, only a few studies have examined quality of life and the burden of symptoms in chronic nonmalignant lung diseases, most of which are in patients who have COPD. Several studies have found that patients who have COPD have a reduced health-related quality of life [27–31]; in most studies, physical, emotional, and social functioning is significantly decreased. Quality of life is also significantly reduced in persons with other lung diseases, such as idiopathic pulmonary fibrosis and sarcoidosis [32,33]. The burden of symptoms in these patients is also high and tends to correlate with larger reductions in quality of life.

Using standardized questionnaires and interviews, Gore and colleagues [34] compared symptoms and morbidity between 50 patients who had severe COPD ($FEV_1 < 0.75$ L and at least one admission for respiratory failure) and 50 patients who had inoperable non–small-cell lung cancer. The authors found that the patients who had COPD had significantly worse physical, social, and emotional functioning ($P < .05$) and more anxiety and depression (90% versus 52%, respectively) than the patients who had cancer. Only 4% of patients in each group reported having been assessed or treated for mental health issues. Eighty-two percent of the patients who had COPD were housebound, and 36% were chairbound, compared with 36% and 10% of patients who had lung cancer, respectively.

As part of the US-based SUPPORT project (Study to Understand Prognoses and Preferences for Outcomes and Risks of Treatments) [35], Lynn and colleagues [36] studied a cohort of 426 patients who had COPD who died within 1 year of their index hospital admission for a COPD exacerbation. Nearly 40% of patients had three or more comorbid illnesses, and between 15% and 25% of the patients' last 6 months of life were spent in a hospital. Twenty-five percent of patients had serious pain throughout their last 6 months of life, and 66% had serious dyspnea. Families were also substantially impacted. In another study from SUPPORT that examined burden of symptoms, Claessens and colleagues [37] compared patients who had severe COPD to patients who had advanced non–small-cell lung cancer. These authors found that pain and breathlessness were common symptoms in both groups. Among patients who had COPD, 56% had severe dyspnea and 21% had severe pain, whereas among patients who had lung cancer, 32% had severe dyspnea and 28% had severe pain.

In a recent retrospective study in the United Kingdom by Elkington and colleagues [38], proxies of patients who died from COPD were queried about their loved ones' symptoms in the last year of life. Breathlessness was present in 98% of patients; fatigue, weakness, low mood, and pain were also common. Finally, Solano and colleagues [39] recently published a systematic review of studies reporting the prevalence of physical symptoms in patients with five progressive diseases (advanced cancer, AIDS, heart disease, COPD, and renal disease). Three common symptoms were present in more than 50% of patients across all five diseases: pain, breathlessness, and fatigue.

Together, the literature on the experiences of patients who have COPD suggests that they have a reduced quality of life and a heavy burden of symptoms that is at least as great—if not greater—than patients who have advanced lung cancer. The most common symptoms are dyspnea, pain, fatigue, and depression (discussed separately later in this article). Although this information is informative and definitely applies to older patients who have lung diseases (the average age of patients in these studies was 70 years), there are other symptomatic considerations in the geriatric population. Not surprisingly, older patients may differ from younger patients medically and psychosocially, and they have a higher likelihood of having particular syndromes, such as dementia or delirium [40].

The prevalence of dementia is estimated to be 1% in persons aged 60 to 65 and increases to 40% in persons older than 80 years [41]. One recent study by Evers and colleagues [42] compared palliative care consultations in patients older than 80 years to those in younger patients. The authors found that patients over age 80 had a much higher prevalence of dementia and incapacity for decision making and a lower prevalence of cancer. Dementia, especially as it progresses, is often associated with a reduced life span, particularly when combined with another event such as a hip fracture or pneumonia [43]. Concomitant dementia affects the prognosis of other chronic illnesses and medical decision making; because many patients with dementia are unable to make their own decisions, involvement of and communication with loved ones and family members are crucial.

Delirium is also common in older patients. It is present is approximately 30% of all hospitalized older adults and 50% of all older adults undergoing surgery [44]. More than half of nursing home patients and more than 80% of dying patients develop delirium [45,46]. Delirium often happens during acute illness, and a subsequent prolonged period of cognitive impairment can follow [47]. Delirium is also a risk factor for mortality, functional decline, and institutionalization [48–50].

Overall, physical symptoms, such as pain and dyspnea, are highly prevalent in older patients with lung disease, as are syndromes such as dementia and delirium. These symptoms and conditions in older patients are major causes of suffering and play a significant role in morbidity. It seems that they may be underrecognized and undertreated in this group of patients.

Palliative care, communication, and decision making about end-of-life issues

Several studies have suggested that the quality of and access to palliative care is not adequate for patients who have chronic lung disease, particularly COPD. The SUPPORT study found that patients who had COPD were significantly more likely to die in the ICU and be on mechanical ventilation compared with patients with lung cancer, despite generally wanting care that focused on comfort [37]. In the study by Gore and colleagues [34], which compared patients who had advanced COPD to persons who had inoperable lung cancer, none of the patients who had COPD was offered or received input from palliative care specialists, whereas 30% of the patients who had cancer received such care and 56% were aware of these services. Au and colleagues [51] recently published a large cohort study that compared health care use at the end of life

between US veterans who had COPD and lung cancer. During the last 6 months of life, patients who had COPD were twice as likely to be admitted to the ICU, were five times more likely to be in an ICU longer than 2 weeks, and received fewer palliative medications.

Although it seems that patients with nonmalignant lung diseases receive less palliative care than patients who have cancer, the reasons for this discrepancy are not entirely clear. Whereas patients who have cancer often predictably decline until death, patients with chronic respiratory diseases, such as COPD, usually deteriorate slowly until an unpredictable exacerbation changes prognosis or leads to death [52]. Some authors have suggested that the differences may be caused by physicians' inability to provide accurate prognostic information toward the end of life in patients who have COPD because estimating life expectancy is difficult in chronic lung disease [53]. The SUPPORT study found that physicians and prediction models were poor at predicting death in patients who had COPD, even 5 days before death [37]. Although disease-specific predictive models for death in patients who have COPD at the population level have been developed [54,55], it is likely that accurate prognostication in an individual will remain difficult because of the variability inherent with chronic lung diseases. This fact has led to the proposal that educating patients and families about the uncertainty in prognosis of lung diseases must be an essential feature of end-of-life care and decision making [53].

Research has shown that physician-patient communication about end-of-life issues and treatment preferences is commonly inadequate. Heffner and colleagues [56] asked 105 patients who had chronic lung disease about their attitudes regarding advanced directives. Less than half of the patients had completed an advanced directive, and although nearly all participants wanted information about advanced directives and life support, less than 20% had had such discussions with their doctors and less than 15% felt that their doctors understood their wishes. In a study of 115 patients who had oxygen-dependent COPD, Curtis and colleagues [57] found that only one third of patients had discussed end-of-life care with their physicians. Most patients reported that their physicians did not discuss how long the patients had to live, what dying might be like, or patients' spirituality. In a qualitative study, Curtis and colleagues [58] also found that in comparison to patients who had AIDS and cancer, patients who had COPD were more likely to be troubled about the lack of education they received about their disease and were more likely to want more information from their physicians about several topics, including prognosis, advanced care planning, and what dying might be like.

Because patient-physician communication about the end-of-life care seems to be insufficient and leaves many patients with unmet needs, it is important that we understand the barriers to effective communication. Two studies have investigated such barriers—one a US study of perceptions of patients and physicians [59] and the other a UK study of the views of general practitioners [60]. Barriers for patients to communicating about palliative care include wanting to focus on staying alive, unwillingness to discuss being sick, changing treatment preferences, and lack of knowledge about the type of care and who the treating physician will be in the event of an acute illness. Barriers for physicians include feeling ill prepared to discuss the issue adequately, lack of accurate prognostic information, lack of time, and difficulty in starting these discussions with patients.

Even when communication between physicians and patients does occur, there may be a mismatch of expectations when making decisions about end-of-life treatment preferences. In a study of more than 5000 seriously ill patients (one third had COPD or respiratory failure), Wenger and colleagues [61] found that 64% of patients wished to receive cardiopulmonary resuscitation (CPR) and 36% of patients wanted to forgo it. When patients wanted to receive CPR, physicians clearly understood their preferences 86% of the time; however, physicians only understood patients' wishes 46% of the time among patients wanting to forgo CPR. As a result of this misunderstanding, many patients who wished to forgo CPR in this study underwent a resuscitation attempt, and most of them died in the hospital.

One aspect of communication with older adults that is important for physicians to understand is the increased importance that older adults place on the burden of treatments. For younger adults, the burden of treatments is relatively less important, but it becomes a much more important issue with increased age [62,63]. Consequently, physicians should include the potential burdens of short- and long-term mechanical ventilation in their discussions of treatment preferences with older adults.

Current available data indicate that palliative care for patients with lung diseases is often inadequate. This inadequacy may be largely caused by poor or infrequent patient-physician communication about end-of-life care and treatment preferences. Many barriers to effective communication exist, and understanding these barriers is likely an important step toward improving communication.

Role of depression in decision making

Depression frequently complicates the care of older patients and patients with chronic lung diseases. Approximately 2% of older people in the community and 9% of older chronically ill adults are depressed, compared with 6% of the general adult population [64]. Geriatric inpatients and nursing home residents have a much higher prevalence of depression, estimated to be between 36% and 47% [65,66]. Using the Geriatric Depression Scale and the Medical Outcome Survey–Short Form 36 (SF-36) to assess depression in 109 patients who had severe COPD (mean age, 71 years), Lacasse and colleagues [67] found that 57% of patients had significant depressive symptoms and that 18% were severely depressed. Only 6% of patients who met the criteria for depression were taking an antidepressant drug. In another investigation, van Manen and colleagues [68] examined depressive symptoms in patients who had COPD and in controls and found that the prevalence of depression was 25% in patients who had severe COPD ($FEV_1 < 50\%$ predicted), 17.5% in controls, and 19.6% in patients who had mild to moderate COPD.

We examined 101 patients who had oxygen-dependent COPD (mean age, 67.4 years), and 45% of patients had symptoms suggestive of depression as measured by the Center for Epidemiologic Study – Depression survey [69]. We found that a higher burden of depressive symptoms in these patients was significantly associated with a preference against CPR. These findings are similar to two other studies, neither of which specifically investigated patients who had COPD [70,71]. A prior report from the same group of patients showed that patients who were depressed rated the quality of patient-physician communication about end-of-life care significantly lower than patients who were not depressed [57]. It is not clear whether this finding reflects an effect of depression on patients' ratings of the quality of communication or whether the quality of patient-physician communication is negatively influenced by depression.

The fact that depression may influence decision making about life-sustaining therapies implies that treatment of depression might change end-of-life treatment preferences for these patients, and several studies have examined this hypothesis. The SUPPORT study found that among patients who initially preferred do-not-resuscitate status, persons whose depression score improved substantially over 2 months of follow-up were five times more likely to change treatment preferences to wanting CPR than patients whose depression scores did not improve [71]. Ganzini and colleagues [72] examined the treatment preferences of 43 elderly depressed patients before and after treatment of the depression and found a clinically evident change in the preferences of the 11 patients who initially were rated as more severely depressed. Eggar and colleagues [73] also investigated the CPR preferences of 49 older depressed patients before and after depression treatment and found that 16 of 17 patients who initially declined CPR accepted CPR after treatment for depression.

Coexisting depression plays a significant role in decision making at the end of life because it seems that depression may influence treatment preferences for life-sustaining therapies. Because prior research suggested that clinical depression among patients who have severe COPD responds to antidepressant therapy [74], clinicians who care for older patients with lung diseases should evaluate patients for depression and realize that spontaneous or therapy-induced improvement in depressive symptoms should warrant a reassessment of patients' treatment preferences.

Talking about end-of-life care with patients and their families

When should we talk about end-of-life care with patients and families?

It is difficult to be prescriptive about the "right" time to discuss end-of-life care with older patients who have chronic lung disease, except to say that we should talk about it as soon as possible and earlier than we usually do. Often, clinicians fail to discuss end-of-life issues and treatment preferences while their patients are relatively well and able to participate in decision making. If these discussions do not take place,

goals of care are not established, and a patient requires hospitalization or even an ICU stay in which he or she may be unable to communicate wishes, the burden of decision making then falls on family members and loved ones who may not know a patient's preferences. A potential solution to these difficulties is to begin discussions with patients who have chronic lung diseases early in the course of their care. These discussions can occur over the course of several outpatient visits during which the focus can be on prognosis, goals of therapy, minimally acceptable quality of life, and the patient's values and attitudes toward medical therapy. These discussions may foreshadow or set the stage for subsequent discussions about withholding life-sustaining treatments, depending on each patient's wishes.

How should we talk about end-of-life care?

Because discussing end-of-life care with patients and families is an important part of providing high-quality medical care, we should approach these discussions with the same care and planning that we approach other important medical procedures. Box 1 outlines some of the steps that may facilitate good communication about end-of-life care (described in more detail later).

Making preparations before a discussion

A common mistake is to embark on a discussion about end-of-life care with a patient and family without having prepared for the discussion. Clinicians should review the medical record and the patient's disease process, including the prognosis, treatment options, and likely outcomes. It is also important for clinicians to review what they know about the patient and family, including their attitudes toward illness, treatment, and death. It is also useful for clinicians to consider their own feelings of anxiety or guilt. Acknowledging these feelings explicitly to oneself can help clinicians avoid projecting feelings or biases onto patients or family. Finally, if a patient has many health care providers, the clinician leading the discussion should attempt to ensure that all appropriate clinicians are consulted about their opinions of the patient's prognosis. It also may be appropriate to invite other providers to be present at one or more of the discussions about end-of-life care.

Holding a discussion about end-of-life care

These discussions often start with opening comments and introductions followed by an

---

Box 1. Components of a discussion about end-of-life care

I. Making preparations before a discussion about end-of-life care:
- Review previous knowledge of the patient and/or family
- Review knowledge of the disease, prognosis, and treatment options
- Examine clinician's own personal feelings, attitudes, and biases

II. Holding a discussion about end-of-life care:
- Introduce everyone present
- If appropriate, set the tone in a nonthreatening way: "This is a conversation I like to have with all of my patients and their families..."
- Find out what the patient or family understands
- Discuss a prognosis frankly in a way that is meaningful to the patient and demonstrates that the clinician cares for the patient and family
- Avoid temptation to give too much medical detail
- If the discussion leads to wishes to withhold life-sustaining treatment, make it clear that deciding to withhold such treatment is NOT withholding caring
- Use active listening and allow the patient and family adequate time to speak
- Acknowledge strong emotions and use reflection to encourage patients or families to talk about these emotions
- Respond empathetically to tears or other grief behavior
- Tolerate silence

III. Finishing a discussion of end-of-life care:
- Achieve common understanding of the disease and treatment issues
- Make a recommendation about treatment
- Ask if there are any questions
- Ensure a basic follow-up plan and make sure the patient and/or family knows how to reach the clinician for questions

---

exchange of information in which a clinician updates patients and family about a patient's illness and treatments and the clinician, in turn, is made aware of the patient's values. The conversation often turns to discussion of the future, including prognosis for survival and quality of life. If a patient's illness is advanced and survival is limited, this is also the time when the discussion of death and what dying might be like occurs. Finally, there is often a discussion of the decisions to be made—either at this conference or in the future—and closing comments are made by the patient and clinicians.

If multiple family members are present during the information exchange, not everyone will have the same level of understanding of the patient's condition. It is often helpful to first find out what a patient or family understands of the patient's illness. This can be a useful way for the clinician to determine how much information can be given, the level of detail that can be understood, and the amount of technical language that can be used. Clinicians should be careful to avoid unnecessary technical jargon. It is important to avoid the

temptation to give too much detail about the physiology or pathophysiology as a way to avoid our own discomfort, but we should be aware that some patients or families may want to hear this type of detail.

During these discussions, it is important to discuss prognosis in an honest way that is meaningful to patients and their families. For example, median survival is not meaningful to most patients. Most experts recommend that clinicians use quantitative estimates of prognosis (such as 50% chance of surviving 1 year) rather than qualitative statements (such as a "poor" prognosis) because it increases the chances that patients will understand. In discussing prognosis, clinicians also should be honest about the degree of uncertainty in the prognosis, but it can be helpful to provide this information in a way that makes it clear that the clinician cares for the patient and the family.

It is important in discussions about end-of-life care that the patient and family understand that if the decision is made to withhold life-sustaining treatment, such as mechanical ventilation, clinicians themselves are not withholding from "caring" for the patient. This information may seem obvious to some clinicians, but it should be stated explicitly to patients and families to avoid any misunderstanding. Patients and families want to know that no matter what treatment preferences they may have, they will be cared for, comfortable, and not abandoned by their health care providers.

After discussing prognosis and treatment options, it is important to spend some time exploring patients' reactions to what was discussed. It can be helpful to repeat what a patient has said as a way to show that the clinician has heard him or her. This form of active listening can be particularly useful when clinicians and patients have differing views. Second, it is important to acknowledge emotions that come up in these discussions. It is useful for clinicians to acknowledge emotions in a way that allows the person with the emotion to talk about his or her feelings. In acknowledging such emotions, it can be useful for clinicians to use reflection to show empathy and encourage discussion about the emotion. For example, a clinician can say "It seems to me that you are very scared of getting sicker. Can you tell me more about that?" as a way to show some empathy and to allow a patient to talk about his or her feelings. It also can be helpful for clinicians to provide support for decisions that patients make by acknowledging the difficulty of the situation and valuing patients' comments. Finally, another technique clinicians can use in discussions with patients is tolerating silences. Sometimes after what seems like a long silence, patients or family members ask a particularly difficult question or express a difficult emotion.

How should we finish a discussion about end-of-life care?

Before finishing a discussion about end-of-life care, there are several steps that clinicians should make. First, it is important that clinicians make recommendations during the discussion. With the increasing emphasis on patient autonomy, there may be a tendency for some clinicians to describe the treatment options without making a recommendation. On the contrary, it is important that clinicians offer their expertise to patients, and part of offering their expertise is making a recommendation. Second, it is important to remind patients that their decisions are not permanent and can be changed at any time if they wish.

Before finishing a discussion about end-of-life care, clinicians should summarize the major points and ask patients if they have any questions. This is a good time to tolerate silence, because it may take a while for the uncomfortable questions to surface. Before completing a discussion about end-of-life care, clinicians also should ensure that there is an adequate follow-up plan, which often means a plan for ongoing discussions at future visits. Finally, it is important to outline the steps that patients should take to make their wishes known and recorded so that these wishes can be performed in the event that their condition deteriorates (see following discussion).

How can we help patients with the decision to withhold cardiopulmonary resuscitation or mechanical ventilation?

Frequently, part of the decision for patients with lung disease is whether they want to receive CPR in the event of cardiac arrest. In our opinion, in helping patients make this decision, it is important that advanced cardiac life support not be broken into components but rather presented as a package. Breaking advanced cardiac life support into components (chest compressions, antiarrhythmic drugs, vasopressor agents, intubation) makes these decisions unnecessarily complex and can lead to an absurd resuscitation status, such as compressions and all drugs but no intubation. With regard to mechanical ventilation in the event of respiratory failure, the procedures of intubation and mechanical ventilation should be explained to patients in understandable terms.

How can we help patients carry out their wishes?

Once patients have decided on their wishes for end-of-life care, several important steps must be taken that should be explained to the patient. First, clinicians should advise patients to legally designate a durable power of attorney for health care, who should be a person a patient trusts to carry out his or her wishes at the end of life. This decision is particularly important if a person the patient would choose is not the person designated by state law. Second, patients should clearly communicate their wishes to this power of attorney so that they are well understood. These wishes should be clearly communicated with the patients' health care providers. Finally, if the decision has been made to forgo CPR, the patient should complete an advanced directive and tell the power of attorney where it is kept so that it can be found at a later date if needed.

Understanding clinicians' own discomfort discussing death

Discomfort discussing death is universal. This is not a problem unique to physicians, nurses, or other health care professionals but has its roots in our society's denial of dying and death. With many medical schools, nursing schools, and health care textbooks providing little education about end-of-life care, it is not surprising that many clinicians have difficulty discussing this topic with their patients and families. Clinicians also may feel that a patient's eventual death reflects poorly on their skills as health care providers and represents a failure on their part to save a patient's life.

It is important for clinicians to recognize the difficulty they have discussing dying and death. If clinicians acknowledge this difficulty, they can work to minimize some of the common effects that such discomfort can take. For example, discomfort discussing death may cause clinicians to give mixed messages about a patient's prognosis or use euphemisms for dying and death. This discomfort in discussing dying and death even can cause clinicians to avoid speaking with a patient or family. Recognizing this discomfort and being willing to confront it are the first steps in overcoming these barriers to effective communication about dying and death with patients and their families.

Summary

The intent of palliative care is to prevent and relieve suffering and support a reasonable quality of life for patients and their loved ones. Over the past few decades, palliative care measures have focused largely on patients who have cancer. Malignancy-based palliative care models, however, have not been applied effectively to patients who have chronic lung disease.

Patients with lung disease have a reduced quality of life and a burden of symptoms that is at least as great as—if not greater than—patients who have cancer. Patients with lung disease commonly experience significant pain, dyspnea, and fatigue. Dementia and delirium also can play a significant role in older patients. Research suggests that patients who have COPD receive suboptimal palliative care, which may be caused by inadequate communication with their physicians. When patients have made decisions about life-sustaining therapies, physicians often either do not know patients' wishes or misunderstand them. Depression, which is common in older patients with chronic illness, may influence patients' decisions about end-of-life care. Clinicians should realize that most patients want more information about end-of-life care and that efforts to initiate and improve communication with patients are important. Further research that investigates and defines interventions to improve and optimize communication and delivery of high-quality palliative care is sorely needed for patients with chronic lung disease.

Discussing end-of-life care and death with patients and their families is an important part of providing good quality medical care. Although there is little empiric research to guide clinicians in the most effective way to have these conversations, there is increasing emphasis on making it an important part of the care we provide. Much like other medical procedures or skills, providing sensitive and effective communication about end-of-life care requires training, practice, and preparation. Different clinicians may have different approaches and should change their approach to match the needs of individual patients and their families.

References

[1] World Health Organization. Active aging: a policy framework. Geneva (Switzerland): World Health Organization; 2002.

[2] National Vital Statistics Report, National Center for Health Statistics, Centers for Disease Control and Prevention, Department of Health and Human Services. Volume 55, Number 19. Available at: http://www.cdc.gov/nchs/data/nvsr/nvsr55/nvsr55_19.pdf. Accessed August 21, 2007.

[3] Murray CJ, Lopez AD. Mortality by cause for eight regions of the world: Global Burden of Disease Study. Lancet 1997;349(9061):1269–76.

[4] Cartwright A. Changes in life and care in the year before death: 1969-1987. J Public Health Med 1991;13(2):81–7.

[5] Rao JK, Anderson LA, Smith SM. End of life is a public health issue. Am J Prev Med 2002;23(3):215–20.

[6] National Heart, Lung, and Blood Institute. Data fact sheet: chronic obstructive pulmonary disease. NIH publication 30-5229. Bethesda (MD): National Heart, Lung, and Blood Institute; 2003.

[7] Hurd S. The impact of COPD on lung health worldwide: epidemiology and incidence. Chest 2000;117 (2 Suppl):1S–4S.

[8] Jemal A, Ward E, Hao Y, et al. Trends in the leading causes of death in the United States, 1970-2002. JAMA 2005;294(10):1255–9.

[9] Pauwels RA, Buist AS, Calverley PM, et al. Global strategy for the diagnosis, management, and prevention of chronic obstructive pulmonary disease: NHLBI/WHO global initiative for chronic obstructive lung disease (GOLD) workshop summary. Am J Respir Crit Care Med 2001;163(5):1256–76.

[10] Lopez AD, Mathers CD, Ezzati M, et al. Global and regional burden of disease and risk factors, 2001: systematic analysis of population health data. Lancet 2006;367(9524):1747–57.

[11] Ries LAG, Melbert D, Krapcho M, et al. SEER cancer statistics review, 1975-2004, National Cancer Institute. Bethesda (MD): National Cancer Institute. Available at: http://seer.cancer.gov/csr/1975_2004/. based on November 2006 SEER data submission, posted to the SEER web site, 2007. Accessed June 29, 2007.

[12] Spiro SG, Silvestri GA. One hundred years of lung cancer. Am J Respir Crit Care Med 2005;172(5):523–9.

[13] Soriano JB, Maier WC, Egger P, et al. Recent trends in physician diagnosed COPD in women and men in the UK. Thorax 2000;55(9):789–94.

[14] Mannino DM, Homa DM, Akinbami LJ, et al. Chronic obstructive pulmonary disease surveillance: United States, 1971-2000. Respir Care 2002;47(10):1184–99.

[15] Holguin F, Folch E, Redd SC, et al. Comorbidity and mortality in COPD-related hospitalizations in the United States, 1979 to 2001. Chest 2005;128(4):2005–11.

[16] Foster TS, Miller JD, Marton JP, et al. Assessment of the economic burden of COPD in the US: a review and synthesis of the literature. COPD 2006;3(4):211–8.

[17] Morrison RS, Meier DE. Clinical practice: palliative care. N Engl J Med 2004;350(25):2582–90.

[18] American Thoracic Society, statement on home care for patients with respiratory disorders. Am J Respir Crit Care Med 2005;171(12):1443–64.

[19] O'Donnell DE, Aaron S, Bourbeau J, et al. State of the art compendium: Canadian Thoracic Society recommendations for the management of chronic obstructive pulmonary disease. Can Respir J 2004;11(Suppl B):7B–59B.

[20] Ringdal GI, Jordhoy MS, Kaasa S. Family satisfaction with end-of-life care for cancer patients in a cluster randomized trial. J Pain Symptom Manage 2002;24(1):53–63.

[21] Higginson IJ, Finlay IG, Goodwin DM, et al. Is there evidence that palliative care teams alter end-of-life experiences of patients and their caregivers? J Pain Symptom Manage 2003;25(2):150–68.

[22] Jordhoy MS, Fayers P, Loge JH, et al. Quality of life in palliative cancer care: results from a cluster randomized trial. J Clin Oncol 2001;19(18):3884–94.

[23] Rabow MW, Petersen J, Schanche K, et al. The comprehensive care team: a description of a controlled trial of care at the beginning of the end of life. J Palliat Med 2003;6(3):489–99.

[24] Teno JM, Clarridge BR, Casey V, et al. Family perspectives on end-of-life care at the last place of care. JAMA 2004;291(1):88–93.

[25] Penrod JD, Deb P, Luhrs C, et al. Cost and utilization outcomes of patients receiving hospital-based palliative care consultation. J Palliat Med 2006;9(4):855–60.

[26] Higginson I. Palliative care: a review of past changes and future trends. J Public Health Med 1993;15(1):3–8.

[27] Engstrom CP, Persson LO, Larsson S, et al. Functional status and well being in chronic obstructive pulmonary disease with regard to clinical parameters and smoking: a descriptive and comparative study. Thorax 1996;51(8):825–30.

[28] McSweeny AJ, Grant I, Heaton RK, et al. Life quality of patients with chronic obstructive pulmonary disease. Arch Intern Med 1982;142(3):473–8.

[29] Ferrer M, Alonso J, Morera J, et al. Chronic obstructive pulmonary disease stage and health-related quality of life: the Quality of Life of Chronic Obstructive Pulmonary Disease Study Group. Ann Intern Med 1997;127(12):1072–9.

[30] Okubadejo AA, Jones PW, Wedzicha JA. Quality of life in patients with chronic obstructive pulmonary disease and severe hypoxaemia. Thorax 1996;51(1):44–7.

[31] Prigatano GP, Wright EC, Levin D. Quality of life and its predictors in patients with mild hypoxemia and chronic obstructive pulmonary disease. Arch Intern Med 1984;144(8):1613–9.

[32] Swigris JJ, Kuschner WG, Jacobs SS, et al. Health-related quality of life in patients with idiopathic pulmonary fibrosis: a systematic review. Thorax 2005;60(7):588–94.

[33] De Vries J, Drent M. Quality of life and health status in interstitial lung diseases. Curr Opin Pulm Med 2006;12(5):354–8.

[34] Gore JM, Brophy CJ, Greenstone MA. How well do we care for patients with end stage chronic obstructive pulmonary disease (COPD)? A comparison of palliative care and quality of life in COPD and lung cancer. Thorax 2000;55(12):1000–6.

[35] The SUPPORT Principal Investigators. A controlled trial to improve care for seriously ill hospitalized patients: the study to understand prognoses and preferences for outcomes and risks of treatments (SUPPORT). JAMA 1995;274(20):1591–8.

[36] Lynn J, Ely EW, Zhong Z, et al. Living and dying with chronic obstructive pulmonary disease. J Am Geriatr Soc 2000;48(5 Suppl):S91–100.

[37] Claessens MT, Lynn J, Zhong Z, et al. Dying with lung cancer or chronic obstructive pulmonary

disease: insights from SUPPORT (Study to Understand Prognoses and Preferences for Outcomes and
Risks of Treatments). J Am Geriatr Soc 2000;48
(5 Suppl):S146–53.

[38] Elkington H, White P, Addington-Hall J, et al. The
healthcare needs of chronic obstructive pulmonary
disease patients in the last year of life. Palliat Med
2005;19(6):485–91.

[39] Solano JP, Gomes B, Higginson IJ. A comparison of
symptom prevalence in far advanced cancer, AIDS,
heart disease, chronic obstructive pulmonary disease
and renal disease. J Pain Symptom Manage 2006;
31(1):58–69.

[40] Kapo J, Morrison LJ, Liao S. Palliative care for the
older adult. J Palliat Med 2007;10(1):185–209.

[41] von Strauss E, Viitanen M, De Ronchi D, et al. Aging and the occurrence of dementia: findings from
a population-based cohort with a large sample of
nonagenarians. Arch Neurol 1999;56(5):587–92.

[42] Evers MM, Meier DE, Morrison RS. Assessing differences in care needs and service utilization in geriatric palliative care patients. J Pain Symptom
Manage 2002;23(5):424–32.

[43] Morrison RS, Siu AL. Survival in end-stage dementia following acute illness. JAMA 2000;284(1):
47–52.

[44] Dyer CB, Ashton CM, Teasdale TA. Postoperative
delirium: a review of 80 primary data-collection
studies. Arch Intern Med 1995;155(5):461–5.

[45] Kiely DK, Bergmann MA, Jones RN, et al. Characteristics associated with delirium persistence among
newly admitted post-acute facility patients. J Gerontol A Biol Sci Med Sci 2004;59(4):344–9.

[46] Casarett DJ, Inouye SK. Diagnosis and management of delirium near the end of life. Ann Intern
Med 2001;135(1):32–40.

[47] McCusker J, Cole M, Dendukuri N, et al. The course
of delirium in older medical inpatients: a prospective
study. J Gen Intern Med 2003;18(9):696–704.

[48] Leslie DL, Zhang Y, Holford TR, et al. Premature
death associated with delirium at 1-year follow-up.
Arch Intern Med 2005;165(14):1657–62.

[49] Marcantonio ER, Flacker JM, Michaels M, et al.
Delirium is independently associated with poor
functional recovery after hip fracture. J Am Geriatr
Soc 2000;48(6):618–24.

[50] Inouye SK, Rushing JT, Foreman MD, et al. A
three-site epidemiologic study. J Gen Intern Med
1998;13(4):234–42.

[51] Au DH, Udris EM, Fihn SD, et al. Differences in
health care utilization at the end of life among patients with chronic obstructive pulmonary disease
and patients with lung cancer. Arch Intern Med
2006;166(3):326–31.

[52] Simonds AK. Living and dying with respiratory failure: facilitating decision making. Chron Respir Dis
2004;1(1):56–9.

[53] Curtis JR, Engelberg RA, Wenrich MD, et al. Communication about palliative care for patients with

chronic obstructive pulmonary disease. J Palliat
Care 2005;21(3):157–64.

[54] Fan VS, Curtis JR, Tu SP, et al. Using quality of life
to predict hospitalization and mortality in patients
with obstructive lung diseases. Chest 2002;122(2):
429–36.

[55] Celli BR, Cote CG, Marin JM, et al. The body-mass
index, airflow obstruction, dyspnea, and exercise
capacity index in chronic obstructive pulmonary
disease. N Engl J Med 2004;350(10):1005–12.

[56] Heffner JE, Fahy B, Hilling L, et al. Attitudes regarding advance directives among patients in pulmonary rehabilitation. Am J Respir Crit Care Med
1996;154(6 Pt 1):1735–40.

[57] Curtis JR, Engelberg RA, Nielsen EL, et al. Patient-
physician communication about end-of-life care for
patients with severe COPD. Eur Respir J 2004;
24(2):200–5.

[58] Curtis JR, Wenrich MD, Carline JD, et al. Patients'
perspectives on physician skill in end-of-life care: differences between patients with COPD, cancer, and
AIDS. Chest 2002;122(1):356–62.

[59] Knauft E, Nielsen EL, Engelberg RA, et al. Barriers and facilitators to end-of-life care communication for patients with COPD. Chest 2005;127(6):
2188–96.

[60] Elkington H, White P, Higgs R, et al. GPs' views of
discussions of prognosis in severe COPD. Fam Pract
2001;18(4):440–4.

[61] Wenger NS, Phillips RS, Teno JM, et al. Physician
understanding of patient resuscitation preferences:
insights and clinical implications. J Am Geriatr
Soc 2000;48(5 Suppl):S44–51.

[62] Fried TR, Bradley EH, Towle VR, et al. Understanding the treatment preferences of seriously ill
patients. N Engl J Med 2002;346(14):1061–6.

[63] Fried TR, Bradley EH. What matters to seriously ill
older persons making end-of-life treatment decisions? A qualitative study. J Palliat Med 2003;6(2):
237–44.

[64] Hybels CF, Blazer DG. Epidemiology of late-life
mental disorders. Clin Geriatr Med 2003;19(4):
663–96 v.

[65] Burke WJ, Wengel SP. Late-life mood disorders.
Clin Geriatr Med 2003;19(4):777–97 vii.

[66] Gebretsadik M, Jayaprabhu S, Grossberg GT.
Mood disorders in the elderly. Med Clin North
Am 2006;90(5):789–805.

[67] Lacasse Y, Rousseau L, Maltais F. Prevalence of depressive symptoms and depression in patients with
severe oxygen-dependent chronic obstructive pulmonary disease. J Cardiopulm Rehabil 2001;21(2):
80–6.

[68] van Manen JG, Bindels PJ, Dekker FW, et al. Risk
of depression in patients with chronic obstructive
pulmonary disease and its determinants. Thorax
2002;57(5):412–6.

[69] Stapleton RD, Nielsen EL, Engelberg RA, et al. Association of depression and life-sustaining treatment

preferences in patients with COPD. Chest 2005; 127(1):328–34.

[70] Blank K, Robison J, Doherty E, et al. Life-sustaining treatment and assisted death choices in depressed older patients. J Am Geriatr Soc 2001;49(2):153–61.

[71] Rosenfeld KE, Wenger NS, Phillips RS, et al. Factors associated with change in resuscitation preference of seriously ill patients: the SUPPORT Investigators (Study to Understand Prognoses and Preferences for Outcomes and Risks of Treatments). Arch Intern Med 1996;156(14):1558–64.

[72] Ganzini L, Lee MA, Heintz RT, et al. The effect of depression treatment on elderly patients' preferences for life-sustaining medical therapy. Am J Psychiatry 1994;151(11):1631–6.

[73] Eggar R, Spencer A, Anderson D, et al. Views of elderly patients on cardiopulmonary resuscitation before and after treatment for depression. Int J Geriatr Psychiatry 2002;17(2):170–4.

[74] Borson S, Claypoole K, McDonald GJ. Depression and chronic obstructive pulmonary disease: treatment trials. Semin Clin Neuropsychiatry 1998;3(2):115–30.

ELSEVIER
SAUNDERS

Clin Chest Med 28 (2007) 813–817

CLINICS
IN CHEST
MEDICINE

Index

Note: Page numbers of article titles are in **boldface** type.

A

Acute cardiogenic pulmonary edema/CHF, NPPV for, in older adults with acute respiratory failure, 797

Acute lung injury, in older adults
  causes of, 784
  incidence of, 784
  treatment of, 784–787
    corticosteroids in, 786
    mechanical ventilation in, 784–786
      weaning from, 786–787

Acute respiratory distress syndrome (ARDS), in older adults, **783–791**
  causes of, 784
  incidence of, 784
  outcomes following, 787–789
  treatment of, 784–787
    corticosteroids in, 786
    mechanical ventilation in, 784–786
      weaning from, 786–787

Acute respiratory failure
  in older adults, noninvasive ventilation in, **793–800**
    NPPV, 793–794
      control of, 794–795
      critical illness use, 794
      in acute cardiogenic pulmonary edema/CHF, 797
      in do-not-intubate patients, 798
      in obstructive lung diseases, 795–797
      in pneumonia, 797–798
      mask interface in, 798
      mechanism of action of, 794
      respiratory mechanics of, 794–795
    in the elderly, 784

Aerosol formulations and delivery devices, in COPD management, 705–706

Age
  as factor in allergy and immunology of lung, **663–672**
  as factor in respiratory function, 783–784
  as factor in sleep changes, 673

Aging
  circadian rhythms and, 673–674
  lung immunity and, 667–668
  sleep disturbance and, causes of, 674

Airway obstruction, asthma in older adults and, 688–689

Allergy(ies), of aging lung, **663–672.** See also *Lung(s).*

Antibiotic(s), for pneumonia in older adults, 763

Anti-inflammatory drugs, for asthma management in older adults, 694–695

Anxiety, COPD and, 707–708

Aortic stenosis, in older adults, 724–725

ARDS. See *Acute respiratory distress syndrome (ARDS).*

Asthma
  atopic, 689–690
  defined, 685–686
  described, 685
  histopathologic findings in, 687
  in older adults
    airway obstruction and, 688–689
    atopy and, 689–690
    bronchial hyperresponsiveness in, 688
    clinical characteristics of, 690–692
    epidemiology of, 686
    histopathologic findings in, 687
    management of, 692–697
      anti-inflammatory agents in, 694–695
      assessment in, 693
      bronchodilators in, 695–697
      clinical outcome in, 697–698
      controlling triggers in, 693–694
      education in, 697
      general considerations in, 693
      goals in, 692–693

0272-5231/07/$ - see front matter © 2007 Elsevier Inc. All rights reserved.
doi:10.1016/S0272-5231(07)00105-0

chestmed.theclinics.com

Asthma (*continued*)
 monitoring in, 693
  pharmacologic, 694–697
 neurogenic influences in, 687–688
 pathophysiology of, 687–689
 prognosis of, 697–698
 nonatopic, 690

Atopy, asthma in older adults and, 689–690

B

Breathing, sleep-disordered, 676–678

Bronchial hyperresponsiveness, asthma in older
 adults and, 688

Bronchodilator(s)
 in asthma management in older adults,
  695–697
 in COPD management, 705
 inhaled corticosteroids and, in COPD
  management, 705

C

Cancer, lung, in older adults, treatment of,
 735–749. See also *Lung cancer, in older adults,
 treatment of.*

Chemotherapy, for NSCLC, 741–743

CHF. See *Congestive heart failure (CHF).*

Chronic obstructive pulmonary disease (COPD)
 anxiety and, 707–708
 comorbidities in, 707–708
 death due to, 703
 depression and, 707–708
 described, 703
 diagnosis of, 704
 in older adults, **703–715**
 management of
  care-giver issues in, 708–709
  end-of-life care in, 708–709
  palliative care for, 708–709
 per-patient costs of, 703
 prevalence of, 704
 prognosis of, 708
 quality of life and, 708
 risk factors for, 703–704
 stable, management of, 704–707
  drugs in, 705–706
  immunizations in, 706
  long-term oxygen therapy in, 706
  nonpharmacologic, 706–707
  nutrition in, 706–707
  pulmonary rehabilitation in, 706
  smoking cessation in, 704–705

Circadian rhythms, aging and, 673–674

Communication, in end-of-life considerations,
 803–804
 family and patient conversations, 805–807

Congenital heart disease–associated pulmonary
 arterial hypertension, in older adults, 720

Congestive heart failure (CHF), NPPV for, in
 older adults with acute respiratory failure,
 797

Connective tissue–associated pulmonary arterial
 hypertension, in older adults, 719–720

COPD. See *Chronic obstructive pulmonary disease
 (COPD).*

Corticosteroid(s)
 for acute lung injury and ARDS in older
  adults, 786
 inhaled
  bronchodilators and, in COPD
   management, 705
  in COPD management, 705

D

Depression
 COPD and, 707–708
 in decision making related to end-of-life
  considerations in older adults with lung
  disease, 803

Do-not-intubate patients, NPPV in, 798

Drug(s)
 in asthma management in older adults,
  694–697
 in COPD management, 705–706

E

Education, asthma-related, in older adults, 697

Elderly, acute respiratory failure in, 784

Embolic disease, pulmonary hypertension due to,
 726

End-of-life considerations, in older adults with
 lung disease, **801–811**. See also *Lung disease,
 older adults with, end-of-life considerations in.*

H

Heart disease, left, pulmonary hypertension and,
 in older adults, 720–725

Hyperresponsiveness, bronchial, asthma in older
 adults and, 688

Hypertension, pulmonary, in older adults, **717–733.** See also *Pulmonary hypertension, in older adults.*

Hypoxemia, pulmonary hypertension associated with, 725–726

I

Idiopathic pulmonary hypertension, in older adults, 718–719

Immunity
  adaptive, of lung, 665–667
  innate, of lung, 664–665
  lung, aging and, 667–668
  overview of, 663–664

Immunization(s), in COPD management, 706

Immunology, of aging lung, **663–672**

Infectious Diseases Society of America/American Thoracic Society (IDS/ATS), 757

Influenza vaccination, in pneumonia prevention, 766

Insomnia, 674–676

L

Left heart disease–related pulmonary hypertension, in older adults, 720–725

Lung(s)
  aging, allergy and immunology of, **663–672**
  immunity of
    adaptive, 665–667
    aging and, 667–668
    innate, 663–664

Lung cancer
  deaths due to, 735
  in older adults, treatment of, **735–749**
    NSCLC, 736–743. See also *Non–small-cell lung cancer (NSCLC), in older adults, treatment of.*
    SCLC, 743–745
  prevalence of, 735

Lung disease, older adults with
  end-of-life considerations in, **801–811**
    clinicians' own discomfort discussing death in, 808
    communication and, 803–804
    decision making related to, 803–804
    depression in, 803
    palliative care and, 803–804
    patient and family communication related to, 805–807

quality of life of, 802–803
    symptoms in, burden of, 802–803

M

Mask interface, NPPV and, 798

Mechanical ventilation
  for acute lung injury and ARDS in older adults, 784–786
    weaning from, 786–787
  in older adults, **783–791**

Mitral valve disease, in older adults, 724–725

Mycobacterial infections, nontuberculous, in older adults, **776–778.** See also *Nontuberculous mycobacterial infections, in older adults.*

Mycobacterium avium complex (MAC)
  diagnosis of, 777
  in older adults, treatment of, 777–778

N

Noninvasive positive pressure ventilation (NPPV), in older adults with acute respiratory failure, 793–795. See also *Acute respiratory failure, older adults with, noninvasive ventilation in, NPPV.*

Noninvasive ventilation, in older adults with acute respiratory failure, **793–800.** See also *Acute respiratory failure, older adults with, noninvasive ventilation in.*

Non–small-cell lung cancer (NSCLC), in older adults, treatment of, 736–743
  chemotherapy, 741–743
  medical, 740–743
  radiotherapy in, 739–740
  surgical, 736–739

Nontuberculous mycobacterial infections, in older adults, **776–778**
  clinical syndromes, 776–777
  diagnosis of, 777
  epidemiology of, 776
  treatment of, 777–778

NPPV. See *Noninvasive positive pressure ventilation (NPPV).*

Nutrition, in COPD management, 706–707

O

Obstructive lung diseases, NPPV in, 795–797

Older adults

Older adults (*continued*)
  acute respiratory failure in, noninvasive
    ventilation in, **793–800.** See also *Acute
    respiratory failure, older adults with,
    noninvasive ventilation in.*
  ARDS in, **783–791.** See also *Acute respiratory
    distress syndrome (ARDS), in older adults.*
  asthma in, 687–698. See also *Asthma, in older
    adults.*
  COPD in, **703–715.** See also *Chronic obstructive
    pulmonary disease (COPD).*
  lung cancer in, treatment of, **735–749.** See also
    Lung cancer, in older adults, treatment of.
  lung disease in, end-of-life considerations in,
    801–811. See also *Lung disease, older adults
    with, end-of-life considerations in.*
  mechanical ventilation in, **783–791**
  pneumonia in, **751–771.** See also *Pneumonia(s),
    in older adults.*
  pulmonary hypertension in, **717–733.** See also
    Pulmonary hypertension, in older adults.
  sleep in, **673–684.** See also *Sleep, in older adults.*
  tuberculosis in, **773–776.** See also *Tuberculosis,
    in older adults.*

Oxygen therapy, long-term, in COPD
  management, 706

P

Palliative care, in end-of-life considerations,
  803–804

Periodic leg movements, during sleep,
  678–679

Pneumococcal vaccination, in pneumonia
  prevention, 766–767

Pneumonia(s)
  community-acquired, treatment, empiric
    therapy in, 760–763
  health care–associated, in older adults,
    treatment of, 764–765
  in older adults, **751–771**
    bacteriology in, 755–757
    causative organisms, 755–757
    clinical presentation of, 754–755
    course of, 754–755
    diagnostic testing for, 757–758
    hospitalization for, determining factors for,
      759–760
    ICU admission for, 760
    pathophysiology of, 752–754
    prevention of, 766–767
    prognostic factors for, 758–760
    risk factors for, 752

    risk stratification for, 758–760
    treatment of, 760–766
      antibiotics in, 763
      empiric therapy in, 760–763
      general approach to, 760
      quinolones in, 763–764
      resolution and response to, 765–766
  NPPV for, in older adults with acute
    respiratory failure, 797–798

Portopulmonary-associated pulmonary arterial
  hypertension, in older adults, 720

Pulmonary arterial hypertension, in older adults
  congenital heart disease–associated, 720
  connective tissue–associated, 719–720
  portopulmonary-associated, 720

Pulmonary hypertension
  idiopathic, in older adults, 718–719
  in older adults, **717–733**
    causes of, 726
    chronic thrombotic disease and, 726
    classification of, 718–727
    hypoxia and, 725–726
    mortality related to, 717–718
    prevalence of, 717–718
    respiratory system–related, 725–726
    treatment of, 726–727
  left heart disease–related, in older adults,
    720–725

Pulmonary rehabilitation, in COPD management,
  706

Q

Quality of life
  COPD and, 708
  in older adults with lung disease,
    802–803

Quinolone(s), for pneumonia in older adults,
  763–764

R

Radiotherapy, for NSCLC, 739–740

Rapid eye movement sleep behavior disorder
  (RBD), 679–680

RBD. See *Rapid eye movement sleep behavior
  disorder (RBD).*

Rehabilitation, pulmonary, in COPD
  management, 706

Respiratory failure, acute
  in the elderly, 784

older adults with, noninvasive ventilation in, **793–800.** See also *Acute respiratory failure, older adults with, noninvasive ventilation in.*

Respiratory system
function of, age as factor in, 783–784
pulmonary hypertension associated with, 725–726

Restless legs syndrome, 678–679

Rhythm(s), circadian, aging and, 673–674

S

Sleep. See also *Insomnia.*
in older adults, **673–684**
age-related changes, 673
architecture of, 673
periodic leg movements during, 678–679
restless legs syndrome during, 678–679

Sleep disturbance, aging and, causes of, 674

Sleep-disorder breathing, 676–678

Small-cell lung cancer (SCLC), in older adults, treatment of, 743–745

Smoking cessation, in COPD management, 704–705

Stenosis(es), aortic, in older adults, 724–725

T

Thrombotic disease, chronic, pulmonary hypertension due to, 726

Tuberculosis, in older adults, **773–776**
clinical presentation of, 774
diagnosis of, 774–775
epidemiology of, 773–774
prevalence of, 773
treatment of, 775–776

V

Vaccination(s)
influenza, in pneumonia prevention, 766
pneumococcal, in pneumonia prevention, 766–767

Ventilation
mechanical. See *Mechanical ventilation.*
noninvasive, for older adults with acute respiratory failure, **793–800.** See also *Acute respiratory failure, older adults with, noninvasive ventilation in.*

W

World Health Organization (WHO), classification scheme for pulmonary hypertension, 718–727

Moving?

Make sure your subscription moves with you!

To notify us of your new address, find your **Clinics Account Number** (located on your mailing label above your name), and contact customer service at:

E-mail: elspcs@elsevier.com

800-654-2452 (subscribers in the U.S. & Canada)
407-345-4000 (subscribers outside of the U.S. & Canada)

Fax number: 407-363-9661

Elsevier Periodicals Customer Service
6277 Sea Harbor Drive
Orlando, FL 32887-4800

*To ensure uninterrupted delivery of your subscription, please notify us at least 4 weeks in advance of move.

United States Postal Service

Statement of Ownership, Management, and Circulation
(All Periodicals Publications Except Requestor Publications)

1. Publication Title	2. Publication Number	3. Filing Date
Clinics in Chest Medicine	0 0 0 - 7 0 6	9/14/07

4. Issue Frequency	5. Number of Issues Published Annually	6. Annual Subscription Price
Mar, Jun, Sep, Dec	4	$211.00

7. Complete Mailing Address of Known Office of Publication (Not printer) (Street, city, county, state, and ZIP+4)

Elsevier Inc.
360 Park Avenue South
New York, NY 10010-1710

Contact Person: Stephen Bushing
Telephone (Include area code): 215-239-3688

8. Complete Mailing Address of Headquarters or General Business Office of Publisher (Not printer)

Elsevier Inc., 360 Park Avenue South, New York, NY 10010-1710

9. Full Names and Complete Mailing Addresses of Publisher, Editor, and Managing Editor (Do not leave blank)

Publisher (Name and complete mailing address)

John Schrefer, Elsevier, Inc., 1600 John F. Kennedy Blvd. Suite 1800, Philadelphia, PA 19103-2899

Editor (Name and complete mailing address)

Sarah Barth, Elsevier, Inc., 1600 John F. Kennedy Blvd. Suite 1800, Philadelphia, PA 19103-2899

Managing Editor (Name and complete mailing address)

Catherine Bewick, Elsevier, Inc., 1600 John F. Kennedy Blvd. Suite 1800, Philadelphia, PA 19103-2899

10. Owner (Do not leave blank. If the publication is owned by a corporation, give the name and address of the corporation immediately followed by the names and addresses of all stockholders owning or holding 1 percent or more of the total amount of stock. If not owned by a corporation, give the names and addresses of the individual owners. If owned by a partnership or other unincorporated firm, give its name and address as well as those of each individual owner. If the publication is published by a nonprofit organization, give its name and address.)

Full Name	Complete Mailing Address
Wholly owned subsidiary of	4520 East-West Highway
Reed/Elsevier, US holdings	Bethesda, MD 20814

11. Known Bondholders, Mortgagees, and Other Security Holders Owning or Holding 1 Percent or More of Total Amount of Bonds, Mortgages, or Other Securities. If none, check box ☐ None

Full Name	Complete Mailing Address
N/A	

12. Tax Status (For completion by nonprofit organizations authorized to mail at nonprofit rates) (Check one)
The purpose, function, and nonprofit status of this organization and the exempt status for federal income tax purposes:
☐ Has Not Changed During Preceding 12 Months
☐ Has Changed During Preceding 12 Months (Publisher must submit explanation of change with this statement)

PS Form 3526, September 2006 (Page 1 of 3 (Instructions Page 3)) PSN 7530-01-000-9931 PRIVACY NOTICE: See our Privacy policy in www.usps.com

---

13. Publication Title	14. Issue Date for Circulation Data Below
Clinics in Chest Medicine	September 2007

15. Extent and Nature of Circulation			Average No. Copies Each Issue During Preceding 12 Months	No. Copies of Single Issue Published Nearest to Filing Date
a. Total Number of Copies (Net press run)			3850	3300
b. Paid Circulation (By Mail and Outside the Mail)	(1)	Mailed Outside-County Paid Subscriptions Stated on PS Form 3541. (Include paid distribution above nominal rate, advertiser's proof copies, and exchange copies)	1936	1834
	(2)	Mailed In-County Paid Subscriptions Stated on PS Form 3541 (Include paid distribution above nominal rate, advertiser's proof copies, and exchange copies)		
	(3)	Paid Distribution Outside the Mails Including Sales Through Dealers and Carriers, Street Vendors, Counter Sales, and Other Paid Distribution Outside USPS®	973	895
	(4)	Paid Distribution by Other Classes Mailed Through the USPS (e.g. First-Class Mail®)		
c. Total Paid Distribution (Sum of 15b (1), (2), (3), and (4))		►	2909	2729
d. Free or Nominal Rate Distribution (By Mail and Outside the Mail)	(1)	Free or Nominal Rate Outside-County Copies Included on PS Form 3541	101	71
	(2)	Free or Nominal Rate In-County Copies Included on PS Form 3541		
	(3)	Free or Nominal Rate Copies Mailed at Other Classes Mailed Through the USPS (e.g. First-Class Mail)		
	(4)	Free or Nominal Rate Distribution Outside the Mail (Carriers or other means)		
e. Total Free or Nominal Rate Distribution (Sum of 15d (1), (2), (3) and (4))		►	101	71
f. Total Distribution (Sum of 15c and 15e)		►	3010	2800
g. Copies not Distributed (See instructions to publishers #4 (page #3))		►	840	500
h. Total (Sum of 15f and g)		►	3850	3300
i. Percent Paid (15c divided by 15f times 100)			96.64%	97.46%

16. Publication of Statement of Ownership
☐ If the publication is a general publication, publication of this statement is required. Will be printed in the December 2007 issue of this publication. ☐ Publication not required

17. Signature and Title of Editor, Publisher, Business Manager, or Owner

[signature] James Panucci – Executive Director of Subscription Services

Date: September 14, 2007

I certify that all information furnished on this form is true and complete. I understand that anyone who furnishes false or misleading information on this form or who omits material or information requested on the form may be subject to criminal sanctions (including fines and imprisonment) and/or civil sanctions (including civil penalties).

PS Form 3526, September 2006 (Page 2 of 3)